SECOND EDITION
PATIENT EDUCATION

JOHN MURTAGH

AM, MB BS, MD, BSc, BEd
FRACGP, DipObstRCOG

Professor of General Practice
Head of Department of Community
Medicine and General Practice
Monash University

McGRAW-HILL BOOK COMPANY Sydney

New York   San Francisco   Auckland   Bogotá
Caracas   Lisbon   London   Madrid   Mexico City
Milan   New Delhi   San Juan   Singapore
Toronto   Kuala Lumpur

To my wife, Jill, and our children, Paul, Julie, Caroline, Luke and Clare, for their understanding, patience and support.

First edition 1992
Reprinted 1992, 1993, 1994
Second edition 1996

Text © 1996 John Murtagh
Illustrations and design © 1996 McGraw-Hill Book Company Australia Pty Limited
Additional owners of copyright material are credited on the Acknowledgments page or are named in on-page credits.

National Library of Australia Cataloguing-in-Publication data:

Murtagh, John.
  Patient education.

  2nd ed.
  Includes index.
  ISBN 0 07 470296 3.

  1. Family medicine. 2. Patient education. I. Title.

615.507

Published in Australia by
McGraw-Hill Book Company Australia Pty Limited
4 Barcoo Street, Roseville NSW 2069, Australia
Typeset in Australia by Midland Typesetters Pty Ltd
Printed in Australia by McPherson's Printing Group Ltd

Publisher: John Rowe
Production editors: Robyn Wilkie and Caroline Hunter
Designer: George Sirett
Technical illustrators: Chris Sorrell and Mary Ferguson

Foreword

During my student days in the late 1940s the idea of educating patients about their illnesses was never discussed. From memory I am not aware that this omission was even noticed, although it may have been by those students who were wiser and more broadly educated than myself. When later I began medical practice as a solo general practitioner, I remember being surprised by the number of patients who had had major surgical procedures (as judged by their obvious scars) and who were quite ignorant of these procedures or what organs they no longer possessed. I found this lack of available information often interfered with the process of diagnosis due to incomplete, and often highly relevant, past medical history.

Another memory of my early years in practice was the number of times I was called out of bed because a child had a fever, only to be met on arrival at the home by a mildly ill child playing with a box of toys. This provided sufficient motivation to start teaching the family about the relative unimportance of a single sign in assessing illness severity, and the need to look at the whole child and not just the thermometer reading. Within two years, despite an increasing population of children in a new suburb, there were two observable results. First, the number of such requests for night and weekend calls had markedly reduced and, second, there was positive feedback from patients, such as 'Thank you for giving your time to explain things to me'. At the time many general practitioners were learning that this educational role was a legitimate and important part of being a competent general practitioner, which is not surprising since the word 'doctor' originally meant 'teacher'.

When I moved to academia, I then had a chance, together with my colleagues, to develop these ideas further and to formalise patient education as an essential part of patient management in the context of today's society. Patient education now forms a major part of a formal undergraduate teaching program embracing a number of consulting skills. In addition to the verbal communication skills of this program we have developed a matching series of take-home pamphlets to reinforce these educational messages.

John Murtagh has taken up the concept of extending the consultation by writing patient hand-outs focusing on illnesses and their management. These have been published over many years in *Australian Family Physician*, and adopted for use by many general practitioners during the consultation. They have been gathered together and rewritten in this format for use by doctors and other health professionals as an aid to improving quality of care, reducing its costs and encouraging a greater input by patients in the management of their own illnesses. The unique objective of this publication is the author's wish to encourage doctors to use the material and to photocopy or even modify those hand-outs considered most useful. A logical extension of this information is to use it in an electronic format; *Patient Education* is also available on computer software.

Many doctors, especially younger doctors and medical students, have claimed that *Patient Education* has been a helpful form of doctor education and very useful in preparation for examinations, both undergraduate and for the fellowship of the Royal Australian College of General Practitioners.

In a society where informed consent is increasingly expected by the public, and the legal profession in particular, it is important for doctors to be aware of the need to provide patients and families with much more information than in the past. Professor Murtagh is to be congratulated for producing the important messages in non-technical language within the confines of a single page. This no doubt is a result of many years of experience in general practice, where he has learned the skills of effective communication.

EMERITUS PROFESSOR NEIL CARSON

Contents

Preface

In modern medicine patient education has become a very important and expected method of patient care. People are more interested than ever before in the cause and management of their problems, and for this reason access to information in easy-to-follow presentation is very beneficial. Furthermore, patients need and deserve the best possible access to information about their health. The material presented in this book is not intended to be used as an alternative to the verbal explanations given by the doctor during the consultation but as complementary information to be taken home. Experience has shown that better understanding of a problem or potential health problem leads to better co-operation and compliance with treatment.

The author has produced patient education information to fit onto one sheet, which can be handed to the patient or person seeking health information. Medical practitioners often refer to this information as 'doctor education' as well as 'patient education'. Such practitioners are invited to use this information for a variety of purposes, such as a basis for their own patient education or for computer information programs. These sheets should have considerable value in undergraduate courses for doctors, nurses and other health professionals.

The catalyst for the initial production of this material came from two sources. The Royal Australian College of General Practitioners, through its official publication *Australian Family Physician* (*AFP*), encouraged the author to write patient education material as a service to general practitioners and their patients. The strategy was to present information on the commonest problems presenting to general practitioners, each on a single A4 sheet and in the lay person's language. Patient education sheets have been a feature of monthly publications of *AFP* since 1979, and doctors have ordered them in vast quantities. We have not simply featured illnesses, but have also used preventive advice and health promotion wherever possible.

The other impetus for this project came from the members of the Monash University Department of Community Medicine and General Practice, who realised the importance of this material for the education of medical students. Apart from providing valuable learning material for the students, it gave them the basis for illness and preventive advice to patients during the consulting skills learning program.

The author believes that the subject matter in this book covers common everyday problems encountered by doctors and hopes that the dissemination of this information will benefit both health care providers and people who are interested in their health.

Acknowledgments

The author would like to thank the Publication Division of the Royal Australian College of General Practitioners for encouraging the concept of patient education and for their permission to reproduce much of the material that has appeared in *Australian Family Physician*. Also, my colleagues in the Department of Community Medicine, Monash University, have provided valuable assistance. Professor Neil Carson's far-reaching vision of general practice training includes the value of this educational medium.

Other educational organisations that have provided ideas and material are the Paediatric Health Education Unit, Westmead Hospital, NSW, and the Parks Community Health Centre, Angle Park, SA. Colleagues who have given considerable advice are Malcolm Fredman, James Kiepert, Don Lewis, Robin Marks, Wendy Rosier and Abe Rubinfeld. The main reference was the *Macmillan Guide to Family Health* (1982) edited by Dr Tony Smith.

Individual contributions, including full or part authorship, have come from the following practitioners, to whom I am indebted:

Lisa Amir (Establishing breastfeeding), Michael Axtens and Lou Sanderson (Common cold), Tim Bajraszewski (Osteoporosis), Bruce Barker (Angina, Diverticular disease, Hepatitis A, Osteoarthritis), Jenny Barry (Dysmenorrhoea), Robin Beattie (Stress: coping with stress), Grant Connoley (Melanoma), Joan Curtis (Autism), Denise Findlay (Self-examination of breasts), David Fonda (Incontinence of urine), John Goldsmid (Lice: head lice, Lice: pubic lice, Scabies), Jenny Gunn and Pat Phillips (Diabetes: blood glucose monitoring at home, Diabetes: healthy diet for diabetics), Anthony Hall (Warts), Judith Hammond (Premenstrual syndrome), Rod Kruger (Ear: otitis externa, Ear: wax in your ear, Eye: foreign body in the eye), Deirdre Lewis (Hirsutism), Jim McDonald (Haemorrhoids), Peter Macisaac (Travel: guide for travellers), Ian McKenzie (Child accident prevention in the home), Jane Offer (Understanding your menstrual cycle), William Phillips (Foreskin hygiene), Jill Rosenblatt (Dysmenorrhoea, Menopause, Vaginal thrush), Chris Silagy (Smoking—quitting), John Tiller (Sleep problems), Cynthia Welling (Incontinence of urine), Richard Williams (Exercises for your knee, Exercises for your shoulder).

Special thanks are given to Chris Sorrell and Levent Efe for permission to use much of their art illustration as appeared in *Australian Family Physician*. The illustrations on pages 5, 7, 23, 43, 59, 60, 77, 93, 94, 99, 115, 121, 123, 129, 130 (Using a spacer), 131, 134, 153, 158, 170, 181 and 190 were drawn by Mary Ferguson.

Finally, thanks go to Nicki Cooper and Caroline Murtagh for typing the manuscript.

PART I

Stages of human development

1 Marriage

Making your marriage work

When a couple marry, a bond of love is invariably present; this bond will at times be put to the test, because marriage is no 'bed of roses'. For most couples this bond will grow, mature and become a wonderful source of joy despite the rough times. However, others may not cope well with the problems of living together. To split up is a terrible loss in every respect, especially for any children of the marriage.

Many troubled couples have achieved great happiness by following some basic rules of sharing.

> The two big secrets of marital success
> are
> *caring* and *responsibility*.

Some common causes of marital trouble

- selfishness
- financial problems/meanness
- sickness (e.g. depression)
- 'playing games' with each other
- poor communication
- unrealistic expectations
- not listening to each other
- drug or alcohol excess
- jealousy, especially in men
- fault-finding
- driving ambition
- immaturity

Some important facts

- Research has shown that we tend to choose partners who are similar to our parents and that we may take our childish and selfish attitudes into our marriage.
- The trouble spots listed above reflect this childishness; we often expect our partners to change and meet our needs.
- If we take proper care and responsibility, we can keep these problems to a minimum.
- Physical passion is not enough to hold a marriage together—'when it burns out, only ashes will be left'.
- While a good sexual relationship is great, most experts agree that what goes on *out* of bed counts for more.
- When we do something wrong, it is most important that we feel forgiven by our partner.

Positive guidelines for success

1. *Know yourself.* The better you know yourself, the better you will know your mate. Learn about sex and reproduction.

2. *Share interests and goals.* Do not become too independent of each other. Develop mutual friends, interests and hobbies. Tell your partner 'I love you' regularly at the right moments.

3. *Continue courtship after marriage.* Spouses should continue to court and desire each other. Going out regularly for romantic evenings and giving unexpected gifts (such as flowers) are ways to help this love relationship. Engage in some high-energy fun activities such as massaging and dancing.

4. *Make love, not war.* A good sexual relationship can take years to develop, so work at making it better. Explore the techniques of lovemaking without feeling shy or inhibited. This can be helped by books such as *The Joy of Sex* and videos on lovemaking. Good grooming and a clean body are important.

5. *Cherish your mate.* Be proud of each other, not competitive or ambitious at the other's expense. Talk kindly about your spouse to others—do not put him or her down.

6. *Prepare yourself for parenthood.* Plan your family wisely and learn about child bearing and rearing. Learn about family planning methods and avoid the anxieties of an unplanned pregnancy. The best environment for a child is a happy marriage.

7. *Seek proper help when necessary.* If difficulties arise and are causing problems, seek help. Your general practitioner will be able to help. Stress-related problems and depression in particular can be lethal in a marriage—they must be 'nipped in the bud'.

8. *Do unto your mate as you would have your mate do unto you.* This gets back to the unconscious childhood needs. Be aware of each other's feelings and be sensitive to each other's needs. Any marriage based on this rule has an excellent chance of success.

The Be Attitudes (virtues to help achieve success)

BE honest.	**BE** loyal.
BE loving.	**BE** desiring.
BE patient.	**BE** fun to live with.
BE forgiving.	**BE** one.
BE generous.	**BE** caring.

Making lists—a practical task

Make lists for each other to compare and discuss.
- List qualities (desirable and undesirable) of your parents.
- List qualities of each other.
- List examples of behaviour each would like the other to change.
- List things you would like the other to do for you.

Put aside special quiet times each week to share these things.

---

2 Pregnancy and postnatal care

About your pregnancy

Congratulations on becoming an expectant parent—this is a very exciting time in your life, even though you may be inclined to feel flat and sick at first. Your baby is very special and deserves every opportunity to get a flying start in life by growing healthily in your womb. Pregnancy is a very normal event in the life cycle and usually goes very smoothly, especially if you have regular medical care.

Why have regular checks?

Antenatal care is considered to be the best opportunity in life for preventive medicine. It is important to check the many things that can cause problems—these are uncommon, but preventable. A special possible problem is *pregnancy-induced hypertension*, a condition of weight gain, high blood pressure and kidney stress, which shows up as protein in the urine.

Areas that need to be checked include:
- blood count
- blood grouping and Rhesus antibodies (Rh factor)
- immunity against infections that may affect the baby (e.g. rubella, hepatitis B)
- number of babies (one or more)
- size and state of your pelvis
- blood pressure
- urine (for evidence of diabetes or pre-eclampsia)
- cervix (smear test)
- progress of the baby (e.g. size of uterus, heartbeat)
- mother's progress, including emotional state

When should you be checked?

The recommended routine is as early as possible and then every 4 to 6 weeks until 28 weeks of gestation, then every 2 weeks until 36 weeks, and then weekly until the baby arrives (usually 40 weeks).

What common things can cause problems in the baby?

- infections such as rubella
- diabetes (can develop in pregnancy)
- high blood pressure
- smoking—retards growth and should be stopped (if impossible, limit to 3–6 smokes per day)
- alcohol—causes abnormalities, including mental retardation, and should not be taken (if you must, drink 1–2 glasses of beer per day maximum)
- other social drugs
- aspirin and various other drugs (check with your doctor)

What is usually prescribed?

No tablets are needed if you have a healthy diet and do not have severe morning sickness.

What important areas should you attend to?

Nutrition
A healthy diet is very important and should contain at least the following *daily* allowances:

1. Eat most:
   - fruit and vegetables (at least 4 serves)
   - cereals and bread (4–6 serves)

2. Eat moderately:
   - dairy products—3 cups (600 mL) of milk or equivalent in yoghurt or cheese
   - lean meat, poultry or fish—1 or 2 serves (at least 2 serves of red meat per week)

3. Eat least:
   - sugar and refined carbohydrates (e.g. sweets, cakes, biscuits, soft drinks)
   - polyunsaturated margarine, butter, oil and cream

Bran with cereal helps prevent constipation of pregnancy.

Antenatal classes
Trained therapists will advise on antenatal exercises, back care, postural advice, relaxation skills, pain relief in labour, general exercises and beneficial activities such as swimming.

Breastfeeding and nursing mothers
Breastfeeding is highly recommended. Contact a local nursing mothers group for support and guidance if you need help.

Employment and travel
Check with your doctor. Avoid standing in trains. Avoid international air travel after 28 weeks.

Normal activities
You should continue your normal activities. Housework and other activities should be performed to just short of feeling tired. However, get sufficient rest and sleep.

When should you contact your doctor or the hospital?

Contact your doctor or seek medical help:
- if contractions, unusual pain or bleeding occur before the baby is due
- if the baby is less active than usual
- if membranes rupture and a large amount of fluid comes out
- when you are getting regular contractions 5–10 minutes apart

Help is only a telephone call away.

John Murtagh, *Patient Education*, Second edition, McGraw-Hill Book Company

Breastfeeding and milk supply

Difficulties with breastfeeding are common, especially in the first week after birth. As a rule, the milk, which is present all the time, 'comes in' at any time from 24 hours after birth. It is common for the breasts to become engorged early on, but in some there is insufficient supply.

Engorged breasts

What is engorgement?

In some women, a few days after delivery the milk supply comes on so quickly that the breasts become swollen, hard and sore. This is called *engorgement*. There is an increased supply of blood and other fluids in the breast as well as milk.

What will you notice?

The breasts and nipples may be so swollen that the baby is unable to latch on and suckle. The soreness makes it difficult for you to relax and enjoy your baby.

How are engorged breasts managed?

- Feed your baby on demand from day 1 until he or she has had enough.
- Finish the first breast completely; maybe use one side per feed rather than some from each breast. Offer the second breast if the baby appears hungry.
- Soften the breasts before feeds or expressing with a warm washer or shower, which will help get the milk flowing.
- Avoid giving the baby other fluids.
- Express a little milk before putting the baby to your breast (a must if the baby has trouble latching on) and express a little after feeding from the other side if it is too uncomfortable.
- Massage any breast lumps gently towards the nipple while feeding.
- Apply cold packs after feeding and cool washed cabbage leaves (left in the refrigerator) between feeds. Change the leaves every 2 hours.
- Wake your baby for a feed if your breasts are uncomfortable or if the baby is sleeping longer than 4 hours.

- Use a good, comfortable brassiere.
- Remove your bra completely before feeding.
- Take paracetamol regularly for severe discomfort.

Remember that regular feeding is the best treatment for your engorged breasts. Follow your demand and your baby's demand. As your breasts are used in this way, they gradually become softer and more comfortable.

Insufficient supply

This is sometimes a problem in mothers who tend to be under a lot of stress and find it hard to relax. A 'let down' reflex is necessary to get the milk supply going, and sometimes this reflex is slow. If there is insufficient supply, the baby tends to demand frequent feeds, may continually suck his or her hand and will be slow in gaining weight.

Remember that there is always some milk present in your breasts.

What should you do?

- Try to practise relaxation techniques to help condition your 'let down' reflex.
- Put the baby to your breast as often as he or she demands, using the 'chest to chest, chin on breast' method.
- Express after feeds, because the emptier the breasts are, the more milk will be produced.
- Make sure you get adequate rest, but if you feel overly tired go to your doctor for a checkup.

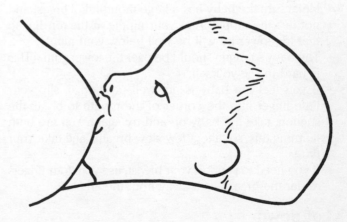

Establishing breastfeeding

There are three important things that you should know about breastfeeding:

1. positioning the baby on the breast
2. the 'let down'
3. supply and demand

Occasionally some women experience engorged breasts or insufficient milk supply until breastfeeding is fully established.

Positioning

Your posture
- Make yourself comfortable.
- Sit upright, but let your shoulders relax.
- Support yourself with cushions or a footstool, if necessary.

Your baby
- Unwrap the baby's arms.
- Turn the baby's body towards yours.
- Have the baby's mouth at the same level as your nipple.
- Support the baby's body well.
- Hold the baby close to you.

Latching on
- Support your baby across the back of the shoulder.
- Tickle the baby's lips with your nipple until the mouth opens wide.
- Quickly move the baby on to the breast when the mouth is wide open. (Do not try to bring your breast to the baby.)
- Make sure the baby has a large mouthful of breast and not just the nipple. Aim your nipple at the top lip, so that the lower lip will be well below your nipple.
- The baby's tongue should be over the lower gum. (This is hard to see yourself.)
- If you feel the baby is not well positioned, slip your little finger into the corner of the mouth to break the suction, take the baby off and try again. You are both learning this, so take a few slow breaths and take your time.
- If you need to support your breast, use your four fingers under the breast, well away from the areola.

Let down

When your baby is feeding, the nerves in the nipple start a reflex action that allows the milk-producing alveoli to be squeezed, which pushes milk along the ducts towards

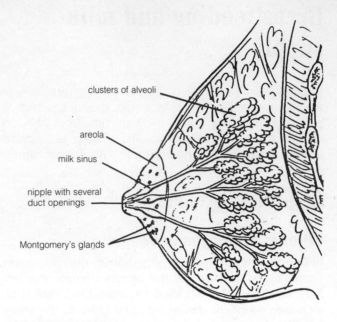

clusters of alveoli

areola

milk sinus

nipple with several
duct openings

Montgomery's glands

Anatomy of the breast

the nipple. This is called the *'let down' reflex*. Some women notice a tingling or a pins-and-needles sensation or a fullness when this occurs. Others notice leaking from the other breast or nothing at all. You may notice that the baby changes from sucking quickly at the breast to a slower suck–swallow–suck–swallow pattern.

The milk higher up in the breast (the *hindmilk*) is rich in fat and calories. It is important that you have a 'let down', so that the baby does not get only foremilk.

If you are anxious, in pain, or embarrassed, your 'let down' may be slow. Eliminate these factors before feeding if you can. Once breastfeeding is well established, you will be able to breastfeed anywhere, but in the early days you need a supportive environment.

Supply and demand

Your breasts produce milk on the principle of supply and demand. This means that the more the breasts are emptied, the more milk is made. When breasts are allowed to remain full, they get the message to slow down milk production.

Your baby automatically controls his or her food intake by taking as much as needed. When the baby needs to increase your supply, he or she will feed more frequently for a couple of days.

If your supply is low, you can easily increase it by expressing milk after feeds. You can offer this milk to your baby after the next feed or in the evening. Usually your breasts will feel fuller after a few days of resting and expressing.

John Murtagh, *Patient Education*, Second edition, McGraw-Hill Book Company

Mastitis with breastfeeding

What is mastitis?

Mastitis is an area of inflammation of breast tissue, in particular the milk ducts and glands of the nursing mother. It is caused by a cracked nipple or blockage of the ducts due to a problem with drainage of the milk. Germs from the outside get into and grow in the stagnant milk.

What are the symptoms?

You may feel a lump and then a sore breast at first. Then follows a red, tender area (see diagram) with fever, tiredness, weakness and muscle aches and pains (like having influenza).

What are the risks?

If treated early and properly, mastitis starts to improve within 48 hours. Doctors regard it as a serious and rather urgent problem, because a breast abscess can quickly develop without treatment and the abscess may require surgical drainage. Apart from the bacterial infection, infection with Candida (thrush) may occur, especially after the use of antibiotics. Candida infection usually causes severe breast pain—a feeling like a hot knife or hot shooting pains, especially during and after feeding.

What is the treatment?

- Antibiotics: your doctor will prescribe a course of antibiotics, usually for 10 days. If you are allergic to penicillin, tell your doctor.
- Pain-killers: take aspirin or paracetamol when necessary for pain and fever.
- Keep the affected breast well drained.
- Keep breastfeeding: do this frequently and start with the sore side.
- Make sure the baby is latched on properly and change feeding positions to drain the milk.
- Heat the sore area of the breast before feeding: have a hot shower or use a hot face washer or hot-water bottle.

- Cool the breast after feeding: use a cold face washer from the freezer.
- Apply cool washed cabbage leaves over the affected side between feeds.
- Massage any breast lump gently towards the nipple while feeding.
- Empty the breast well: hand express if necessary.
- Get sufficient rest: rest when you feel the need to do so and get help in the home.
- Keep to a nutritious diet and drink plenty of fluids.

How can it be prevented?

Breast engorgement and cracked nipples must be attended to. It is important to make sure your milk drains well. Faulty drainage can be caused by an oversupply of milk, missed feeds, the breast not being fully emptied (e.g. from rushed feeding, poor attachment or wrong feeding positions), exhaustion, poor nutrition and too much pressure on the breast (e.g. bra too tight and sleeping face downwards).

Keep the breasts draining by expression or by waking the baby for a feed if he or she sleeps for long periods. For an oversupply, try feeding from one breast only at each feed. Avoiding caffeine and smoking may also help.

Note: It is quite safe to continue breastfeeding with the affected breast unless your doctor advises otherwise.

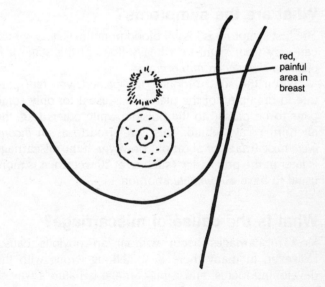

red, painful area in breast

Miscarriage

After your miscarriage you will undoubtedly be confused and wondering why this sad event happened to you. The main thing is to remember that it was nothing that you did wrong, and so you should not feel any sense of blame or guilt.

What is a miscarriage?

A miscarriage, which is called a *spontaneous abortion* in medical terms, is the spontaneous ending of pregnancy before the baby (foetus) can survive outside the womb. Sometimes it is *complete* (when both foetus and afterbirth are expelled); other times it is *incomplete* (when only part of the pregnancy is expelled).

What are the surprising facts?

- About 1 in 4 pregnancies are 'lost'.
- Many are lost soon after conception; in such a case the woman may not be aware of anything except a small alteration in her period.
- Most are lost in the first 14 weeks and are obvious to the mother.

What are the symptoms?

The first symptom is loss of blood from the vagina, which can vary from slight to a heavy flow. At this stage it is called a *threatened miscarriage*.

When the solid products are passed, you feel pain due to cramping of the uterus. It is usual for only some parts to be passed to the outside, while others (e.g. the afterbirth) stay behind. This is referred to as an *incomplete* miscarriage or abortion. However, if the miscarriage is later in the pregnancy (such as at 20 weeks), it is more usual to have a *complete* abortion.

What is the cause of miscarriage?

Most miscarriages occur without an obvious cause. However, in many there is something wrong with the developing foetus, and a miscarriage is nature's way of handling the problem.

This abnormality may be caused by a genetic disorder, or by a viral infection that has affected the foetus in the first 12 weeks. Often the mother is unaware that she has picked up a serious infection (such as rubella, influenza or cytomegalovirus), but it is harmful to the delicate growing tissues of the foetus.

In other cases, abnormalities of the uterus may not allow the fertilised egg to attach to its lining, or it may reject the developing foetus later on.

What are the risks?

There is usually no risk to the mother's health. If the miscarriage is incomplete and not attended to, infection or anaemia from blood loss could occur. If you get fever, heavy bleeding, severe pain or an offensive discharge, contact your doctor. You may feel emotionally upset or depressed with feelings of loss and grief. If so, you will require help.

Will it happen again?

You are no more likely to have a repeat miscarriage than any other pregnant woman. The odds favour your next pregnancy being successful. There is no special treatment to prevent any further miscarriages, and it is best left to natural means. However, it is advisable to keep healthy and not indulge in alcohol, smoking or the use of other drugs.

What is the treatment?

It is usual to have a surgical cleaning of your uterus, especially if the miscarriage was early in the pregnancy and bleeding continues. This is called a *dilation and curettage* (D&C).

Other aspects of treatment include:
- basic pain medication such as paracetamol
- blood tests and possible ultrasound examination
- checking for Rhesus blood grouping (a Rhesus negative person may be given immunoglobulin)
- reduced activity and rest for at least 48 hours

Pay attention to any adverse emotional reactions—make sure you talk about any unusual feelings. Talk over your feelings with your partner and family.

You will need at least a week off work.

How soon should you wait before trying again?

You can safely start trying to get pregnant again very soon. It is best to wait until you have had at least one normal period. Your next period may be heavy and abnormal. Use sanitary towels and not tampons for the next 4 weeks.

Make sure that your body is ready before having sex again. It usually takes a while to become interested in sex again, and therefore partners have to be very patient and understanding.

John Murtagh, *Patient Education*, Second edition, McGraw-Hill Book Company

Nipple problems while breastfeeding

Sore nipples

Sore nipples are a common problem and are considered to be caused by the baby not taking the nipple into its mouth properly, often because of breast engorgement. The problem is preventable with careful attention to the position of the baby at the breast and the baby's sucking technique.

How are sore nipples managed?

It is important to be as relaxed and comfortable as possible (with your back well supported) and for your baby to suck gently, so:

- Try to use the 'chest to chest, chin on breast' feeding position.
- Vary the feeding positions. (Make sure each position is correct.)
- Start feeding from the less painful side first if one nipple is very sore.
- Express some milk first to soften and lubricate the nipple. Avoid drying agents (such as methylated spirits, soap and tincture of benzoin) and moisturising creams and ointments, which may contain unwanted chemicals and germs.
- Gently break the suction with your finger before removing the baby from the breast. (*Never* pull the baby off the nipple.)
- Apply covered ice to the nipple to relieve pain.
- Keep the nipples dry by exposing the breasts to the air and/or using a hair dryer on a low setting.
- If you are wearing a bra, try Cannon breast shields inside the bra. Do not wear a bra at night.

Cracked nipples

Cracked nipples are usually caused by the baby clamping on the end of the nipple rather than applying the jaw behind the whole nipple. Not drying the nipples thoroughly after each feed and wearing soggy breast pads are other contributing factors. Untreated sore nipples may progress to painful cracks.

What are the symptoms?

At first, the crack may be so small that you cannot see it. The crack is either on the skin of the nipple or where it joins the flat, dark part of the nipple (the *areola*). A sharp pain in your nipple with sucking probably means a crack has developed. Feeding is usually very painful, and bleeding can occur.

How are cracked nipples managed?

Cracked nipples nearly always heal when you get the baby to latch onto the breast fully and properly. It usually takes only 1–2 days to heal.

- Follow the same rules as for sore nipples.
- Do not feed from the affected breast—rest the nipple for 1–2 feeds.
- Express milk from that breast by hand.
- Feed that expressed milk to the baby.
- Start feeding gradually with short feeds.
- A sympathetic expert such as an experienced nursing mother will be a great help if you are having trouble coping.
- A pliable nipple shield may be used for a short period.
- Contact your doctor if the problem is not resolving.
- Take paracetamol just before nursing to relieve pain.

Inverted nipples

What is an inverted nipple?

It is a nipple that inverts or moves into the breast instead of pointing outwards when a baby tries to suck from it. When the areola is squeezed, the nipple retracts inwards.

What is the treatment?

During pregnancy, rolling and stretching the nipple by hand can be helpful. Your partner can assist with gentle oral and manual stimulation of your breasts and nipples.

A simple treatment, which should start at the beginning of the seventh month of pregnancy, is the Hoffman technique:

1. Draw an imaginary cross on the breast with the vertical and horizontal lines crossing at the nipple.

2. Place the thumbs or the forefingers opposite each other at the edge of the areola on the imaginary horizontal line. Press in firmly and then pull the thumbs (or fingers) back and forth to stretch the areola.

3. In the vertical position, pull the thumbs or fingers upwards and downwards.

Repeat this procedure about 5 times each morning. The nipple will become erect and is then easier to grasp, so that it can be slowly and gently drawn out.

After baby is born, try to breastfeed early while the sucking reflex is strong and your breasts are soft.

Before breastfeeding, draw the nipple out by hand or with a breast pump. Check that your baby is correctly positioned on the breast. Usually, with time, inverted nipples will be corrected by the baby's sucking.

John Murtagh, *Patient Education*, Second edition, McGraw-Hill Book Company

Postnatal depression

It is quite common for women to feel emotional and flat after childbirth; this is apparently due to hormonal changes and to the anticlimax after the long-awaited event. There are two separate important problems:
1. postnatal blues
2. postnatal (or postpartum) depression

Postnatal blues

'The blues' are a very common problem that arises in the first 2 weeks (usually from day 3 to day 5) after childbirth.

What are the symptoms?
- feeling flat or depressed
- mood swings
- irritability
- feeling emotional (e.g. crying easily)
- tiredness
- insomnia
- lacking confidence (e.g. in bathing and feeding the baby)
- aches and pains (e.g. headache)

What is the outcome?
Fortunately 'the blues' are a passing phase and last only a few days. It is important to get plenty of help and rest until they go away and you feel normal.

What should you do?
All you really need is encouragement and support from your partner, family and friends, so tell them how you feel.
- Avoid getting overtired: rest as much as possible.
- Talk over your problems with a good listener (perhaps another mother with a baby).
- Accept help from others in the house.
- Allow your partner to take turns getting up to attend to the baby.

If the blues last longer than 4 days, it is very important to contact your doctor for advice.

Postnatal depression

Some women develop a very severe depression within the first 6–12 months (usually in the first 6 months) after childbirth. They seem to get 'the blues' and cannot snap out of it.

What are the symptoms?
Some or all of the following may occur:
- a feeling that you cannot cope with life (e.g. hopelessness, helplessness)
- continual tiredness
- feeling a failure as a mother
- sleeping problems
- eating problems (e.g. poor appetite or overeating)
- loss of interest (e.g. in sex)
- difficulty in concentrating
- tension and anxiety
- feeling irritable, angry or fearful
- getting angry with the baby
- feeling rejected
- marital problems (e.g. feeling rejected or paranoid)

What is the outcome?
This is a very serious problem if not treated, and you cannot shake it off by yourself. There is a real risk of a marriage breakdown because you can be a very miserable person to live with, especially if your husband does not understand what is going on. If it is severe, there is a risk of suicide and even of killing the baby.

What should you do?
You must be open and tell everyone how you feel. You need help. Take your baby to the childhood centre for review. It is most important to consult your doctor and explain exactly how you feel. Your problem can be treated and cured with antidepressant medicine.

Support groups
There are some excellent support groups for women with postnatal depression, and it is worth asking about them and joining them for therapy.

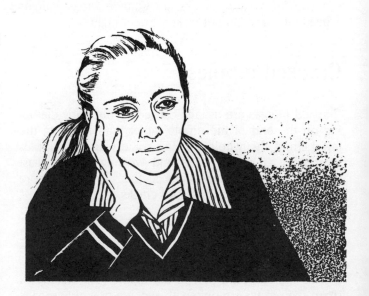

John Murtagh, *Patient Education*, Second edition, McGraw-Hill Book Company

3 Children's health

Allergy in your baby

What is allergy?

Allergies are sensitive reactions that occur when the body's immune system reacts in any unusual way to foods, airborne dust, animal hair and pollens. This results in conditions such as hay fever, eczema, hives and bowel problems. The condition is also called *atopy*.

Allergies are common in babies and children. They usually disappear as the child grows older, but sometimes can continue into adult life.

Unlike most of the common illnesses (such as measles and chickenpox) an allergy can have many symptoms, and these vary widely from child to child. Allergies are not infectious.

How to tell if a baby has an allergy

An allergic reaction might take hours or even days to develop and can affect almost any part of the body. Symptoms may be any of the following:

1. *Digestive system (includes stomach and intestines)*: nausea, vomiting and spitting up of food, colicky behaviour in the young baby (including pulling away from the breast), stomach pain, diarrhoea, poor appetite, slow weight gain.

2. *Respiratory system (includes nose, throat and lungs)*: runny nose, sneezing, wheezing, asthma, recurring attacks of bronchitis or croup, persistent cough.

3. *Skin*: eczema, hives, other rashes.

What are the causes?

Common causes of allergic reaction are foods and airborne irritants. Soaps and detergents might aggravate some skin conditions.

- Foods that commonly cause allergic reactions include milk and other dairy products, eggs, peanut butter; sometimes oranges, soya beans, chocolate, tomatoes, fish and wheat.
- Airborne particles linked with allergic reactions include dust mites, pollens, animal hair and moulds.

Some reactions are caused by food additives such as colourings, flavourings and preservatives. Additives are found in many prepared foods (e.g. lollies, sauces, ice-cream, cordial, soft drinks, biscuits, savoury snacks and processed meats).

The allergic reaction to dairy products has almost the same symptoms (stomach pain and diarrhoea) as those that occur when a baby has *lactose intolerance*, which is when he or she cannot digest the sugar (lactose) in dairy products. The correct diagnosis is a matter for your doctor.

Is allergy inherited?

Allergy cannot be passed from generation to generation, but children from families that have a tendency to allergy have a greater chance of becoming allergic. However, anyone can become allergic.

What is the management?
Feeding

Breastfeeding of allergy-prone babies for the first 6 months might diminish eczema and other allergic disorders during infancy.

If breastfeeding is not possible, choose a breast milk substitute (formula) carefully. Get advice from your doctor or infant welfare nurse.

What happens when solids are introduced?

If possible, do not start solids until the baby is 5 or 6 months old. Start one food at a time, in small amounts. The quantity can be increased the next day if no reaction occurs.

New foods should be introduced at least several days apart. Particular care should be taken when starting foods that most commonly cause allergic reactions (dairy products, eggs, citrus fruits and peanut butter). They should be avoided during the first 6–9 months.

Be alert!

If possible, prepare the baby's food using fresh ingredients. For example, a child with cows milk allergy should avoid cows milk in any form. Read labels carefully to check ingredients in products.

Other allergies

Many babies and children develop allergies to house dust and animal hair. Vacuuming regularly and keeping pets outside will reduce the problem.

Bedding should be aired regularly. Damp and poorly ventilated homes are subject to mould, which can cause allergy. Both the mould and its cause should be eliminated.

Other things that can be done
- Cotton clothing is best for babies and children with skin problems.
- Avoid strong soaps, detergents and nappy wash solutions.
- Boil the baby's bottles rather than use chemical solutions.
- Use household chemicals such as strong fly sprays, perfumes and disinfectants sparingly, and air the house thoroughly afterwards.
- Do not smoke or allow others to smoke when your baby is in the room.

Atopic eczema

What is atopic eczema?

Eczema refers to a red, scaly, itchy, sometimes weeping skin condition. *Atopy* refers to an allergic condition that tends to run in families and includes problems such as asthma, hay fever, atopic eczema and skin sensitivities. However, anyone can become allergic.

Atopic eczema is common and affects about 5% of the population. It is not contagious. No particular cause has been found.

What are the symptoms?

In mild cases the skin is slightly red, scaly and itchy and covers small areas. In infants it usually starts on the face and scalp; in severe cases it can cover large areas, is very itchy and starts to weep and become crusted. The children may be very irritable and uncomfortable.

What ages are affected?

Eczema usually starts in infants from any age. It tends to improve from 1 to 2 years, but the rash may persist in certain areas, such as the flexures of the elbows and knees, the face and neck, and the fingers and toes. It tends to be coarse, dry and itchy at this stage. Many children have outgrown it by late childhood, most by puberty, but a few have it all their lives.

What are the risks?

It is not a dangerous disease, but infection can occur from scratching, especially if the skin is raw. Contact with herpes simplex (cold sores) can produce nasty reactions. Patients have a tendency to develop asthma and other 'atopies' later.

What things appear to aggravate eczema?

- sand, especially sandpits
- dust
- soaps and detergents
- rough and woollen clothes
- scratching and rubbing
- frequent washing with soap, especially in winter
- drying preparations such as calamine lotion
- extremes of temperature, especially cold weather with low humidity
- stress and emotional upsets
- teething
- certain foods (which parents may identify)

Note: The relationship of diet to eczema is controversial and uncertain. It may be worthwhile avoiding certain suspect foods for a 3–4 week trial—these include cows milk, fish, eggs, wheat, oranges and peanuts.

What about skin tests and injections?

The value of allergy testing is doubtful, and 'desensitisation' injections may make the eczema worse.

What is the treatment?

Self-help

- Avoid soap and perfumed products—use a bland bath oil in the bath and aqueous cream for the skin to keep it moisturised (e.g. Sorbolene, Aquasol).
- Older children and adults should have short, tepid showers.
- Avoid rubbing and scratching—use gauze bandages with hand splints for infants.
- Avoid sudden changes of temperature, especially those that cause sweating.
- Wear light, soft, loose clothes such as cotton clothing, which should always be worn next to the skin.
- Avoid dusty conditions and sand, especially sandpits.

Medical help

Your doctor, who should be consulted if you are concerned, may prescribe antihistamine medicine for the allergy and sedation, special moisturising creams and lotions, antibiotics for infection (if present) and milder dilute corticosteroid creams, which can be very effective.

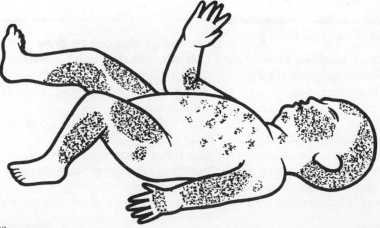

Typical sites of infantile eczema

John Murtagh, *Patient Education*, Second edition, McGraw-Hill Book Company

Autism

What is autism?

Autism, described first by Kanner in 1943, is a developmental disorder commencing in early childhood. It affects at least 4 children in 10 000; boys are 4 times more likely than girls to be affected. The main features are:

- inability of the child to form normal social relationships, even with his or her own parents
- delayed and disordered language development (about one-half of all autistic children never learn to speak effectively)
- obsessive and ritualistic behaviours such as hand flapping, spinning, twiddling pieces of stick or string and hoarding unusual objects
- restricted range of interests
- lack of imagination and difficulty in development of play
- anxiety over changes in routine

What is the cause?

The cause of autism is unknown and no one particular anatomical, biochemical or genetic disorder has been found in those who suffer from it. The problem appears to lie in that part of the brain responsible for the development of language.

What are the symptoms?

Many autistic children appear physically healthy and well developed. However, they may show many disturbed behaviours. As infants they may cry a lot and need little sleep. They resist change in routine and often refuse to progress from milk and baby food to a solid diet. They avoid eye contact and often behave as if they are deaf. Normal bonding between mother and child does not occur and prolonged bouts of crying do not respond to cuddling. As the children get older and more agile they may show frequent tantrum behaviour, destructiveness, hyperactivity and a disregard for danger, requiring constant supervision to prevent harm to themselves or their environment.

What is the treatment?

There is no medical treatment for autism, although some medications may help for some of the symptoms. If there is a deterioration in behaviour or skills, a thorough medical check is required because the autistic child does not indicate pain or communicate clearly. Best results are obtained by early diagnosis, followed by a firm and consistent home management and early intervention program. Later the child will benefit from remedial education, either in a specialised facility or in a regular school with specialist backup. Speech therapy can help with language development, and non-speaking children can be taught alternative methods of communication.

Most difficult behaviours can be reduced or eliminated by a program of firm and consistent management.

What is the outlook?

Behavioural and emotional problems may get worse in adolescence, especially during sexual development. Most autistic children have some degree of mental retardation, although some may have normal or superior intelligence. Only about 5% will progress to the stage of independent living and open employment as adults. Most require at least some degree of lifelong support in order to remain within the community and enjoy a good quality of life. As their life expectancy is normal, this represents a considerable commitment from their families and community support services.

Autistic persons have an increased risk of developing epilepsy, and many suffer psychiatric complications such as anxiety, depression and obsessive-compulsive disorder as they get older. These require appropriate medical treatment.

Where to seek advice

Consult your general practitioner, who may refer you to a paediatrician or child psychiatrist. Assistance can also be obtained from Autism Associations in each state, which can provide full information regarding assessment and diagnostic services, management programs and family support services.

Bed-wetting (enuresis)

What is *nocturnal* enuresis (bed-wetting)?

It refers to bed-wetting at night in children (or adults) at a time when control of urine could be reasonably expected.

What is normal?

Bed-wetting at night is common in children up to the age of 5. About 50% of 3-year-olds wet their beds, as do 20% of 4-year-olds and 10% of 5-year-olds. It is considered a problem if regular bed-wetting occurs in children 6 years and older, although many boys do not become dry until 8 years. Bed-wetting after a long period of good toilet training with dryness is called *secondary enuresis*.

What causes it?

There is usually no obvious cause, and most of the children are normal in every respect but seem to have a delay in development of bladder control. Others may have a small bladder capacity or a sensitive bladder. It tends to be more common in boys and seems to run in families. Most bed-wetting episodes occur in a deep sleep, and so the child cannot help it. The cause of secondary enuresis can be psychological; it commonly occurs during a period of stress or anxiety, such as separation from a parent or the arrival of a new baby. In a small number of cases there is an underlying physical cause, such as an abnormality of the urinary tract. Diabetes and urinary tract infections may also be responsible.

Should the child be checked by your doctor?

Yes; this is quite important, as it will exclude the rare possibility of any underlying physical problem (such as a faulty valve in the bladder) that might cause bed-wetting.

How should parents treat the child?

If no cause is found, reassure the child that there is nothing wrong, and that it is a common problem that will eventually go away. There are some important ways of helping the child adjust to the problem:
• Do not scold or punish the child.
• Praise the child often, when appropriate.
• Do not stop the child drinking after the evening meal.
• Do not wake the child at night to visit the toilet.
• Use a night light to help the child who wakes.
• Some parents use a nappy to keep the bed dry, but try using special absorbent pads beneath the bottom sheet rather than a nappy.
• Make sure the child has a shower or bath before going to kindergarten or school.

When should you seek professional help?

Seek help if there is:
• continued bed-wetting by children aged 6 or 7 years that is causing distress
• ongoing wetting during the daytime
• bed-wetting starting after a year's dryness

What are the treatment options?

Many methods have been tried, but the bed-wetting alarm system is generally regarded to be the most effective. If the child has emotional problems, counselling or hypnotherapy may be desirable. Drugs can be used and may be very effective in some children, but they do not always achieve a long-term cure and have limitations.

The bed alarm

There are various types of alarms: some use pads in the pyjama pants and under the bottom sheet, but recently developed alarms use a small bakelite chip, which is attached to the child's briefs by a safety pin. A lead connects to the buzzer outside the bed, which makes a loud noise when urine is passed. The child wakes, switches off the buzzer and visits the toilet. This method works well, especially in older children.

Key points

Bed-wetting:
• is not the child's fault
• rarely has an emotional cause
• gets better naturally
• nearly always clears up before adolescence
• requires a gentle, non-interfering approach
• responds well to an alarm from 7 years

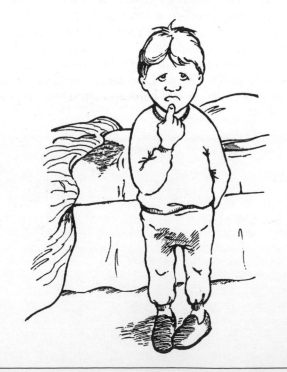

John Murtagh, *Patient Education*, Second edition, McGraw-Hill Book Company

Chickenpox

What is chickenpox?

Chickenpox (varicella) is a mild disease, but is highly contagious and in adults it may result in severe illness. It is caused by a virus that can also cause shingles (herpes zoster). Recovery occurs naturally, because a virus cannot be killed by drugs. Chickenpox affects mainly children under the age of 10.

What are the symptoms?

General

Children are not very sick, but are usually lethargic and have a mild fever. Adults have an influenza-like illness.

The rash

The pocks come out in crops over 3–4 days. At first they resemble red pimples, but in a few hours these form blisters that look like drops of water. The blisters are very fragile and soon burst to leave open sores, which then form a scab and become dry. They can be very itchy.

The site of the rash

The pocks are concentrated on the trunk and head, but spread to the limbs. Do not be alarmed if they appear in or on the mouth, eyes, nose, scalp, vagina or penis.

How infectious is chickenpox?

The disease is very infectious and can spread by droplets from the nose and mouth or by direct contact with the 'raw' pocks. Patients are infectious for 24 hours before the pocks erupt and remain so until all the pocks are covered by scabs and no new ones appear. The incubation period is about 12–21 days, and so the disease appears about 2 weeks after exposure to an infected person. After recovery, lifelong immunity can be expected.

What are the risks?

It is usually a mild illness with complete recovery, but rarely encephalitis and pneumonia occur. Infection of the spots can occur. A severe reaction occurs rarely if aspirin is used in children.

Scarring

Most people worry about this, but usually the spots *do not* scar unless they become infected.

Exclusion from school

Children should be kept at home for 7 days or until all the pocks are dried and covered by scabs. At home it would be sensible to expose other children to the infected person so that the illness can be contracted before adulthood.

What is the treatment?

- The patient should rest in bed or move around quietly until feeling well.
- Give paracetamol for the fever. (Never give aspirin to children.)
- Daub calamine or a similar soothing lotion to relieve itching, although the itch is usually not severe.
- Avoid scratching; clean and cut fingernails of children.
- Keep the diet simple. Drink ample fluids, including orange juice and lemonade.
- Daily bathing is advisable, with sodium bicarbonate added (half a cup to the bath water) or with ordinary soap. Pat dry with a clean, soft towel; do not rub.

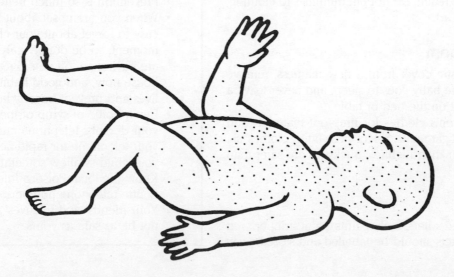

Typical spread of chickenpox

John Murtagh, *Patient Education*, Second edition, McGraw-Hill Book Company

Child accident prevention in the home

In the kitchen

The most dangerous place for children is in the kitchen—poisons and burns are the dangers. Put all spray cleaners, kerosene, pesticides, rat poison and so on out of children's reach, and keep matches in a childproof cupboard.

Electric jugs with cords dangling down are very dangerous, and a cup of tea is just as hot as boiling water. Never drink anything hot while holding a baby, or pass anything hot over a baby's head or body. Do not allow saucepan handles to stick out into the kitchen from the top of the stove. Do not use tablecloths. Always put hot food and drinks in the centre of the table.

Preschool children can easily choke on peanuts and small hard foods.

In the bathroom

Poisons and burns are also the main bathroom hazards, but children do drown in baths. Run cold water before hot into children's baths and always test the water temperature before the child gets in. Never leave children unattended in a bath.

Tablets and medicines may be fatal for children: store tablets and medicines in a childproof place and destroy all leftovers. Toilet cleaners and deodorants also should be locked away.

In the playroom

Any object smaller than a 20-cent piece may choke a child: there should be no beads around or small removable parts on toys. Keep jars containing small items such as buttons out of reach. Do not pin dummies to clothing; tie them on instead.

In the bedroom

Remove the plastic cover from a new mattress, remove the bib before the baby goes to sleep, and never leave a baby unattended on the bed or table.

Check children's clothes for fireproof materials and choose the safest garments. Select close-fitting clothes; ski pyjamas are safer than nighties; tracksuits are safer than dressing gowns.

In the yard

Insecticides, weed-killers, fuels, paints, paint strippers and all garden products should be labelled and stored away from children. They should never be stored in old drink bottles. Children will crawl and fall over veranda edges and steps unless they are fenced off.

Short stakes in the garden should be removed, and keep children inside while mowing the lawn. Do not leave ladders around.

In the pool

Five centimetres of water in a pool can drown a toddler. A pool not in use should be made safe from wandering children—at least covered and preferably fenced off—and children should swim only with adult supervision. Keep pool chemicals, especially acid, locked away.

In the car and on the road

Place your child in the car first, and then walk right around the car before reversing down the drive. All children should be placed in approved child restraints, even to be driven just around the corner.

Train your children to sit in the back on the passenger side so that they get out on the kerb.

In general

Floor-to-ceiling glass doors and windows should have two stickers on them (one at your eye level, the other at toddler eye level) to prevent people walking through.

False plugs should be inserted into all power points that are not in use, especially those within toddlers' reach.

Bar radiators and children do not mix. Any type of fire should have a guard around it.

Remember

- Prevention is so much better than cure.
- When you are upset about something it is easy to forget about your child for a moment, so be doubly careful when you are having an 'off day'. Prepare your house now, and good habits will save lives and prevent tragedy later.
- Buy a bottle of syrup of ipecac and write your doctor's telephone number beside your telephone for rapid action should your child swallow something dangerous. Know the local Poisons Information Centre telephone number.
- Your friends' and relatives' homes may not be as safe as yours.

John Murtagh, *Patient Education*, Second edition, McGraw-Hill Book Company

Circumcision

Who gets circumcised?

Circumcision is performed on baby boys for a number of reasons, but mainly because it is demanded or requested by their parents, often for religious or cultural reasons. It is a routine ritual in some religions or cultures, but in other societies parents tend to be uncertain about the decision to circumcise and may worry a lot about it. Some parents want the operation so that the child can be just like his father. In older boys and some adults, circumcision may be necessary for medical reasons, but this is quite uncommon.

Why are doctors generally against circumcision?

As a rule doctors advise against routine circumcision, mainly because it is unnecessary on medical grounds and any unnecessary operations should be avoided. Any operation carries a risk of complications and some, such as bleeding, can occur during circumcision. The foreskin has a protective function for the delicate glans (tip) of the penis, and many doctors see this as an important feature of the natural order of the human body.

When can the foreskin be fully pulled back?

The foreskin of all newborn babies is tight. As time goes by the foreskin frees up so that by the age of 5 years it can usually be fully retracted. It is not worth trying too hard before this age. When it is pulled back, it is advisable to gently wash away the cheesy material that has built up. If it is not possible to fully pull back the foreskin by the age of 10, it is worthwhile consulting your doctor.

Who needs circumcision?

In some boys the foreskin may be very tight (this is called *phimosis*) and prone to infection. Sometimes an infection can cause the skin to become too tight. This leads to a very small opening, which can cause problems when passing urine (e.g. dribbling or spraying). Redness and discharge as well as pus when passing urine indicate infection. This may well mean that circumcision will be necessary. However, one or two attacks do not mean circumcision is essential. Rarely the foreskin cannot be pulled back easily (and may get stuck) in some older boys, and this may be a reason for circumcision.

The decision to circumcise

It is important to weigh up the pros and cons for circumcision and then discuss it with your doctor. Doctors usually advise against operating on newborn babies and point out that there is no hurry to operate because it is best performed when the baby is not wearing nappies.

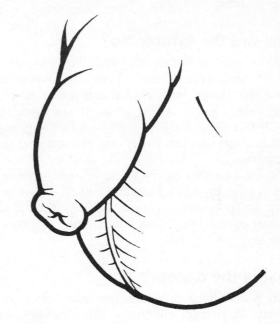

Key points
- Routine circumcision is not recommended.
- It is best avoided on newborn babies.
- It should be considered when there is:
  - very tight foreskin
  - recurring infection of the foreskin
  - difficulty in passing urine
  - foreskin that cannot be pulled back easily

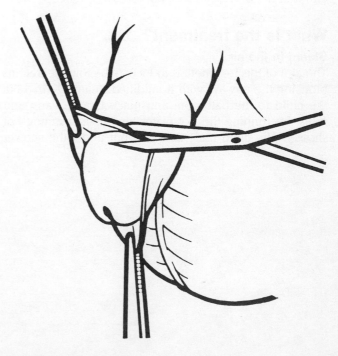

Tight foreskin

Method of circumcision

Croup

What is croup?

Croup is a common viral infection of the upper airway at the level of the throat, namely the voice box (larynx) and windpipe (trachea). It is a special problem in children, who normally have narrow air passages, and usually occurs from 6 months to 3 years of age but can occur up to 6 years or so. The younger the child, the more susceptible he or she is to croup. It tends to occur in the winter months.

What are the symptoms?

A harsh, 'barking' cough and noisy breathing are the main symptoms. Croup usually begins as a normal cold, then a sore throat, hoarse voice and fever follow. The cough, which is dry, hollow sounding and 'barking', is very characteristic. A *stridor* (a high-pitched wheezing or grunting noise with breathing) may develop, and this is a serious sign.

Attacks of croup usually occur at night, causing the child to wake up with a fright and a harsh, brassy cough or stridor. The symptoms are worse if the child is upset and may last for 3 or 4 days, but the first 1 or 2 days are the worst.

What is the danger?

Croup is usually a mild infection and settles nicely; however, in younger children it can sometimes cause complete airway obstruction, which is rapidly fatal. These children need to be in hospital to have a tube inserted.

What is the treatment?

Steam in the air

The aim of this treatment is to loosen the thick secretions blocking the airways with humidified steaming air. Take the child to the bathroom and make the air warm and moist by running the hot water taps or a steaming hot shower. The child must never be put under the shower or left alone in the bathroom with the hot taps running. Nursing the child in this atmosphere will settle mild attacks. It is important to keep the child calm.

The air can also be kept moist and warm by simply boiling a kettle. Special nebulisers that produce a fine mist are available for hire from some pharmacists and can be left by the bed as the child sleeps.

Other treatments

- Give the child paracetamol for fever.
- Antibiotics will not help, because croup is caused by a viral infection; however, they are used for any bacterial infection that develops with the croup.
- Stay by the child's bedside until the child settles.
- Have the child propped up in bed or lying on a few pillows for support. Watching television can help the child relax.
- Wrapping the child in a blanket and walking around outside may help the symptoms to settle.

When should you seek immediate medical help?

Call your doctor or take your child to the hospital urgently if:
- the stridor gets worse and is present when resting or sleeping
- the breathing becomes very difficult
- the child becomes blue and pale
- the breastbone of the chest sucks in on breathing
- the child is floppy and dribbling
- the child becomes very restless or irrational
- the child looks sick and you are most concerned

Key points

- Croup is worse at night.
- Keep the child calm.
- Treat with moist air.
- Croup can be dangerous.
- Get help if you are concerned.

John Murtagh, *Patient Education*, Second edition, McGraw-Hill Book Company

Crying baby

'All noise at one end and no sense of responsibility at the other' is an old saying about infants. However, crying is an important expression to develop a proper interaction between the baby and parent or carer.

What is normal crying?

During the first few weeks, the average baby sleeps a lot and when awake cries loud and often, usually without tears. From 6 weeks onwards, the baby has some wakeful periods without crying, and by 6 months spends 3–4 hours a day playing and gurgling without crying.

What is excessive crying?

Crying is excessive when it lasts for long periods when the baby should be sleeping or playing. It appears to be more common with the first baby and is aggravated by parents getting angry with the baby.

A check list of common causes

- hunger
- wet or soiled nappy
- teething
- infant colic
- loneliness or seeking attention
- infection

You should keep these problems in mind when you check your crying baby.

Feeding problems and hunger

The main feeding problem that causes crying is underfeeding. If so, the baby will be slow in gaining weight and may pass small, firm, dark-green motions. It is important to check this with your doctor or infant welfare nurse.

Passing urine or wet nappies

Wet or dirty nappies may cause discomfort to babies, and so this needs to be checked. Do not fall for the old trap of thinking that passing urine is painful for the baby. It is worth remembering that crying can cause the baby to pass urine.

Teething

Babies usually cut their first teeth between the ages of 6 months and 2 years. The gum is often swollen and sore at the spots where the tooth erupts. This discomfort can make the baby cry, but it does not usually last for longer than a week.

Infant colic

This is one of the commonest causes of unexplained gusty crying in an infant. It is a distressing but harmless problem that some babies develop from as early as 1–2 weeks of age and lasts until 12–16 weeks. It typically develops in the late afternoon and early evening and lasts for about 3 hours in a day and continues for at least 3 weeks.

Loneliness

Some babies may cry because they feel lonely and are looking for comfort and attention. If the baby stops crying when picked up, the cause may well be this lonely feeling.

Infections

Infections are not all that common in infants but will be diagnosed by your doctor. Examples of such infections are a respiratory tract virus, urinary tract infection, gastroenteritis and middle ear infection. A middle ear infection, which can cause much distress, may be indicated by a fever, running nose and the baby pulling at his or her ear.

What should be done?

Simply check out and attend to these common causes. It is important to understand that these crying episodes are not the mother's (or carer's) fault and that the mother needs help to allow her to rest and get over the birth. It is common for some mothers to feel a failure, but nothing could be further from the truth. These crying periods do not usually last very long. Seek advice from your doctor if you are worried and cannot work out the cause or remedy. You must report any unusual symptoms.

Dyslexia and other SLDs

What is a specific learning disability (SLD)?

It is an unexpected and unexplained condition, occurring in a child of average or above average intelligence who has a significant delay in one or more areas of learning. SLDs are commoner than realised and affect about 10% of children.

What learning areas are affected?

- reading
- spelling
- writing
- arithmetic
- language (comprehension and expression)
- attention and organisation
- co-ordination
- social and emotional development

What causes general learning difficulties?

General learning difficulties have many causes, including deafness, immaturity, intellectual handicaps, absence from school, poor teaching, visual handicaps, chronic illness, head injuries, meningitis, language disorders, autism, environmental and emotional disadvantages and SLDs.

What causes SLDs?

SLD is really a descriptive term. The primary cause is unknown. There may be multiple subtle factors causing the SLD.

How are SLDs diagnosed?

If the problem is not picked up by parents, any undisclosed learning problem will soon be picked up in the classroom. Sometimes the disability is not picked up until later (from the age of 8 onwards), when more demanding school work is required. SLDs vary from very mild to quite severe. Speech delays, reading problems and calculation problems are among the first signs. The child will then be assessed medically, including his or her hearing and vision. If a physical problem such as poor vision can be detected, the child will be referred to a specialist in this area.

What effects do SLDs have?

Apart from having delayed learning at school, many children with SLDs have difficulty in coping with life in general. They are subject to ridicule by other children and tend to develop a poor self-image and low self-esteem. The problem may manifest as a behaviour disorder. Both the child and the family suffer, especially if the cause is not clear to them.

What is dyslexia?

Dyslexia is an SLD with reading. A dyslexic child has below average reading skills yet has no physical problems and has a normal IQ. Other SLDs may be present, particularly with spelling, writing and clear speaking.

Dyslexia is a term derived from the Greek for 'difficulty with words'. It was originally called 'word blindness'.

What are the features of dyslexia?

The two main features are reading and spelling difficulties because the child confuses certain letters whose shapes are similar but have different positions, perhaps mirror images. Examples include confusing *b* with *d* and *p* with *q*. This means that the child cannot properly use and interpret the knowledge that he or she has acquired.

Characteristics include:
- a reluctance to read aloud
- a monotonous voice when reading
- following the text with the finger when reading
- difficulty repeating long words

The above features, of course, are seen in all or most learners, but if they persist in a bright child dyslexia should be considered. The most important factor in management is to recognise the problem, and the earlier the better.

What is the management of SLDs?

It is important to build the child's self-esteem by explaining the problem carefully, removing any sense of self-blame and encouraging efforts towards progress. Parents can play an important role in building up their child's self-esteem and in helping learning. Parents are the most important teachers.

Children with SLDs are usually referred to an experienced professional or to a clinic such as a dyslexia clinic for assessment. The management may involve a clinical psychologist, an audiologist, an optometrist or a speech pathologist. A specific method of correcting the problem and promoting learning will be devised. It is also worthwhile seeking the help of a support organisation.

John Murtagh, *Patient Education*, Second edition, McGraw-Hill Book Company

Earache in children

What causes earache in children?

The commonest cause of earache is acute infection of the middle ear (*otitis media*), which usually follows a nose or throat infection such as the common cold.

Another common cause, especially in older children, is infection of the outer ear (*otitis externa*) caused by fungi or bacteria that infect ears blocked with wax, water and sweat. This often occurs after swimming, and so is more prevalent in summer.

An important cause to consider is a foreign body in the ear (e.g. an insect or the child poking something down the ear). This could even cause a ruptured eardrum.

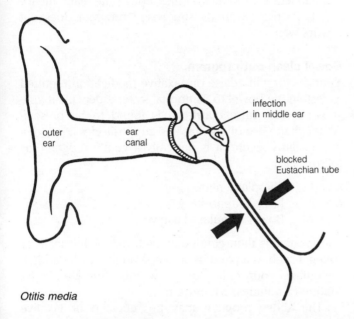

outer ear

ear canal

infection in middle ear

blocked Eustachian tube

Otitis media

Middle ear infection (otitis media)

What is the cause?

Viruses and bacteria can travel up the short and narrow Eustachian tube, which connects the middle ear to the back of the throat. When this tube becomes congested and blocked from a cold, the germs get trapped in the middle ear cavity and cause a painful infection, often with infected fluid (pus). The younger the child, the more likely is infection. The two commonest age groups appear to be between 6–12 months and 5–6 years (when school is commenced).

What are the symptoms?

The main symptoms are:
- earache, often intense pain
- irritability; frequent rubbing or pulling of ear
- fever or general feeling of being unwell
- usually a blocked or runny nose

There may also be:
- poor hearing
- a discharge from the ear

What should you do?

- Place the child in an upright position with pillows or by nursing in your lap.
- Give analgesics such as paracetamol. (It is very important to relieve pain.)
- Give a decongestant to free the Eustachian tube, preferably an oral one but nose drops or spray can be used.
- Contact your doctor, who may prescribe an antibiotic after inspecting the ear.

Glue ears

It is advisable to have your child checked after a middle ear infection to see that the ear has returned to normal. Sometimes a 'glue ear' (*secretory otitis media*) follows acute otitis media. This is the build-up of a sticky glue-like fluid that gets trapped behind the drum when the fluid cannot drain out of the Eustachian tube.

What are the symptoms?

- deafness (usually partial only) and inattentiveness
- earache (usually mild)

What is the treatment?

Glue ears usually get better naturally but can be helped with decongestant medicine and strong nose-blowing exercises. If possible, get the child to pinch the nose and blow out hard against the back of the hand. Sometimes it is necessary to operate to drain the sticky fluid out of the ear by placing small drainage tubes through the drum.

Encopresis

What is encopresis?

Encopresis is the condition in a child over 4 years of age who regularly starts soiling his or her underclothes, after having previously been well toilet trained. Children do not usually have complete bowel control until at least $2\frac{1}{2}$ years of age. About 1–2 children in 100 have the problem and it is 3 times commoner in boys than in girls.

What are some of the features of encopresis?

- Bowel movements occur spontaneously into the underwear.
- The stools may be fully formed or partly formed.
- The soiling has to be present for at least 1 month.
- The child appears to have no control or warning.
- The abdomen may swell.
- Enuresis (bed-wetting) is often present.

Note: Diarrhoea has to be excluded.

What are the causes?

The commonest cause is constipation with false diarrhoea around the clogged up bowel. This may follow a period of resistance to or embarrassment about using toilets at kindergarten or school, on camping trips or outdoors. Rarely it may follow a bad experience visiting a school or other public toilet. School bullying can be a factor.

Sometimes the cause is not apparent. It may develop after a period of being too preoccupied with activities, resulting in bad habits with going to the toilet.

Some apparent causes are:

- a serious illness
- a poor diet, leading to constipation
- painful bowel movements (e.g. an anal fissure)
- stress or an emotional upset (e.g. parental separation)
- child abuse
- negative reaction to parents' obsession about toilet use

What is false (spurious) diarrhoea?

This is a trick played by the body. It occurs when after a period of constipation large amounts of hard faeces build up in the lower bowel and rectum. The fluid faeces from higher up tend to trickle past the obstruction and soil the underwear. The child is unaware of this and control has been lost because the usual anal reflex does not respond.

Parents often think their child has diarrhoea when the problem is really constipation. The doctor can diagnose it by examining the rectum.

What is the management?

Role of parents

- A concerned, understanding and supportive approach is essential.
- Be sensitive to other stresses in your child's life.
- Do not shame or punish the child for 'dirty habits'.
- Ensure your child is not subject to any abuse.
- Approach toilet training sensibly—have realistic expectations. However, a structured toilet program may be advisable for your child; for example, regular sitting on the toilet for 5 minutes 3 times a day (after each meal). A too strict or poorly supervised program does not work well.

Bowel clean out program

Your doctor will advise on laxative medication required to restore the bowel to its normal state, especially if constipation with false diarrhoea is found to be present. Although the use of enemas and suppositories in a 3 day cycle seems severe, it is basically a gentle program, as follows:

Day 1   Microlax enema
Day 2   Rectal suppository
Day 3   Bowel stimulant laxative

The laxative is then continued each day. A lubricant or softener such as a paraffin oil preparation may be added. Encourage your child to follow the structured toilet routine (5 minutes, 3 times a day).

The above program may be repeated or laxative therapy continued until the problem settles. It usually requires supervision for at least 12 months. Sometimes referral to a special clinic may be necessary.

Other pointers for parents

- Get children 5 years and older to clean up themselves.
- Ask for the teacher's co-operation.
- Do not return to napkins.
- Do not allow siblings to tease the child.
- Provide incentives (e.g. time out with parents).

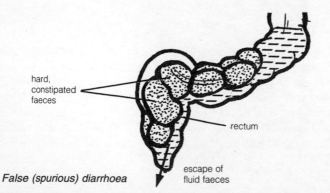

hard,
constipated
faeces

rectum

escape of
fluid faeces

False (spurious) diarrhoea

> **Remember**
> - Praise effort and success.
> - Do not blame, shame or punish for accidents.
> - Do not overreact.
> - Check and correct any stresses.
> - Seek the co-operation of all contacts.
> - Provide a special high fibre diet.
> - Establish good toilet habits.

John Murtagh, *Patient Education*, Second edition, McGraw-Hill Book Company

Febrile convulsions

What are febrile convulsions?

Febrile convulsions are fits or seizures that occur in young children when they have a high fever. A *convulsion* (fit) is a sudden event when the child is not 'quite with it', starts to jerk or twitch and may have difficulty in breathing.

What causes febrile convulsions?

They only occur when the child has a high temperature. The growing brains of little children are more sensitive to fever than are more mature brains, and when the normal brain activity is upset a fit can occur.

The fever is caused by an infection, which is usually a viral infection and often is not obvious. A simple viral infection that would give an adult a heavy cold is the type often responsible. Sometimes an infected ear or throat or bladder may be found by the doctor.

Who gets them?

They are common and can affect any normal child. About 5 in every 100 children will have a fit from a fever. They tend to run in families.

They usually occur in children from 6 months to 3 years of age, the commonest age range being from 9 months to 20 months; they usually stop by 6 years of age.

What are the risks?

Febrile convulsions (whether one or several) in normal children do not usually cause brain damage or epilepsy. Most children are absolutely normal later on.

How do you manage a convulsion?

1. Place the child on his or her side, chest down, with the head turned to one side. Never lie a fitting or unconscious child on his or her back. Do not force anything into the child's mouth.

2. Obtain medical help as soon as possible. Ring or go to your local doctor or to your nearest hospital. Even if the fit stops, have your child checked.

How do you help prevent another episode?

Because some children have further febrile convulsions, it is important to manage any fever as soon as it is noticed. Undress the child down to singlet and under-pants, keep the child cool, give fluids and paracetamol mixture.

Key points

- Febrile convulsions may occur again.
- They usually occur from 6 months to 3 years of age.
- They cause no long-term problems.
- They do not cause death, brain damage or epilepsy.
- They stop by 6 years of age.

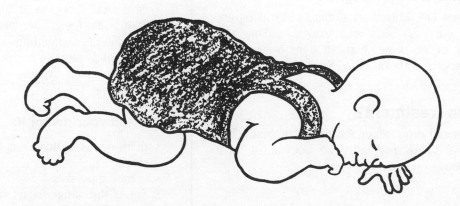

The correct positioning of a child during a fit

Gastroenteritis in children

What is gastroenteritis?

It is an infection of the bowel that causes diarrhoea and sometimes vomiting. It is very common in young children and is mainly caused by viruses.

How is it caught?

The viruses can be easily picked up from other people who may have immunity but pass on the infection. Bacteria, usually on contaminated food and often spread by flies, can also cause the problem.

What are the symptoms?

- diarrhoea—frequent, loose, watery, greenish motions
- vomiting—usually early on
- abdominal pain—colicky pain may be present
- crying—due to pain, hunger, thirst or nausea
- bleeding—uncommon but sometimes seen in motions
- fever—sometimes present
- anal soreness

What is the outcome?

The vomiting usually settles in a day or so. The diarrhoea may last for up to 10 days, but usually lasts only 2 or 3 days.

What are the problems?

The serious problems are loss of water (dehydration) and loss of minerals such as sodium chloride and potassium. The younger the child, the greater the danger. The main cause is persistent vomiting.

What are the danger signs?

The danger signs are listlessness, difficulty in waking up, sunken eyes, very dry skin and tongue, pallor, and passing scanty or no urine. If these signs are present, contact your doctor without delay. Your child may need admission to hospital.

What is the treatment?

There is no special drug treatment for this problem. The inflamed bowel needs rest, and the body must have water and glucose.

Day 1

Give fluids a little at a time and often (e.g. 50 mL every 15 minutes if vomiting a lot). A good method is to give 200 mL (about 1 cup) of fluid every time a watery stool is passed or a big vomit occurs.

The ideal fluid is Gastrolyte, a glucose and mineral powder that you can obtain from your pharmacist and make up according to the directions on the packet. Alternatives to Gastrolyte are:

• lemonade (not low calorie)	1 part to 4 parts water
• sucrose (table sugar)	1 teaspoon to 240 mL (1 cup) water
• glucose	1 teaspoon to 240 mL (1 cup) water
• cordials (not low calorie)	1 part to 16 parts water

Warning: Do *not* use straight lemonade or mix up Gastrolyte with lemonade or fluids other than water.

Days 2 and 3

Reintroduce your baby's usual milk or formula diluted to half strength (i.e. mix equal quantities of milk or formula and water).

Do not worry that your child is not eating food. Solids can be commenced after 24 hours. Start with bread, plain biscuits, jelly, stewed apple, rice, porridge or non-fat potato chips. Avoid fatty foods, fried foods, raw vegetables and fruit, and wholegrain bread.

Day 4

Increase milk to normal strength and gradually reintroduce the usual diet.

Breastfeeding

If your baby is not vomiting, continue breastfeeding but offer extra fluids (preferably Gastrolyte) between feeds. If vomiting is a problem, express breast milk for the time being while you follow the oral fluid program.

Rules to follow for diarrhoea and vomiting

- Give small amounts of fluid often.
- Start bottle feeds after 24 hours.
- Continue breastfeeding.
- Start solids after 24 hours.
- Maintain good hygiene—the problem is infectious.

Consult your doctor if:

- diarrhoea is profuse, e.g. 8–10 watery stools
- vomiting persists
- any of the danger signs are present
- severe abdominal pain develops
- diarrhoea persists or recurs with introduction of milk

John Murtagh, *Patient Education*, Second edition, McGraw-Hill Book Company

Hearing problems in children

What can cause hearing problems?

Your child may be born with a hearing problem, which could have been caused by an infection such as rubella during pregnancy. The commonest cause of hearing problems is a 'glue ear', which is a build-up of sticky fluid in the middle ear following middle ear infections.

The outer ear can get blocked with things such as wax and foreign objects put in there by the child.

How might I know my child is deaf?

Your child may not respond in an expected way to sounds, especially to your voice. Deaf children do not respond to normal conversation or to the television, even if it is turned up loud.

Deafness could show up as unusual problems such as poor speech, disobedience and other behavioural problems and learning problems at school. The kindergarten or school teacher may pick up the problem.

What are the early signs of normal hearing?

The following stages at various ages are useful guides:
- *1 month*: should notice sudden constant sounds (e.g. car motor, vacuum cleaner) by pausing and listening.
- *3 months*: should respond to loud noise (e.g. will stop crying when hands are clapped).
- *4 months*: should turn head to look for source of sound such as mother speaking behind the child.
- *7 months*: should turn instantly to voices or even to quiet noises made across the room.
- *10 months*: should listen out for familiar everyday sounds.
- *12 months*: should show some response to familiar words and commands, including his or her name.

Can hearing tests be done on babies?

Yes. Hearing can be tested at any age. No baby is too young to be tested, and this includes the newborn. If you have any concerns, contact your family doctor, who can arrange a hearing test at an acoustic laboratory. It is most important to diagnose a hearing problem as early as possible. Do not put it off.

Are hearing tests complex?

No; the tests are quite simple. They are not uncomfortable and, as you can imagine, the audiologists are very experienced in dealing with children and getting accurate results.

Remember

- Hearing problems are common in children.
- The earlier deafness is detected the better.
- The commonest cause of hearing difficulties is ear infection leading to 'glue ear'.
- Deafness can cause learning problems at school, poor speech and behaviour problems.
- Any speech or language delay requires investigation.
- Hearing tests are easy to do at any age.

Immunisation of children

The importance of immunisation

The use of vaccines during childhood has dramatically reduced the number of deaths from the basic infectious diseases. At the turn of this century thousands of children died from diphtheria and whooping cough, but immunisation has changed that. However, these infectious diseases are still around and could surface again if we do not immunise. Immunisation is vital preventive medicine, and parents have a responsibility to make sure their children are immunised.

How do the vaccines work?

Whenever we have an infection, our bodies automatically defend themselves by producing substances called *antibodies* that neutralise the infection. These antibodies remain in the body to fight further contact with germs, and this protection is called *immunity*. A vaccine is really an artificial type of infection that stimulates the production of antibodies to give us this immunity.

What diseases do we vaccinate against?

Diphtheria
Diphtheria is a bacterial infection that causes a membrane to grow across the throat and block the airway. It is now rarely seen because of the successful immunisation program.

Whooping cough
Whooping cough (*pertussis*) is a serious bacterial infection of the chest that causes a dramatic cough in children as they struggle to breathe. It is still a common infection in our community, but immunisation has made it a milder disease. Children who have not been immunised can get severe attacks.

Tetanus
This is another bacterial infection; it causes a severe infection known as *lockjaw*. Although cases still occur, it is rare because of our awareness of the problem. Tetanus can be easily picked up in the non-immune person through a simple injury such as a small cut or a nail breaking the skin. The germs live in the soil, especially that fertilised by manure.

Polio
Polio, once a common disease, is a severe viral infection of the nervous system. It causes paralysis of parts of the body. At first the vaccine was given by injection, but now is in the form of small liquid drops given on a spoon.

Measles
Measles is a very serious viral illness that has not been well controlled, mainly because only 70% of Australians get immunised against it. It can cause serious brain damage (due to encephalitis) in its victims. An injection given at 12 months and then a booster at 10 to 16 years provide immunity. The vaccine is now combined with mumps and rubella.

Mumps
Mumps is one of the well-known infectious diseases of childhood that is now being controlled with immunisation. It can infect the brain (meningitis and encephalitis) and the testicles in young men.

Rubella
Rubella or German measles is not a serious disease except if contracted during the first 3 months of pregnancy, when it can cause serious problems in the baby. It is available for all children at 12 months and then during early adolescence for schoolgirls. Being immune to rubella takes a great load off the mind of any expectant mother.

Haemophilus influenza type B (HIB)
This is a serious bacterial infection that caused many deaths from meningitis and epiglottitis. The vaccine was introduced in 1992, and infections are now rarely seen.

Are there any side effects?

The vaccines usually are free of side effects, although a mild reaction can occur. Sometimes an injection can cause the child to be quite ill, and it usually is the whooping cough (pertussis) component. Your doctor will be able to advise about this.

Childhood immunisation schedule (recommended by the National Health and Medical Research Council, Australia)

Age	Vaccine
2 months	DTP [a] haemophilus polio [b]
4 months	DTP haemophilus polio
6 months	DTP haemophilus polio
12 months	measles, mumps, rubella
18 months	DTP haemophilus
Before school entry	DTP polio
10–16 years	measles, mumps, rubella
Before leaving school (15–19 years)	ADT booster [c] polio

(a) diphtheria, tetanus and pertussis (whooping cough), known as 'triple antigen'
(b) sabin vaccine
(c) diphtheria and tetanus, known as 'ADT'—adult diphtheria, tetanus

John Murtagh, *Patient Education*, Second edition, McGraw-Hill Book Company

Infant colic

What is infant colic?

It is the occurrence in a well baby of regular, unexplained periods of inconsolable crying and fretfulness, usually in the late afternoon and evening, especially between 2 weeks and 16 weeks of age. No cause for the abdominal pain can be found, and it lasts for a period of at least 3 weeks.

It is very common and occurs in about one-third of infants.

What are the typical features?

- baby between 2 and 16 weeks old
- prolonged crying—at least 3 hours
- crying worst at around 10 weeks of age
- crying during late afternoon and early evening
- occurrence at least 3 days a week
- child flexing legs and clenching fists because of the 'gut ache'
- child gets better naturally with time

The myths of infant colic

It is important for concerned parents to know that the colic is *not* caused by the mother's or family's anxiety, by artificial feeding or by food allergy.

Unfortunately, the problem does tend to cause tensions in the family, but it must be emphasised that the baby will thrive, the condition will pass away and the parents are not responsible for the colic.

Some cautionary advice

This can be a danger time for child abuse by frustrated parents, and so please speak to someone about any troublesome feelings. Remember that it is no one's fault and it will soon settle. You must avoid using fad diets or herbal treatments for the baby.

What is the treatment?

- Use gentleness (such as subdued lighting where the baby is handled, soft music, speaking softly, quiet feeding times).
- Avoid quick movements that may startle the baby.
- The advice from and close contact with a maternal or child health nurse is most helpful.
- Advice from the Nursing Mothers Association is helpful.
- Make sure the baby is not hungry—underfeeding can make the baby hungry.
- If the baby is breastfed, express the watery foremilk before putting the baby to the breast.
- Provide demand feeding (in time and amount).
- Make sure the baby is burped and give posture feeding.
- Provide comfort from a dummy or pacifier.
- Provide plenty of gentle physical contact.
- Cuddle and carry the baby around (e.g. take a walk around the block).
- A carrying device such as a 'snuggly' or a 'Meh Tai Sling' allows the baby to be carried around at the time of crying.
- Make sure the mother gets plenty of rest during this difficult period.
- Do not worry about leaving a crying child for 10 minutes or so after 15 minutes of trying consolation.

Mother's diet

The breastfeeding mother's diet has been a controversial issue, but some mothers have found that cutting out cows milk, eggs and spicy foods has helped their babies' colic. A trial of avoiding these foods in the diet is worthwhile.

Drug treatment

Drugs are not generally recommended, especially as some may sedate the baby. However, for severe problems your doctor can prescribe something to help. Fortunately the problem is not serious and soon gets better.

Measles

What is measles?

Measles is a highly contagious disease caused by a virus; it can have more serious after-effects than many people realise. The complications can be dangerous, and so the illness should be taken seriously.

What are the symptoms?

For the first three days the patient is miserable with symptoms like a heavy cold—fever, runny nose, red and watering eyes and a dry, hacking cough. By the third day tiny white spots like grains of salt (called *Koplik's spots*) appear inside the mouth. On the fourth and fifth days a blotchy red rash appears. The rash starts behind the ears and on that day spreads to the face, the next day to the body and later to the limbs. By the sixth day the rash is fading, and after a week all the symptoms have disappeared. However, the rash can leave a pinkish red stain.

If a cough and red eyes are not present, the patient is unlikely to have measles.

How is it spread?

The disease is very infectious and is spread to other people usually by kissing, coughing and sneezing. Once inside the body the virus has an incubation period of about 10–14 days, and the patient is infectious for about 5 days before and 5 days after the rash appears.

What are the risks?

Most patients make a good recovery with lifelong immunity from further attacks, but some get complications from bacterial infections affecting the ear or chest.

There is a small but important risk of getting encephalitis (inflammation of the brain), which can lead to permanent brain damage. For this reason, immunisation of all the population is an important aim of health authorities.

What is the treatment?

The patient should rest quietly, avoid bright lights and stay in bed until the fever has settled. Any high fever should be treated with tepid sponging and paracetamol.

The nasty cough can be controlled with a cough linctus. However, there is no specific treatment and no special drug for measles. Antibiotics are not effective against viral infections, but are used if complications such as ear infections and pneumonia develop.

School exclusion

Children should be kept away from school until they have recovered or for at least 7 days from the appearance of the rash.

What should you do?

- Notify your doctor if any unusual problems develop, including severe constant headache, a stiff neck, convulsions, breathing problems, unusual drowsiness or earache.
- Notify school authorities.

How can measles be prevented?

A vaccine against measles is available and recommended to be given to children at 12 months and once more between 10 and 16 years. It is combined with the mumps and rubella vaccines.

> All children should be vaccinated against measles. The vaccine is free.

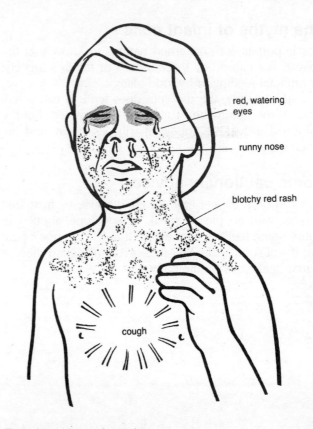

red, watering eyes

runny nose

blotchy red rash

cough

Typical symptoms of measles

John Murtagh, *Patient Education*, Second edition, McGraw-Hill Book Company

Mumps

Mumps

Mumps is a viral infection of the salivary glands, especially the *parotid gland*, which lies in front of and below the ear. It was one of the common infectious diseases of childhood, but is not seen as often now because of the immunisation program.

What are the symptoms?

- swollen and tender glands—one parotid gland swells first, and in 70% of cases the opposite side swells after 1 or 2 days (other glands that lie just below the jaw may also be infected)
- fever
- weakness and lethargy
- dry mouth
- discomfort upon eating or opening the mouth

How is it spread?

Mumps is spread by coughing or sneezing. The virus takes about 18 days to incubate after contact. Mumps is only a moderately infectious disease. It is infectious from 2 days before its onset up to the time the swellings disappear (usually after 6 days but up to 12 days).

The patient should be isolated, especially from adults who have not had mumps.

What are the risks?

Mumps usually is a mild illness, but an uncommon complication is swelling or inflammation of the testes in a male or of the ovaries in a female. It affects adolescents and adults, especially males. Swelling usually affects one side only, coming on 3–4 days after the neck swelling.

The swelling, which can be very painful for a day or so, subsides after a few days. Sterility is rare, and occurs only if both testes are affected. Like any viral infectious disease, it can very rarely cause meningitis and encephalitis (inflammation of the brain).

What is the treatment?

There is no special treatment because the illness has to run its course. General measures are:

- Take paracetamol for pain or high fever.
- Rest until the fever settles.
- Follow a normal soft diet and take ample fluids. Drinking through a straw may be more comfortable.
- Apply heat to the glands (e.g. hot washers or towels) to help relieve any pain.

School exclusion

Fourteen days is recommended, or up to the obvious disappearance of the swollen glands.

What should you do?

Notify your doctor:

- if a boy gets pain or swelling in the testes or a girl complains of low abdominal pains
- if the patient appears very sick (e.g. severe vomiting or headache), is delirious or has a stiff neck
- if the hearing seems affected

Notify school authorities.

How can mumps be prevented?

Mumps can be prevented by a vaccine, which in Australia is recommended to be given to children at 12 months and once more between 10 and 16 years. It is combined with the measles and rubella vaccines.

Nappy rash

What is nappy rash?

It is a red, irritating skin rash corresponding to the area covered by the nappy. It affects the genitals, buttocks, groin and thighs, but usually spares the creases not in contact with the nappy.

What are the symptoms?

The skin is red, spotty and moist. It is irritated when urine is passed, and so causes the baby to cry.

What causes nappy rash?

It is basically caused by excessive contact of the skin with urine or faeces. It is common—most babies have nappy rash at some time, but the skin of some babies is more *sensitive* than others. The appearance of nappy rash does not mean that the carer/s have been neglectful.

The main cause is *dampness* due to urine and faeces, especially from a chemical formed from the urine in the nappy.

Other causes or aggravating factors are:
- a tendency of the baby to eczema
- a tendency of the baby to seborrhoea
- infection, especially monilia (thrush)
- rough-textured nappies
- detergents and other chemicals in the nappies
- plastic pants (aggravate wetness)
- excessive washing of the skin with soap
- too much powder over the nappy area

What is the treatment?

1. Keep the area dry. Change wet or soiled nappies frequently and as soon as you notice them.

2. After changing, gently remove any urine or moisture with diluted sorbolene cream or warm water.

3. Wash gently with warm water, pat dry (do not rub) and then apply any prescribed cream or ointment to help heal and protect the area. Lanoline or zinc cream applied lightly will do.

4. Expose the bare skin to fresh air whenever possible. Leave the nappy off several times a day, especially if the rash is severe.

5. *Do not wash in soap or bath too often*—once or twice a week is enough.

6. *Avoid powder and plastic pants.*

7. Use special soft nappy liners that help protect the sensitive skin.

How to care for nappies

1. Rinse soiled nappies immediately in cold water and rinse out any disinfectants or bleaches used *before* washing.

2. Wash the nappies in a normal hot wash in the washing machine.

3. Make sure the nappies are rinsed to remove chemicals used and *then* dried.

Key points
- Keep the skin dry.
- Expose the skin to air and sunlight where possible.
- Use protective creams.
- Do not use soap or plastic covers.
- Do not bath the baby too much.
- Visit your doctor if the rash is not responding after 4 days.

John Murtagh, *Patient Education*, Second edition, McGraw-Hill Book Company

Rearing a happy child

As parents we want our children to be happy and to grow to be well adjusted. We want to give them the best possible opportunities. We cannot guarantee that our children will be happy, but they have certain basic needs and dreams that we should try to fulfil.

Our children did not ask to be born. God has worked with us to give this gift to the world, and we have to treat this special person with love, care and due responsibility. We must realise that children are not all alike, and that each is an individual with his or her own special personality and needs. However, every person has the same basic needs that require attention. These needs include comfort, security, food, activity, warmth and proper sleep.

Being a good parent is one of the hardest and most challenging jobs in the world, and most parents do a wonderful job in raising children. Some important basic needs of children follow.

Children need love

> Love is to a child what sunlight is to a flower.

Children are not 'spoiled' by too much love, but rather by too little. The little 'brat' is usually the child who is neglected in some way and is seeking attention.

Children have 'antennae'—they can sense feelings towards them. The child who is loved knows it and develops into a contented, mature adult.

Love has to be unconditional—no strings attached. Children have to receive genuine love, for their own sake—not because they are pretty or talented or have great personalities. No matter who they are, or what they look like, or how they perform at school or sport, they all need encouragement and praise so that they have a healthy self-esteem.

Love is not being possessive and clinging to children with smothering affection or showering gifts on them. Love is common sense.

Children need security

A feeling of security is vital to children. It comes not only from being loved but also from growing up in a secure home that is free from fighting parents, child abuse, over-interference from brothers and sisters and the problems of drugs (such as alcohol abuse). A warm bed, sufficient food and clothing are all part of the feeling of security.

Children need play

Children need to be active and creative; they need to be given the opportunity to express themselves freely. 'Make believe' play is important, so that they can work through their fantasies and frustrations.

Some rules for healthy and happy play are:
- Play with parents.
- Play in a supervised playground.
- Have playmates.
- Imitate the jobs of parents /other adults.
- Play with sand and water (a sandpit is great).

Children need discipline

Children need the security of firm, loving discipline. They need to be protected from dangerous toys, games and situations. We must draw the line between wholesome freedom and allowing them to do as they like. It is important for children to learn early that there are certain limits in behaviour. They must learn to respect their own and other people's possessions.

Be consistent with your discipline. Never make threats that you cannot or will not carry out. Taking away certain privileges for a while (rather than physical punishment) when children are naughty seems to work well.

Children need honesty

It is important to be honest with children. They learn to resent incorrect and illogical decisions and comments from their parents. This means being honest when explaining things that hurt, such as an injection or a visit to the dentist. We must also be fair in our comments about others, including their race and religion.

Remember
- Parents are heroes and role models for their children. Don't let your children down.
- Parents are the best teachers.
- At times parents need the wisdom of Solomon.

Reflux in infants

What is gastro-oesophageal reflux?

Reflux is where the food in the stomach overflows back into the oesophagus (gullet). It often causes a baby to bring up or vomit milk after a feed.

A mild degree of reflux is normal in babies, especially after they burp; this condition is called *posseting*. However, the reflux can be quite severe in some babies, who appear to vomit after their bottle or breastfeeding.

What are the symptoms?

Milk will flow freely from the mouth soon after feeding, even after the baby has been put down for a sleep. Sometimes the flow will be forceful and may even be out of the nose.

Despite this vomiting or regurgitation, the babies usually are comfortable and thrive. Some infants will cry, presumably because of heartburn.

What is the outlook?

Reflux gradually improves with time and usually ceases soon after solids are introduced into the diet. Most cases clear up completely by the age of 9 or 10 months, when the baby is sitting. Severe cases tend to persist until 18 months of age.

Contact your doctor should any unusual symptoms appear (such as green or blood-stained vomit or projectile vomiting), or if your baby is distressed after feeds or stops putting on weight.

What is the treatment?

Simple home measures

The baby's stomach can empty more quickly if you elevate the head of the cot by about 10–20 degrees and place the baby on his or her left side for sleeping. Also, you could place the child upright in a suspended 'swing' for periods of about 30–60 minutes after feeds when awake. The old 'bucket' method, in which the child is placed in a bucket, is not necessary.

Feeding

It is better to give small feeds quite often rather than large infrequent feeds. It is best to avoid fatty and spicy foods in older children.

Thickening of feeds

Giving the baby thicker feeds usually helps those with more severe reflux. The old-fashioned remedy of using cornflour blended with milk in bottles is still useful.

Bottle-fed babies (powdered milk formula)

Carobel: Add slightly less than 1 full scoop per bottle.

Gaviscon: Mix slightly less than ½ teaspoon of Infant Gaviscon Powder with 120 mL of formula in the bottle.

Cornflour: Mix 1 teaspoon with each 120 mL of formula. Check with your doctor or nurse for the proper method.

Karicare: This formulation is easy to use but is more expensive. Give according to the manufacturer's instructions.

Breastfed babies

Carobel: Add slightly less than 1 full scoop to 20 mL cool boiled water or 20 mL expressed breast milk and give just before the feed.

Gaviscon: Mix slightly less than ½ teaspoon of Infant Gaviscon Powder with 20 mL cool boiled water or expressed breast milk and give just after the feed.

Key points

Reflux:
- is common
- improves with age
- usually clears up by 9 months of age
- is helped by elevating the cot
- is helped by thickening the feeds
- is helped by frequent small feeds
- is helped by propping up the baby after feeds

John Murtagh, *Patient Education*, Second edition, McGraw-Hill Book Company

Rubella (German measles)

What is rubella?

Rubella is an infectious disease caused by a virus called the *rubella virus*. It is also called *German measles*, because the disease was first described in Germany. It is usually a very mild illness and causes no more trouble than a common cold. However, it has very serious consequences for a woman who gets infected in the first 3 months of her pregnancy. Her baby may be born with blindness, deafness and an abnormal heart. This is called *congenital rubella*.

What are the symptoms?

The patient usually feels unwell, has a slight fever, possibly a runny nose, and swollen glands behind the ears and in the neck.

A rash appears on the first or second day and consists of reddish-pink spots that appear first on the face and neck and then spread rapidly to the body, especially to the chest. The rash lasts for about 2–3 days, and by the fourth or fifth day all symptoms have faded away.

It is possible to have picked up the rubella virus and have no obvious symptoms. This applies to about one-quarter of all patients, who fortunately become immune from further infection.

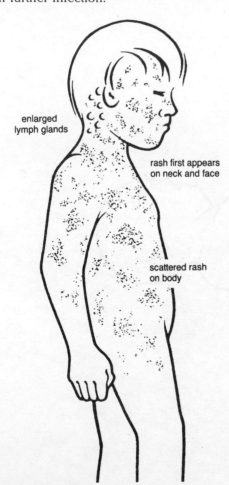

enlarged lymph glands

rash first appears on neck and face

scattered rash on body

Typical symptoms of rubella

How is it spread?

The disease is moderately infectious and is spread by droplets from the nose and throat. Once inside the body, the virus has an incubation period of about 14–21 days before it starts to cause symptoms (if at all).

What are the risks?

The main risk is to an unborn baby. A more common complication, especially in adults, is stiff, swollen joints (arthritis), which is usually short lived. Rarely (1 case in 5000) it carries a risk of encephalitis (inflammation of the brain).

What is the treatment?

Because rubella is such a mild disease, there is no specific treatment. However, patients should rest quietly until they feel well and take paracetamol for fever or aching joints.

School exclusion

The child is usually excluded until fully recovered or for at least 4 days from the onset of the rash.

What should you do?

- Notify your doctor immediately if the patient has a convulsion.
- Notify school authorities.
- Contact any pregnant women who have been exposed to the patient.
- If visiting the doctor, telephone beforehand in order to avoid exposure to pregnant women in the waiting room (if you think rubella is the diagnosis).

How can rubella be prevented?

The rubella vaccine should be given to all women before puberty. In Australia, it is routinely given to children at 12 months (combined with mumps and measles vaccines) and given again between the ages of 10 and 16. Older girls and women of child-bearing age who have not had rubella should be immunised at least 3 months before becoming pregnant. In Australia, most women aged 15–45 are immune and therefore protected from rubella. However, the only way to tell is to have a special blood test.

Seborrhoea in infants

What is seborrhoea?

Seborrhoeic dermatitis is a common skin inflammation that occurs mainly in the hair-bearing areas of the body, especially the scalp and eyebrows. It can appear on the face, neck, armpits and groin. In particular, it can cause nappy rash.

What are the symptoms?

Seborrhoeic dermatitis usually appears as red patches or blotches with areas of scaling. This becomes redder when the baby cries or gets hot. Cradle cap may appear in the scalp. A flaky, scurf-like dandruff appears first, and then a yellow, greasy, scaly crust forms. This scurf is usually associated with reddening of the skin.

Unlike eczema, it does not usually itch and irritate the child, who is usually comfortable, in good health and does not scratch. However, the dermatitis can become infected, especially in the napkin area, and this becomes difficult to clear up. If untreated, it often spreads to many areas of the body. It is said that 'cradle cap and nappy rash may meet in the middle'.

At what age does it occur?

Seborrhoeic dermatitis tends to occur during the first year of life, especially during the first 3 months. Many cases begin in the first month of life. It is rare to see it begin after 2 years.

What is the treatment?

Self-help

Seborrhoeic dermatitis can heal naturally by following a few basic rules. It is most important to keep the areas clean and dry by bathing in warm water, patting the area dry with a soft cloth and keeping the skin exposed to the air and sun (moderate amounts) as much as possible. Avoid using soap for washing.

For cradle cap, rub the scales gently with baby oil and then wash away the loose scales.

For nappy rash, change wet or soiled nappies often, as soon as noticed. Keep the area dry and clean, exposing it to the air and sun for short periods several times a day. Do not wash in soap, use excessive powder or plastic pants.

For the body, apply a thin smear of zinc cream to help mild areas heal and to prevent spread.

Medical help

If the problem is not settling with basic care, consult your doctor, who may prescribe a cream containing sulphur or a special stronger cream if necessary.

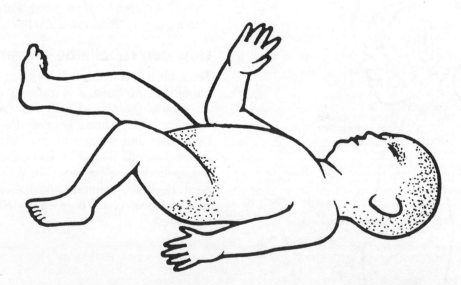

Typical distribution of the rash of seborrhoea

John Murtagh, *Patient Education*, Second edition, McGraw-Hill Book Company

Snuffling infant

What is the cause of snuffling?

Snuffling is usually caused by a viral infection that infects the upper respiratory tract (airways), particularly the nose. This is called *rhinitis*, which is a common minor infection in adults but in children it causes considerable discomfort because the nasal passages are so small. The infection makes it difficult to breathe through the nose.

The virus is usually one that causes the common cold.

What are the symptoms?

- nose blockage with yellow or green mucus
- coughing
- irritability with crying
- feeding difficulty caused by the nose blockage

What are the risks?

It is usually not a serious problem and appears worse than it actually is, although you may not think so at the moment. Sometimes infection with bacteria can develop, and so you should contact your doctor if there is:
- loss of activity
- swelling and infection of the eye
- wheezing or other breathing difficulty
- neck stiffness
- an unusually high fever
- other unusual symptoms

A robust crying child is not as big a cause for concern as is a whimpering, pale, inactive child.

What is the treatment?

Since the problem is caused by a virus, antibiotics do not cure it and so they are not prescribed unless a bacterial infection such as a middle ear infection complicates the problem. Your doctor will be able to check your child's ears, throat and chest to discover any such infections.

Pain-killers

To ease your child's discomfort when he or she seems uncomfortable or distressed, give paracetamol mixture or drops according to the recommended age dosage.

Clean the nose

Cleaning the infected mucus from the nose is quite an easy task for parents. Make a salt solution by mixing a teaspoon of salt with 500 mL of boiled water. Using a cotton bud, gently clear out the secretions from the nose about every 2 waking hours.

Nose drops

When the nose has been cleaned instil saline nose drops or spray (e.g. Narium nasal mist). An alternative is a paediatric decongestant nose drop or spray preparation (such as Vasylox Junior or Otrivin) if the saline drops are not effective and if there is a problem with feeding. These stronger drops should only be used for 4 to 5 days.

Teething

When does teething occur?

Baby teeth (milk or deciduous teeth)
- Babies usually cut their teeth from age 6 months until 2–3 years.
- New teeth continually erupt during this time.
- The first teeth to appear are the lower incisors (during the first year). These seldom give much trouble.
- The first and second molars (between ages 1 and 3) tend to cause problems.
- Usually the first set (20 teeth) is complete soon after the second birthday.
- Be prepared for variations—some babies have teeth (1 or 2) at birth, while others have none at 1 year. This has no significance.
- These teeth are lost between 6 and 12 years.

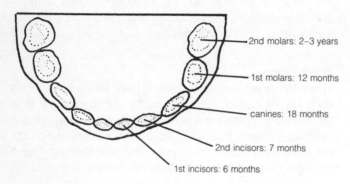

Lower set of 10 'baby' teeth and times when they usually appear

2nd molars: 2–3 years
1st molars: 12 months
canines: 18 months
2nd incisors: 7 months
1st incisors: 6 months

Adult teeth
- Permanent teeth may appear as soon as the baby teeth fall out.
- If they appear before this, the dentist may have to extract the baby teeth.
- Permanent molars appear later, about 12 years.
- A full set is 32 teeth.

What are the symptoms of teething?
- The gum is slightly swollen and red. This may cause little or no discomfort, or may be quite painful.
- The baby is more clinging and fretful than normal.
- The baby dribbles more than usual.
- The baby wants to chew on something (such as fingers).
- The baby is irritable and crying (on and off for no more than a few days).
- The baby has difficulty with sleeping.

The problem usually settles quickly and it is important not to link coincidental illnesses such as fever, diarrhoea, vomiting, earache, convulsions, nappy rash and cough with teething.

Are pitted, dark teeth a problem?

Some children who are breastfed for long periods (such as 3 years) may develop unsightly pitting of the front surface of their teeth. This will not go away, but the parents should be reassured that the adult teeth will be normal when they appear.

What is the treatment?

Soothing methods
- Gentle massaging of the gum with the forefinger wrapped in a soft cloth or gauze pad is comforting. A gel such as Orosed can be massaged into the gums every 3 hours if the problem appears to be extremely troublesome.
- Place a face washer in the freezer and allow the baby to chew on the cool washer.
- Allow the baby to chew on a clean, cold, lightly moistened face washer. (A piece of apple can be placed inside the face washer.)
- Give the baby a teething ring (kept cold in the refrigerator) or a teething biscuit.

Medication
Medicine is usually not necessary for teething. Paracetamol mixture should be used for any discomfort. For more severe problems, especially if they are affecting sleep, an antihistamine or a combined mixture of antihistamine and analgesic can be given at night. Your doctor can advise you about this.

Other measures
- Cleaning the teeth at first with a face washer and then with a small soft toothbrush can commence when they appear, especially after the 8 incisors have erupted.
- Regular dental visits are advisable from about 3 years.
- Explain to children what they can expect about losing their first teeth.

John Murtagh, *Patient Education*, Second edition, McGraw-Hill Book Company

Thumb sucking

What does thumb sucking involve?

It involves placing the thumb or finger on the roof of the mouth behind the teeth (hard palate) and sucking with the mouth closed. It is basically a habit and should not be regarded as an abnormal disorder. It is one of the first pleasurable acts that the infant can manage.

How common is thumb sucking?

It is very common and occurs in children of both sexes up to the age of 12 years, but is commonest in children under the age of 4 years.

What can bring on thumb sucking?

It usually starts for no apparent reason. The child tends to suck the thumb when relaxing, such as when watching television or when put to bed before going to sleep. It also tends to occur when the child is ill, hungry or tired.

Insecurity, such as the arrival of a sibling in the family, can increase thumb sucking; it can be related to an apparent withdrawal of parents' attention.

What are the risks?

Thumb sucking should be regarded as normal and usually settles by the age of 6 or 7. However, if it persists beyond this age it can cause problems with the permanent teeth, which begin to appear at about the age of 7. One effect is that the pressure on the front teeth may cause protrusion of these teeth (i.e. buck teeth).

How can it be prevented?

It is best to provide other comfort measures in infants if this habit is developing. Giving the infant a dummy (pacifier) is preferable. If the habit persists, avoid making it an issue and thus drawing attention to it.

What is the treatment?

No special medicine or diet is necessary.

What to avoid
- nagging
- punishment
- scolding
- gloves, mittens or arm splints
- bad-tasting chemicals on the thumb or finger

What to do (for a child over 6 years)
- Carefully observe things that provoke thumb sucking.
- Find ways of avoiding these trigger factors.
- Provide extra attention.
- Organise pleasant distractions.
- Give praise and rewards for efforts to stop.

When to seek help
- if the problem persists after 6 years, especially if it is excessive and persistent
- if the child wishes to stop but cannot despite good efforts (even when offered rewards for good attempts to stop)

In such situations special counselling may be required. Sometimes the help of the dentist to fit a special training device in the mouth may be required.

> **Remember**
>
> Thumb sucking is usually a passing habit that most children grow out of by school age. Special treatment is rarely necessary. Avoid giving attention to the problem, but give plenty of attention to the child.

Umbilical hernia

Umbilical hernias are very common in babies.

What is an umbilical hernia?

It is a bulge of soft tissue covered by skin in the *umbilicus* (navel) of a baby. It is the site where the blood vessels in the umbilical cord joined mother to baby.

What are the symptoms?

The hernia rarely causes any problems to the baby. Parents may be concerned when the hernia bulges further with crying.

What are the risks?

Because the opening is wide, there is hardly any risk of strangulation.

What happens normally?

The hernia gradually becomes smaller as the baby grows and the hole becomes smaller. Most hernias have disappeared within 12 months, while the larger ones usually disappear by the age of 4. If the hernia has not disappeared by the age of 4, a minor operation to remove it may be necessary.

What is the treatment?

No special treatment is required and the hernia is left to settle naturally. The old-fashioned method of taping a coin over the lump is not necessary and is not advised.

The operation

If the hernia is still present at 4 years, surgery is advisable. The operation involves simply placing a stitch (rather like a purse string) in the hole to close it over. The scar will hardly be noticeable and is usually invisible in adults.

There are no stitches to be removed afterwards. The child comes in as a day patient and will not have to stay overnight under normal circumstances. Children cope and recover much better than do adults with these operations and will be able to carry on with their normal activities the day after the operation.

Key points

Umbilical hernias:
- are common in infants
- do not require treatment
- usually go away by 4 years of age
- can be corrected by a simple operation if necessary

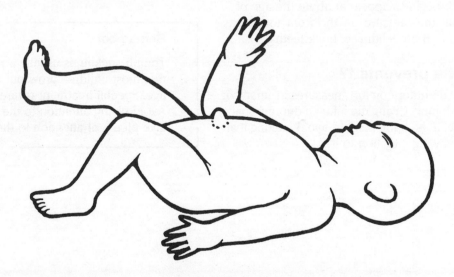

Umbilical hernia

John Murtagh, *Patient Education*, Second edition, McGraw-Hill Book Company

Viral skin rashes in children

What are viral skin rashes?

A viral skin rash is an acute outbreak of a red rash on the body. The rash is part of the illness associated with a generalised viral infection.

In the past, a red rash in a child was usually due to one of the 'big three'—rubella virus, measles virus or scarlet fever. Now the rashes are commonly caused by other viruses.

What are the effects on the child?

The rashes described here—not measles, rubella (German measles) or scarlet fever—are usually mild and do not cause any distress to the child. The rash usually lasts for a few days before disappearing without any ill effects.

Apart from having the rash, the child may feel unwell with fever and display a lack of interest and loss of energy. Sometimes diarrhoea and a snuffly nose can occur.

What are the risks?

Complications of these infections are very rare in healthy children and almost always the problem is mild. Most children go about their normal play as though nothing is wrong.

Is the problem contagious?

These virus illnesses are mildly contagious, especially *fifth disease* (slapped face syndrome), which can occur in outbreaks at schools and among members of the same family. The virus usually spreads from person to person by close contact, mainly by the breath.

What are the main types?

There are three main types, which are simply called *fourth, fifth* and *sixth disease*. The term 'disease' is not a good one, as they are not really diseases.

Fourth disease

This common problem can be caused by a number of viruses, especially those affecting the bowel. The rash is so much like rubella that it is often misdiagnosed as rubella. However, unlike rubella, it is not concentrated on the face and neck. It mainly occurs on the trunk (body), is usually not itchy and often fades after 2 days. It tends to occur in preschool children.

Fifth disease

This is an interesting problem, and is also called *erythema infectiosum* or *slapped face syndrome*. A bright red rash appears on the face first (giving a slapped face appearance), and then after a day or so appears on the arms and legs. The rash lasts for only a few days but may recur on and off for a few weeks. It is a mild illness but can

have serious effects on the foetus if acquired during pregnancy. The infection usually occurs in young school-aged children.

Sixth disease

Sixth disease (also known as *roseola infantum*) usually affects infants at the age of 6–18 months. It has a classic feature in that the child develops a high fever and runny nose and as soon as the fever settles a bright red rash appears, mainly on the trunk. It is uncommon on the face and limbs. The rash lasts only about 2 days.

What is the treatment?

Treatment is very simple. Give paracetamol for the fever. The rash does not require any special treatment as it tends to fade rapidly. If the rash appears to cause discomfort, soothe the child with a tepid bath with Pinetarsol or sodium bicarbonate (half a cup to the bath water).

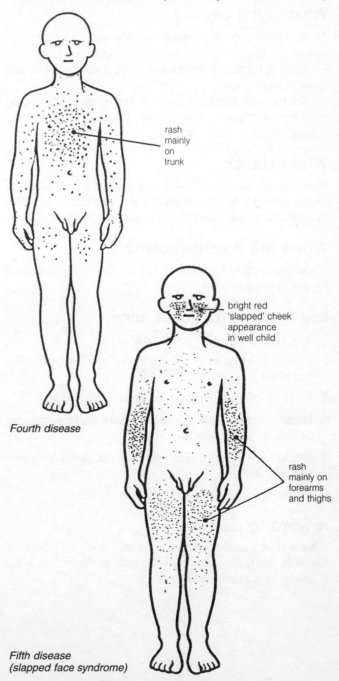

rash mainly on trunk

Fourth disease

bright red 'slapped' cheek appearance in well child

rash mainly on forearms and thighs

Fifth disease (slapped face syndrome)

4 Adolescent health

Acne

What is acne?

Acne is inflammation of the *sebaceous* (oil) glands of the skin. At first these glands become blocked (blackheads and whiteheads) and then inflammation can lead to red bumps (*papules*), yellowheads (*pustules*), and even deep, tender cysts.

Acne is a common disorder of adolescence. It appears usually on the face, but can extend onto the neck, chest and back.

What is the cause?

Acne is related to the increase in the levels of male hormones during puberty in both sexes. Although the increase in hormone levels is normal, some people seem more sensitive to it.

Bacteria on the skin grow in the blocked gland and release fatty acids, which are irritating and set up inflammation.

Who gets it?

Most young men aged 13–18 will get acne. It is worse in males aged 18–19. It is slightly less common in girls; for them it is worse around 14 years and around period time.

When will it settle down?

It usually settles by the age of 20, but may continue longer in severe cases.

Important facts about acne

1. It is not usually affected by diet.

2. It is not caused by oily hair or hair touching the forehead.

3. It is not infectious from one person to another.

4. Ordinary chemicals (including chlorine in swimming pools) do not make it worse.

5. Blackheads are not dirt, and will not dissolve in hot, soapy water.

6. It may flare up with excessive stress.

A word to parents

Your son or daughter hates acne and finds it embarrassing. It is not due to the way the skin is washed or what is eaten—it just happens.

It will not help if you are overanxious and nag your child; give support and encouragement instead, especially in following your doctor's instructions.

Treatment

This varies according to the severity and persistence of the problem and the person's skin type.

Diet

Avoid any foods that seem to aggravate your acne (such as chocolate or milk), but special diets are not advised. However, have a sensible, nutritious diet.

Soap and washing

Special soaps are unhelpful. Use a normal soap and wash gently and often—do not scrub.

Cosmetics

Avoid oily or creamy cosmetics and all moisturisers. Use cosmetics sparingly. Water-based lotion-style cosmetics are preferred.

Hair washing and shampoos

These make no difference.

Blackhead removal

This is not recommended; avoid picking and squeezing.

Exercise

This is not of proven value.

Ultraviolet light

This can be very beneficial (includes sunlight and controlled artificial ultraviolet light). However, avoid extreme exposure to ultraviolet light. (This includes avoiding sunburn.)

Lotions, creams and gels

Many preparations are useful. These include sulphur, salicylic acid, benzoyl peroxide and retinoic (tretinoin) lotions.

Antibiotics

Those taken by mouth are of proven value, especially long-term tetracyclines. Topical antibiotic preparations are also effective.

The pill

Women who have acne and require oral contraception can benefit from some pill preparations. Ask your doctor.

John Murtagh, *Patient Education*, Second edition, McGraw-Hill Book Company

Understanding the adolescent

Adolescence is a difficult period in which the young person is trying to cope with the inner conflict of striving for independence while still relying on adult support. There are inevitable clashes with parents, especially during the turbulent years of 13–16.

What are the hallmarks of the adolescent?

- self-consciousness
- self-awareness
- self-centredness
- lack of confidence

These basic features lead to anxieties about the body, and so many adolescents focus on their skin, body shape, weight and hair. Concerns about acne, curly hair, round shoulders and obesity are very common.

There are usually special concerns about boy–girl relationships and maybe guilt or frustration about sexual matters. Many adolescents therefore have a lack of self-worth or a poor body image. They are very private people, and this must be respected. While there are concerns about their identity, parental conflict, school, their peers and the world around them, there is also an innate separation anxiety.

What are the needs of adolescents?

- 'room' to move
- privacy and confidentiality
- security (e.g. stable home)
- acceptance by peers
- someone to 'lean on' (e.g. youth leader)
- special 'heroes'
- establishment of an adult sexual role
- at least one really good personal relationship

How does rebelliousness show?

It is quite normal for normal parents and normal teenagers to clash and get into arguments. Adolescents usually have a suspicion of and rebellion against convention and authority (parents, teachers, politicians, police and so on). This attitude tends to fade after leaving school (at around 18 years of age).

Common signs are:
- criticising and questioning parents
- putting down family members or even friends

- unusual, maybe outrageous, fashions and hairstyles
- experimenting with drugs such as nicotine and alcohol
- bravado and posturing
- unusual, often stormy, love affairs

Signs of out-of-control behaviour are:
- refusal to attend school
- vandalism and theft
- drug abuse
- sexual promiscuity
- eating disorders: anorexia, bulimia, severe obesity
- depression

Note: Beware of suicide if there are signs of depression.

What should parents do?

Wise parenting can be difficult, because one cannot afford to be overprotective or too distant. A successful relationship depends on good communication, which means continuing to show concern and care but being flexible and giving the adolescent 'space' and time.

Important management tips are:
- Treat adolescents with respect.
- Be non-judgmental.
- Stick to reasonable ground rules of behaviour (e.g. regarding alcohol, driving, language).
- Do not cling to them or show too much concern.
- Listen rather than argue.
- Listen to what they are *not* saying.
- Be flexible and consistent.
- Be available to help when requested.
- Give advice about diet and skin care.
- Talk about sex and give good advice, but only when the right opportunity arises.

Healthy distraction

Most authorities say that the best thing to keep adolescents healthy and well adjusted is to be active and interested. Regular participation in sporting activities and other hobbies such as bushwalking, skiing and so on with parents or groups is an excellent way to help them cope with this important stage of their lives.

Remember

Adolescent problems are a passing phase. Some authorities say it ends at 18 or 19, while others claim the 'age of reason' is reached at 23 or 24!

John Murtagh, *Patient Education*, Second edition, McGraw-Hill Book Company

Understanding your menstrual cycle

What is the menstrual cycle?

When we talk about the *menstrual cycle* the first thing many of us think of is 'periods'. The period (*menstruation*) is just part of a continuous cycle of changes in the body that is regulated by hormones.

The cycle usually begins during the teenage years and continues until the menopause, at about the age of 50. The purpose of the menstrual cycle is to prepare the body for reproduction.

What is the normal cycle?

The menstrual cycle can vary from woman to woman. For some it is normal to have a shorter cycle (e.g. 21 days) and for others a longer cycle (e.g. 35 days). The average for all women in the world is 28 days.

This means that the time of ovulation varies, but the average is the 14th day.

The periods can last from 1 to 8 days, with the average being about 4–5 days.

What causes irregularity of the periods?

The cycle will vary in a woman from time to time. This can be the result of emotional stress, illness, travel, sudden weight change or the use of some medicines.

What are some of the problems?

Many women will experience problems with their menstrual cycle at some time. The commonest problems are period pain, premenstrual tension, irregular periods and very heavy periods.

If you have any problems or questions about your menstrual cycle, discuss them with your doctor.

When is pregnancy likely to occur?

You are most likely to get pregnant between the 8th and the 18th day, depending on when you ovulate and how long the sperm remain active. It is useful to know when you ovulate—you may feel a pain in the abdomen and notice that your vaginal mucus changes from jelly-like to watery. Intercourse at this time and for the next 2 days is most likely to cause pregnancy.

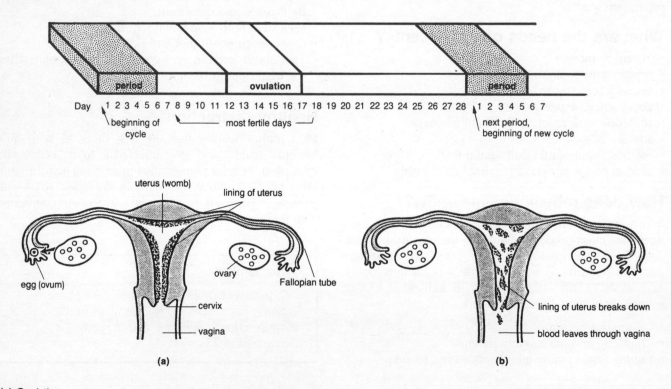

(a) Ovulation
- *Ovulation occurs usually from day 11 to 17 (average day 14)*
- *Up to this time the hormones have been preparing the lining of the uterus to receive the embryo if the egg is fertilised*
- *This lining gets thick and full of blood*

(b) Menstruation
- *If fertilisation (pregnancy) does not occur, the lining of the uterus is no longer required*
- *It is shed through the vagina*
- *This is called the menses*

John Murtagh, *Patient Education*, Second edition, McGraw-Hill Book Company

5 Women's health

Cystitis in women

What is cystitis?

Cystitis is inflammation of the bladder, which is a very common problem; it is suffered by many women at some stage in their lives. The most vulnerable times are starting sexual activity (hence the term 'honeymoon cystitis'), during pregnancy and after menopause.

What causes cystitis?

It is almost always caused by bacteria travelling upwards along the rather short passage (the *urethra*) from the outside into the sterile bladder. This is often caused by intercourse, which pushes this short passage and bacteria upwards. These bacteria, which are present in the bowel, are normally found around the openings of the anus, vagina and urethra. The bladder soon learns to cope with these germs by a type of local immunity, but some women are prone to recurrent infections.

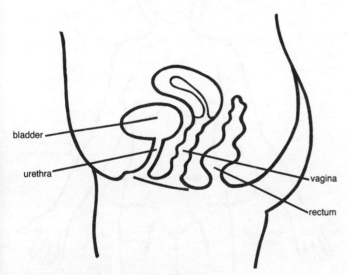

What are the symptoms?

- burning or stinging when passing urine
- an urge to pass urine often
- passing only small amounts of urine
- discoloured and smelly urine
- fever; pain in the back or low abdomen (may be present)
- feeling generally unwell

What are the risks?

Cystitis is very uncomfortable and irritating, but is not a serious problem. An untreated infection can spread up to the kidneys, and this is serious.

What is the treatment?

Self-help

- Keep yourself rested and warm.
- Drink a lot of fluid: try 2–3 cups of water at first, and then 1 cup every 30 minutes.
- Try to empty your bladder completely each time.
- Gently wash or wipe your bottom from the front to the back with soft, moist tissues after going to the toilet.
- Take analgesics such as paracetamol for pain.

You should visit your doctor if the attack lasts more than 24 hours and bring a fresh specimen of urine, which you should collect after washing your vulva with clean cottonwool and water.

Medical help

You will be prescribed a course of antibiotics, which should all be taken. Your doctor may advise making the urine alkaline by using Ural or Citravescent. A follow-up urine test will be necessary. If the antibiotics do not work or if you have more attacks, some special tests (including X-rays) may be necessary to check your urinary tract.

How can you prevent further attacks?

- Get into the habit of drinking plenty of fluids, especially on hot days.
- Pass urine often and when you feel like it—do not let it build up.
- Make sure you empty your bladder each time.
- Wash your bottom gently after each bowel motion, using mild soap and soft tissues.
- Empty your bladder immediately after intercourse.
- If your vagina is dry, use lubrication for intercourse (KY jelly for young women and oestrogen cream after the menopause).
- Wear cotton underwear; avoid tight jeans and vaginal deodorants.

Dysmenorrhoea (painful periods)

What is dysmenorrhoea?

It is the medical term for painful periods. These can occur as part of an otherwise normal menstruation cycle—this is known as *primary dysmenorrhoea.*

On the other hand, painful periods can be caused by a problem that has developed in the womb, such as fibroid tumours or an infection—this is called *secondary dysmenorrhoea.*

What causes primary dysmenorrhoea?

It is caused by high levels of *prostaglandins*, which are natural substances produced by the lining of the womb. One of the actions of prostaglandins is to cause the muscles of the womb to contract tightly, thus producing cramping sensations. The problem is associated with the onset of ovulation, that is when the ovary starts releasing eggs.

What are the symptoms?

Period pains vary a lot in strength and in position. Some women have a dull dragging pain in the abdomen or lower back or in both areas; others have more severe cramping abdominal pain. In some the pain may be felt in front of the thighs.

The pain is worse at the beginning of the period and may even commence up to 12 hours before the menses appear. It usually lasts for 24 hours, but may persist for 2 or 3 days.

Some women may get nausea and vomiting, and in severe cases fainting may occur.

What are the risks?

Dysmenorrhoea is very common, but most cases are mild and do not require medical attention. There is no risk at all unless it is a symptom of an underlying problem such as pelvic infection.

What is the treatment?

For most women pain-killers such as paracetamol relieve the pain. If the pain is severe, your doctor may prescribe a stronger analgesic that neutralises the effect of prostaglandins. Taking the contraceptive pill usually stops dysmenorrhoea. It often disappears after you have a baby or as you get older.

Keeping fit by leading a healthy lifestyle (including avoiding smoking and excessive alcohol and undertaking regular exercise) seems to help, as does practising relaxation techniques such as yoga.

If you get severe pain, rest in bed.

Simple measures such as placing a hot-water bottle over the painful area and curling your knees up to your chest as you lie on your side may provide relief.

When should you consult your doctor?

Consult your general practitioner if the pain worsens or if you develop period pain following 3 or 4 years of relatively pain-free periods.

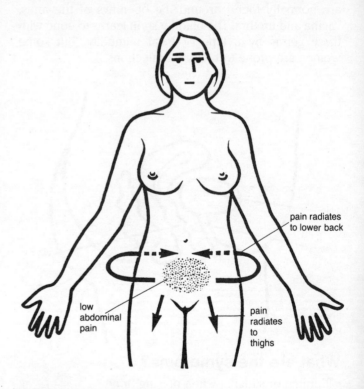

Typical sites of period pain

John Murtagh, *Patient Education*, Second edition, McGraw-Hill Book Company

Endometriosis

What is endometriosis?

The tissue lining your uterus (womb) is called the *endometrium*. Each menstrual cycle part of it grows and becomes engorged with blood and then is shed as a period. *Endometriosis* is a condition in which fragments of the endometrium grow in other places such as the wall of the uterus, the ovaries, the ligaments inside the pelvis, the Fallopian tubes and on other pelvic organs.

Each cycle, the blood from these fragments cannot escape because it is embedded in tissue in the pelvis. Small blood blisters develop and irritate the tissues.

There are many theories about the cause of endometriosis, but we do not fully understand how it comes about.

What are the symptoms?

- painful or heavy periods
- a dragging pain in the back or pelvis or abdomen during periods
- pain during intercourse

You may have only one or two of these symptoms, and they can vary in severity from one person to another.

Many women with endometriosis have no symptoms at all, or have symptoms so mild that they pass unnoticed.

How common is endometriosis?

Endometriosis is a common problem, especially in its mild form. About 1 woman in 10 will have it to some degree, but only 1 in 100 will be affected by it. About 20% of women investigated for infertility will be diagnosed as having endometriosis.

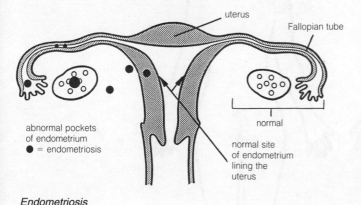

Endometriosis

Who gets endometriosis?

It can occur between puberty and menopause in any woman and appears most often between the ages of 25 and 35. It is more common in women who have not had children. It is not known why endometriosis occurs in some women and not in others. It is more common in some families.

How is it diagnosed?

It is indicated by the symptoms, but the only accurate method of diagnosis is by directly seeing the condition with a small tube called a *laparoscope* passed through a small cut into the abdomen. The spots of endometriosis are seen as small red or black lumps.

What should be done?

If you are suffering from painful periods and other symptoms that suggest endometriosis you will be referred to a gynaecologist, who will probably perform a laparoscopy before making a firm diagnosis.

What are the risks?

Endometriosis is a common cause of infertility. It can cause painful cysts inside the pelvis, and can affect the ovaries or the uterus. An operation may be necessary to remove the cysts, repair the ovaries or remove the uterus, but these measures are not usually necessary.

What is the treatment?

Many women do not require treatment. If necessary, however, endometriosis can be treated with drugs or surgery or both.

Surgical treatment

The ovaries and womb are usually left intact but the endometrial tissue is destroyed by heat or laser and scar tissue is removed. The aim is to reduce symptoms and improve fertility.

Medical treatment

Hormone treatment with one of the contraceptive pills, progestogens or danazol, aims to suppress the menstrual cycle, causing the endometrial cells to shrink and, hopefully, disappear. Hormones are usually taken for 6 to 12 months.

Hirsutism

What is it?

Hirsutism is the presence of excessive body or facial hair. For women, the areas most affected are the 'beard' area (upper lip, chin, front of the ears), the chest, the abdomen and the front of the thighs. The condition varies from being mild and hardly noticeable to being obvious.

What is normal?

Many women feel they are very 'hairy', but if this occurs in the normal female hair-growth areas (such as the armpits, forearms, pubic area and around the nipples) there is no cause for concern. A tendency to be 'hairy' may run in families or be prevalent in some races, such as those from the Mediterranean region. Even if the hair growth seems to be in a male pattern, there is usually no serious underlying cause and the problem can be treated. About 10% of Australian women are affected.

What causes hirsutism?

It is due to excessive hair growth caused by overactive male sex hormones (present in all women) at the hair root. The reason for this is unclear. Often hairiness runs in families or is more common in certain races, such as negroids. It is rare in orientals. Certain medications, such as anti-epilepsy drugs and some oral contraceptive pills, can cause it. Uncommonly, it is caused by cysts or tumours of the ovaries or adrenal glands.

What can be done?

Your doctor will need to take a full medical history and examine you to assess your hair growth. A blood test may be necessary.

What is the treatment?

- Your doctor may be able to reassure you that your hair growth is normal, and therefore no therapy is needed.
- Cosmetic measures (such as bleaching, waxing and shaving) and treatment with depilatory creams or electrolysis (which is the only permanent cosmetic method of hair removal) can help. Your doctor will advise what will suit you. There is no evidence that shaving increases the rate of hair growth, but plucking the hair does stimulate growth. Do not pluck hairs around the lips and chin.
- Medical treatment with drugs such as spironolactone can be used if your hair growth is excessive and causes understandable social embarrassment. It will probably take at least 3 months for you to notice any difference in your hairiness, and for most women the hair grows back once they stop taking the medications.

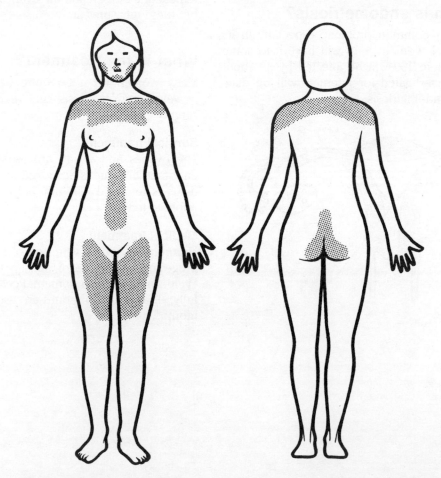

Sites of unwanted hair in women

John Murtagh, *Patient Education*, Second edition, McGraw-Hill Book Company

Incontinence of urine

These exercises are designed to help women with incontinence of urine. *Incontinence* means wetting yourself when you do certain things such as coughing, running, sneezing or laughing, or when your bladder gets full and you pass urine before you reach the toilet.

Pelvic muscle exercises

The muscles around the pelvis (pelvic muscles) are very important in supporting the bladder, urethra, vagina and rectum (see diagram). Following childbirth or with advancing age, these muscles may weaken. They may be strengthened by regularly practising pelvic muscle exercises. If these exercises are practised throughout life, they will reduce the chances of becoming incontinent. An outline of some of these exercises is given here. A physiotherapist may be able to assist in assessing and teaching pelvic muscle exercises.

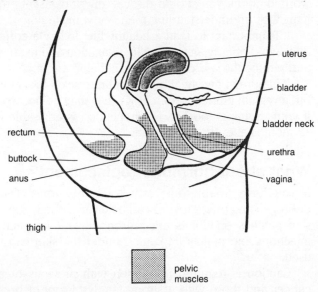

Simplified cross-section of the female pelvis

Stage 1

To identify the correct muscles to exercise, do the following exercises during the first week:

(a) To identify the muscles around your back passage or rectum, sit or stand comfortably and imagine that you are trying to control diarrhoea by consciously tightening the ring of muscles around the back passage. Hold this 'squeeze' for 4 seconds each time.

(b) Go to the toilet and commence passing urine. Now try to stop the flow of urine in midstream. Once this is done, recommence voiding until the bladder has emptied. The muscles used to slow or stop the flow of urine are the front pelvic muscles, which help support the bladder.

(c) Some women find they can identify the correct pelvic muscles by inserting a finger into their vagina, then squeezing the finger by contracting the pelvic muscles. If the finger cannot be felt to be squeezed, probably the wrong muscles are being exercised or the muscles are still very weak. Do not give up, but proceed with the stage 2 exercises.

Please note
- Do *not* bear down as if trying to pass a bowel motion (or as a woman would do during childbirth). This strengthens the wrong muscles and may make the incontinence worse.
- It may take a week or more to begin to identify the muscles that need to be exercised to regain the strength and tone of the pelvic muscles.

Stage 2

Now that the correct muscles have been identified, these are the pelvic exercises to do every day. They should *not* be done while passing urine.

(a) While sitting or standing with thighs slightly apart, contract the muscles around the back passage (rectum) then the front muscles around the vagina. Hold this contraction while counting to 5 slowly. Now relax these muscles. Repeat this 4 times. Try to be aware of the squeezing and lifting sensation in the pelvis that frequently occurs when these exercises are done correctly.

(b) While sitting or standing, tighten the muscles around the front and back passage together. Hold this contraction for just 1 second and relax. Repeat this exercise 5 times in quick succession.

Please note
- These 'slow' and 'quick' exercises are important to strengthen the pelvic muscles properly.
- In stage 2, it is *not* appropriate to do the stage 1 exercise of stopping the flow of urine each time urine is passed at the toilet. This is only a preliminary exercise.
- These exercises ideally can be done every hour, but certainly not less than 4 times every day.
- With practice, the exercises should be quite easy to master, and they can be carried out at any time—while waiting for a bus, standing at the sink or watching television. There is no need to interrupt the daily routine.
- Once every week or two, it is important to return to stage 1 for a quick check that the correct muscles are being used.
- While these exercises are particularly useful for women, they may be helpful also for men, particularly those suffering from dribbling or urgency.

> **Note**
>
> Check with your doctor if you are having persistent problems.

Menopause

What is the menopause?

The *menopause* is the end of menstruation, which in most women occurs between the ages of 45 and 55, with an average age in Australia of 51 years. However, the term is used in a broader sense to describe the months or years before and after the last period, during which the periods become irregular and the body adjusts to reduced levels of female hormones. This may last 2–5 years or sometimes longer.

What causes the menopause?

The female hormones, *oestrogen* and *progestogen*, are no longer produced by the ovary because of a decline and finally a complete absence of maturing eggs (ova).

What are the symptoms?

Due to small amounts of oestrogen being produced in the adrenal glands, symptoms (other than the cessation of periods) may be mild or absent.

Period changes

Periods may stop abruptly or after a prolonged irregular pattern such as lighter periods occurring further apart or heavier frequent periods. Fertility is greatly reduced, far more unpredictable and finally absent.

Hot flushes

These symptoms are a sensation of heat, usually in the face and neck, but can be experienced from head to toe and last from seconds to minutes. They may be accompanied by sweating, palpitations, headache, faintness and disturbed sleep, and can be aggravated by alcohol, hot foods and drinks, and stress.

In themselves they are harmless, but they can cause embarrassment, tiredness and anxiety. They may continue from a few months to many years after the periods cease.

Vagina and bladder symptoms

The normally moist tissue of the vagina and base of the bladder can become dry and inelastic. This can result in uncomfortable intercourse and an increased chance of infection of the bladder or vagina.

Emotional problems

A woman may experience fluctuating levels of energy and concentration with tiredness, irritability, lack of confidence and loss of interest in sexual activity. Occasionally anxiety and depression can be a problem.

Other symptoms may include aches and pains in the muscles or joints, dryness of the skin and hair, and a 'creepy crawling' feeling over the skin.

Is osteoporosis (thinning of bone) a problem?

It has been shown that reduced levels of oestrogen cause increased loss of calcium from bone tissue, which causes osteoporosis of varying degrees. Certain drugs and medical conditions and smoking can aggravate it. Hormone replacement therapy, which may continue for the rest of life, can certainly prevent osteoporosis. If you are slightly built or have a family history of osteoporosis, speak to your doctor about this potential problem.

What should be done?

While it is important to accept that the menopause is a natural fact of life and nothing to be embarrassed or worried about, you should discuss any unpleasant problems with an understanding friend or your doctor.

It is important to lead a healthy life: follow a correct diet, avoid obesity, get adequate relaxation and exercise, and reduce the use of cigarettes, caffeine and alcohol.

It is normal and healthy to continue sexual relations, but a vaginal lubricant such as KY jelly may be necessary if your vagina is too dry. Contraception is advisable for 12 months after the last period.

What about hormone replacement?

If you have troublesome symptoms, hormones (both oestrogen and progestogen) can be given. Usually special skin patches or tablets are prescribed, but long-acting injections and pellets implanted under the skin can be used.

Caution is required in women with previous breast cancer and those with a strong family history of breast cancer (2 first degree relatives).

A vaginal cream or tablet containing oestrogen is available for a dry vagina.

Remember

- Menopause is a normal change representing the end of reproductive life. Be informed and unafraid.
- Report to your doctor if you have a return of unusual bleeding.
- Continuing medical checks for breast examination, Pap smears and general health assessment are important.

John Murtagh, *Patient Education*, Second edition, McGraw-Hill Book Company

Painful breasts

What causes breast pain?

Breast pain (known as *mastalgia*) has several causes. The main type of breast pain is *cyclical mastalgia*, which is a general breast discomfort that occurs in the second half of the menstrual cycle. The pain, which comes on with ovulation, is mainly premenstrual. It obviously is caused by a hormonal effect and is not harmful.

Other causes are:
- pregnancy
- infection (after childbirth)
- tumours
- certain drugs
- weight gain
- bra problems

Note: Early breast cancer is usually painless, but all lumps need careful investigation.

Is it common?

It is a very common problem, with about 2 out of 3 women complaining of breast pain at some stage of their lives. It is most common in the thirties and early forties.

What are the symptoms?

The pain can vary from very mild to severe. It is usually a heaviness or discomfort in the breasts, while some women experience a prickling or stabbing sensation.

The breasts may be so tender that relationships with partners and children are affected because hugging and fondling cause distress. The breasts may feel lumpy or quite normal to touch. The lumpy breast may develop cysts, which your doctor may drain.

What is the treatment?

The first thing to keep in mind is that breast pain is common, and only 1 case in 200 will have cancer as the cause. However, you must continue to practise breast self-examination and report any lumps that do not go away after your periods. You do not have to live with your breast discomfort.

Self-help
- Reduce weight if you are overweight: aim to keep at ideal weight.
- Reduce or cut out caffeine.
- Follow a nutritious diet.
- Wear good quality, comfortable bras.
- Take 2 aspirin or other mild analgesic for pain.
- Exercise aerobically and exercise the upper trunk.

'Natural' medication
Vitamins may help (although this is not scientifically proven):
- Vitamin B_1: 100 mg per day
- Vitamin B_6: 100 mg per day
- Evening primrose oil capsules: 4 g per day

Most women (85%) can be treated with natural methods. Your doctor can prescribe stronger medication to relieve the problem, so report persistent pain or any persistent lumps.

Drug treatment
Adjustment of oral contraception or hormone replacement therapy (if it applies to you) may help mastalgia. However, there are several other hormones that can be prescribed.

Pelvic inflammatory disease

What is pelvic inflammatory disease (PID)?

Pelvic inflammatory disease describes any infection of the reproductive organs of a woman. It occurs when microbes (germs) travel up through the cervix and uterus (womb) and then spread inwards to the Fallopian tubes, ovaries and surrounding tissues in the pelvis. The commonest serious infection is that of the tubes—this is called *salpingitis*.

A pelvic infection can be either *acute*, which causes sudden severe symptoms, or *chronic*, which gradually produces milder symptoms.

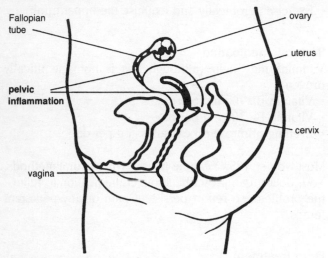

What are the facts?

Here are some basic facts about the disease:
- Sexual intercourse causes up to 75% of cases.
- Minor operations [such as the insertion of an intra-uterine device (IUD)] or procedures of pregnancy (such as a miscarriage, an abortion or even a delivery) can cause PID.
- Up to 10% of young women normally have the microbes, which include chlamydia and gonorrhoea, on their cervix. These women are at special risk of getting PID.
- The commonest cause of infertility in Australia is PID—it affects about 5000 Australian women each year.
- PID is a preventable disease and it is best diagnosed by *laparoscopy* (where a tube is passed through the abdomen).

Who are the women most at risk?

The women most at risk are those who:
- are under 25 years of age
- have abnormal Pap smears when aged between 15 and 35 years

- have multiple sexual partners
- have steady partners who have sex with others
- do not use barrier methods of contraception (e.g. condoms)
- have operations needing the opening of the cervix (e.g. dilation and curettage, and placement of an IUD)

What are the symptoms?

Some patients may feel no symptoms, but others may have symptoms that vary from mild to very severe.

Acute PID
- fever
- severe abdominal pain

Chronic PID
- ache in the lower back
- mild lower abdominal pain

Both acute and chronic
- painful intercourse
- menstrual problems (e.g. painful, heavy or irregular periods)
- unusual, perhaps smelly, vaginal discharge
- painful or frequency of urination

What are the risks?

The main serious risks are subsequent sterility, ectopic pregnancies and further episodes of PID. Occasionally an acute infection may cause a pelvic abscess or cause peritonitis or even blood poisoning by spreading.

How can it be prevented?

- Safe sex is most important. Insist that a partner with a possible sexually transmitted disease (STD) uses a condom.
- Avoid IUDs if you have a history of PID or have a number of sexual partners.
- It is advisable to have antibiotic treatment if a partner has or gets an STD even if you have no symptoms.
- If you get PID, your partner or partners should be treated.
- Those at risk for PID should have regular checkups.

What is the treatment?

A course of antibiotics is given, usually by mouth. Avoid sexual intercourse or manipulation of your vagina (e.g. with hands or tampons) until the infection is cleared. This may take 2–4 weeks.

If you have an IUD, it should be removed.

John Murtagh, *Patient Education*, Second edition, McGraw-Hill Book Company

Pill: the combination pill

What is the combination pill?

It is a combination of two female sex hormones that prevents pregnancy by changing the hormone balance in your body to stop ovulation (the monthly release of the egg from the ovary). There are 28-day and 21-day packets, the only difference being the 7 inactive 'sugar' pills in the 28-day packet.

How effective is the pill?

If taken according to instructions, it is at least 99% safe.

How is it commenced?

This varies according to the type of pill prescribed, so follow the instructions that come with the pill packet. It is usual to start the 28-day pack on the 1st day of bleeding of your next period and the 21-day pack on the 5th day of your cycle or on a particular day (e.g. Saturday) after your next period starts.

When and how is it taken?

The tablet should be swallowed whole with a small amount of water. It does not matter what time of the day you take it, but once a time has been chosen it is important to get into the habit of taking the pill at the same time (e.g. after breakfast or at bedtime). To be effective to stop pregnancy, the pill must be taken at a regular time.

What if a pill is missed or taken late?

The 7 day rule
- Take the forgotten pill as soon as possible, even if it means taking two pills in one day.
- Take the next pill at the usual time and finish the course.
- If you forget to take the missed pill for more than 12 hours after the usual time, there is an increased risk of pregnancy and so you should use another form of contraception (such as condoms) for 7 days.
- If these 7 days run beyond the last hormone pill in the packet, miss out the inactive pills (or 7 day group) and proceed directly to the first hormone pill in the next pack.

How does it affect periods?

Periods tend to become shorter, regular and lighter. The blood loss may be the brownish colour of old blood. The pill also tends to stop painful periods.

Is a break from the pill necessary?

There is no reason to take a break from the pill. It is best to continue on until pregnancy is contemplated.

What if a period is missed?

If you miss a period, stop taking the pill, check with your doctor as soon as possible and use other methods of contraception.

Is it safe during lactation?

The pill can interfere with the quantity and quality of breast milk, and so it is better to use other contraception during breastfeeding. If a pill is used, the most appropriate is a progestogen only pill.

What are the unwanted effects (side effects)?

The most common side effects are nausea (feeling sick), breast tenderness and breakthrough spotting (i.e. bleeding between your usual periods). These side effects tend to disappear after a couple of months on the pill. Other side effects include vaginal thrush (which causes itching), discolouration of the skin and feeling depressed. More serious (although uncommon) effects include migraine headaches, high blood pressure and a tendency to form clots in the veins. To check if you should not take the pill, refer to the instruction leaflet that comes with the pill, or consult your doctor. Some women feel better when taking the pill, and their skin and hair condition can improve. A special pill can be used if you have acne.

What about alcohol and other drugs?

Alcohol in moderation does not appear to interfere with the pill. Medications that can reduce the effectiveness of the pill include antibiotics, vitamin C and drugs to treat epilepsy and tuberculosis. The pill may affect blood-thinning and antidiabetic preparations. Check with your doctor.

If you are taking antibiotics, continue the pill, use another contraceptive method during the course and follow the 7 day rule when the course is finished.

What are the special rules to follow?

- Smoking creates a health risk with the pill, and so you should not smoke.
- Make sure you tell a doctor if you are taking the pill when other medicine is about to be prescribed.
- Diarrhoea and vomiting may reduce the effectiveness of the pill—use additional contraception until you finish that particular course. (Follow the 7 day rule.)
- Report persistent or heavy bleeding between periods.
- Report any onset of blurred vision, severe headache or pain in the chest or limbs.
- Return for a checkup every 6 months while you are on the pill.
- Perform breast self-examination regularly and have a smear test every 2 years.
- Remember that the pill is highly effective, but pregnancy can occur if the pill is taken at irregular times, if intercurrent illnesses such as fever and gastric upsets develop, or if you are taking some other drugs.

Premenstrual syndrome

What is the premenstrual syndrome?

The *premenstrual syndrome*, which is commonly called *premenstrual tension* or *PMT*, is a set of symptoms, both physical and psychological, that some women experience before their periods. These symptoms usually go away when the period starts. The symptoms are caused by hormonal changes in the body before the period and vary from woman to woman. The build-up of fluid in the body at this time is an example of this.

Is it common?

Yes; possibly up to 90% of women experience some symptoms, which can vary from minor to severe. PMT tends to increase with age.

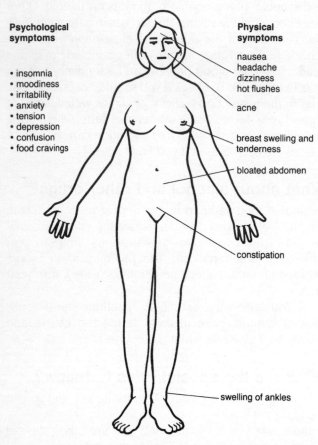

Psychological symptoms

- insomnia
- moodiness
- irritability
- anxiety
- tension
- depression
- confusion
- food cravings

Physical symptoms

nausea
headache
dizziness
hot flushes

acne

breast swelling and tenderness

bloated abdomen

constipation

swelling of ankles

Symptoms of premenstrual tension

What are the symptoms?

The important symptoms are summarised in the diagram, but the commonest symptoms are moodiness, irritability, tension, headache, constipation, sore breasts and bloated feelings.

What can be done about these symptoms?

Insight

Understanding your symptoms and why they occur can be a big help. It is helpful to be open about your problem and tell your family and close friends about these symptoms. Consider joining a support group.

Keep a diary

Keep a list of your main symptoms and note when they occur over a 2–3 month period. Use this information to help plan around your symptoms; for example, avoid too many social events and postpone demanding business appointments.

Lifestyle changes

- *Diet*. Eat regularly and sensibly: eat small rather than large meals; avoid salt, caffeine and excess fluids. If necessary, reduce your weight to ideal level.
- *Exercise*. Regular exercise often helps (e.g. swimming, aerobics, tennis).
- *Relaxation*. Plan to do things that you find relaxing and enjoyable during this time. Stress aggravates PMT, so reduce it wherever possible.
- *Proper dress*. Sensible dressing to cope with breast tenderness and a bloated abdomen is useful (e.g. a firm-fitting bra and loose-fitting clothes around the abdomen).
- *Medicine*. Some medicines may help those with more severe symptoms, so discuss these options with your doctor. Examples of treatment used for premenstrual tension include vitamin B_6 (pyridoxine), evening oil of primrose and oral contraceptives.

John Murtagh, *Patient Education*, Second edition, McGraw-Hill Book Company

Self-examination of breasts

Why examine your breasts?

- Regular breast self-examination (BSE) helps you become familiar with the usual feel of your breasts.
- You will detect any lumps in the breast at an early stage of their development.
- Although only 1 in 10 breast lumps is cancer, 1 in 15 women develops breast cancer at some time.
- Most breast cancers are found (as a lump) by the woman, not by the doctor.

Early detection of a lump—if it is a breast cancer—may mean a better chance of a cure.

By performing regular BSE, you are safeguarding your health.

What is the technique?

There are several BSE methods. No matter which you use, it is important that you examine your breasts regularly and that you cover the breast area completely.

The method outlined here is simple, easy to learn and provides good coverage of the entire breast.

When should it be done?

Breast examination should be done once a month a few days after the end of your period.

Position

- The breast tissue must be spread as flat as possible.
- Lie on your back with one arm behind your head. The right breast is examined by the left hand and vice versa.
- Large-breasted women might need to modify this position. First lie on your side, then bring your shoulders flat onto the bed. Once you have examined as far as the nipple, lie flat on your back to examine the remainder of the breast.

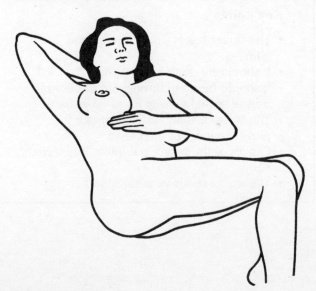

Self-examination of breasts

Boundaries of the 'map'

Your examination must cover the breast tissue area completely. The boundaries are:
- the collarbone
- the brassiere line
- the breastbone
- a line vertical from the middle of the underarm

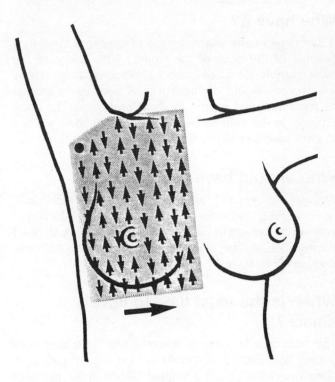

Examination

Vertical strips

Examine up and down the breast in vertical 'strips', beginning from the outer border. At the end of each strip, move the fingers about 2 cm towards the breastbone and examine another vertical strip.

The flat of your fingers

Use the flat part of your fingers, including the fingertip pads, to feel the breast. Move your hand in *slow, circular* movements.

Light and firm pressure

At each spot feel first with *light pressure* (to detect any lump just below the surface), then with a *firm pressure* (to detect any lump near the ribs).

When finished, reverse the position to examine the other breast.

What should you do if you find a lump or thickening?

If you find a lump, dimpling of the skin, or a discharge, make sure you see your doctor as soon as possible. Please do not be afraid or put it off. Most changes are not cancer.

John Murtagh, *Patient Education*, Second edition, McGraw-Hill Book Company

Smear test

What is a smear test?

The *smear test*, also called a *Pap test* (Papanicolaou test), is a simple test that scrapes cells off the surface of your cervix for examination in a laboratory.

Why have it?

It can detect early warning signs of cancer of the cervix (cancer of the neck of the womb). This is one of the most curable forms of cancer if detected early; hardly any women would die from it if all had regular smears as recommended by the medical profession. The early changes in the cells cause no symptoms, and so women in early stages of cervical cancer feel quite healthy.

Who should have it?

Any woman over 15 years of age who has had sex should have a smear test, and it should be performed every 2 years up to the age of 70. Even women who have stopped having periods or stopped having sex should have regular smear tests.

When is the ideal time to have a smear?

The best time to have a smear is any time after your period has finished. It should not be done if you have been douching or using vaginal tablets in the previous 24 hours.

How is the Pap smear done?

It is part of a normal pelvic or vaginal examination.

1. You lie on your back or your side on the couch.

2. An instrument called a *speculum* is slid gently into your vagina and then opened so that the doctor can see the cervix clearly, with the help of a light.

3. The smear is then taken with a thin spatula and a soft brush. It is really a very thin amount of mucus with cells that sit on the surface and the small opening of the cervix. The smear is then placed on a glass slide, which is sent away to be tested.

Does the smear test hurt or take long?

It is a simple test that does not take long (only about 2–3 minutes) and should not hurt. If you are tense, it may feel a little uncomfortable but will not cause any pain. The more relaxed you are the better. Deep breathing will help you relax.

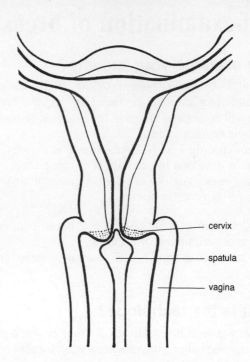

cervix

spatula

vagina

Will I feel embarrassed?

It is quite normal to feel a little embarrassed. Doctors, of course, are used to doing them and perform many each day, so that they understand. Nobody has ever died of embarrassment, but many have died of cancer of the cervix by not having a smear test.

What about the results?

The results take about 1–2 weeks. Ask your doctor when you should ring for the results. The results are almost always normal. Abnormal cells are seen in only about 3 in 1000 smears and do not always mean cancer. The microscopic findings are not infallible, unfortunately, but are improving all the time and are almost 100% accurate. If there is any doubt, you will be recalled for a repeat test. For most women who have abnormal cells, the treatment is simple and effective.

Key points

- The smear test is simple, quick and painless.
- It should be done every 2 years.
- It should be done throughout life from the start of sexual activity up to 70 years.
- The smear test allows your doctor to prevent cancer of the cervix.
- Cancer of the cervix is curable if detected early.
- The smear test is your safeguard.

John Murtagh, *Patient Education*, Second edition, McGraw-Hill Book Company

Tubal ligation

What is tubal ligation?

Tubal ligation is a sterilisation operation in which the Fallopian tubes are cut off or blocked. This stops the sperm reaching the egg in the tube, which is the normal site of fertilisation.

How is the operation done?

Tubal ligation is usually done under a general anaesthetic. It is necessary to get inside the abdomen. This is done by one of several methods, most commonly by a small cut just above the pubic hair line or through a special tube called a *laparoscope*. In the laparoscopic method the tube is passed through a small cut about 1 cm long made just below the navel, and the tubes are located through a powerful light system. Rings or clips can be attached to the two tubes or the tubes can be burnt (*cauterised*) and the ends tied off. The ring or clip method makes reversal easier if necessary later on.

In other methods the surgeon picks up each tube through the wound, removes a section of tube and ties the ends.

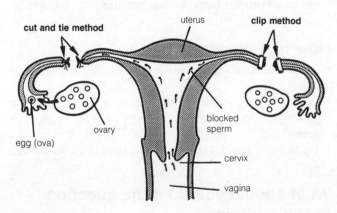

Tubal ligation

How long is the hospital stay?

This is usually 1–2 days, depending on the operation method and the policy of the hospital.

How effective is tubal ligation?

It is very effective, but failures do occur in about 1 in 200 operations. Some methods have a better success rate than others.

Does tubal ligation affect sexual function?

A normal sex life can resume once the effect of the operation is over. Many women find that their sex life is better without the worry about getting pregnant.

Does tubal ligation affect menstruation?

Menstruation continues as usual, but some women report that their periods are heavier, especially if large pieces of tube are removed. However, the modern laparoscopic methods do not appear to cause heavier menstruation.

Does tubal ligation cause weight gain?

No, it does not cause weight gain because it has no effect on hormones or appetite.

Can sterilisation be reversed?

The cut tubes can be rejoined by microsurgery, but there is no guarantee of regaining fertility. The successful pregnancy rates vary between 30 and 80%, depending on the technique used. The simple clip method gives a better chance of reversal.

Tubal ligation, however, should be regarded as permanent and irreversible and not entered into lightly.

Vaginal thrush

Vaginal thrush, sometimes called 'monilia' or a 'yeast' infection, is a common condition caused by an overgrowth of the micro-organism *Candida albicans*.

What are the symptoms?

Symptoms around the genital area
- itching
- irritation
- soreness
- swelling of the vaginal opening

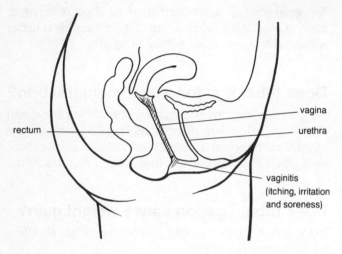

The extent of vaginal thrush

rectum

vagina

urethra

vaginitis (itching, irritation and soreness)

Other symptoms
- cheesy-white discharge
- discomfort during intercourse
- pain when urinating

What is the cause?

Candida is one of a large number of organisms present in the vagina all the time. These organisms do no harm until something upsets their normal balance (and sometimes that trigger factor is not obvious).

Factors likely to cause vaginal thrush
- diabetes
- treatment with antibiotics or cortisone
- pregnancy

Factors that might cause vaginal thrush
- intercourse
- oral contraceptives
- an IUD (intrauterine device)
- tight-fitting jeans
- nylon underwear
- leaving on a wet bathing suit after swimming
- humid weather
- travel (due to prolonged sitting)

What is the treatment?

- See your doctor about a vaginal cream or pessary to insert high up in the vagina.
- Bathe the genital area gently 2 or 3 times a day to relieve the discomfort and itching. Use 1 tablespoon of bicarbonate of soda in 1 litre of warm water.
- Dry the genital area thoroughly after showering or bathing.
- Wear loose-fitting cotton underwear.
- Do not have intercourse while you have thrush.
- Sometimes tablets to take by mouth are prescribed.

Should my partner be treated?

This is a controversial issue but is not recommended as there is no proven benefit from treating your partner.

How is it prevented?

- Wash and thoroughly dry the genital area at least once a day.
- Do not wear panty hose, tight jeans or tight underwear or use tampons. (*Candida* thrives in warm, moist, dark areas.)
- Do not use vaginal douches, powders or deodorants.

What should you do if the infection keeps returning?

- Are you taking antibiotics? Ask your doctor's advice about the thrush.
- If you are using oral contraceptives, you might have to change to another form of contraception.
- See your doctor about checking your urine for sugar (diabetes) or another infection.

John Murtagh, *Patient Education*, Second edition, McGraw-Hill Book Company

6 Men's health

Foreskin hygiene

The normal foreskin in infants and children does not need special care and should not be retracted for cleaning from birth to 5 years of age.

Why is foreskin hygiene important?

If you have a foreskin, you owe it to yourself to practise correct hygiene because the failure to do this can result in an unpleasant smell, soreness, irritation and infection. Poor hygiene is associated with a greater risk of getting cancer of the penis and possibly with sexually transmitted diseases. A man who neglects his foreskin may end up with a smelly and sore penis that could affect his sex life, for it will be obvious to his partner.

It is important to retract the foreskin and wash all of the area at least once a week. All males should practise proper hygiene from the age of 6 or 7.

Foreskin hygiene is very simple!

When you have your shower or bath, follow these steps:

1. Slide your foreskin back towards your body (diagrams (a)–(c)). A male older than 5 years should be able to slide his foreskin back. If you cannot, check with your doctor.

2. Wash the end of your penis and foreskin with soap and water. (Do not let soap get in the opening—it stings!)

3. After your shower or bath, *dry* the end of your penis and foreskin properly and *replace* the foreskin (diagrams (d)–(f)).

Do not forget to replace the foreskin, or it could get trapped back and cause unpleasant problems.

Also, when you urinate, slide the foreskin back just enough so that the urine does not get on the foreskin—this helps to keep it clean.

Do not forget—if you have any problems, see your doctor.

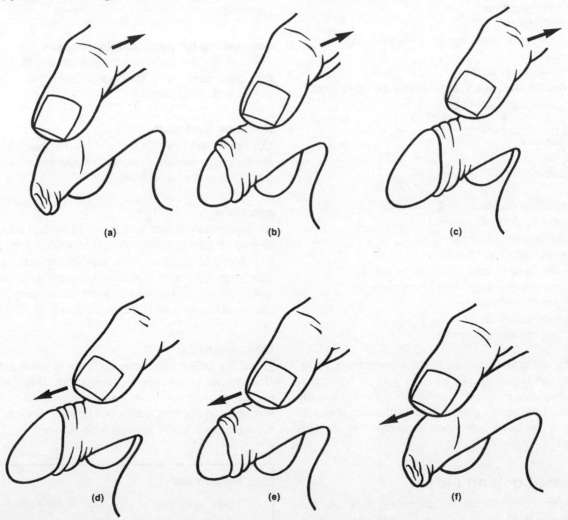

(a)　　　(b)　　　(c)

(d)　　　(e)　　　(f)

Cleaning the foreskin

Impotence (erectile dysfunction)

What is erectile dysfunction?

Erectile dysfunction refers to the inability of a man to get or maintain an erection of the penis sufficiently to have sexual intercourse. Most adult men have probably experienced a short period of temporary impotence at some time. This is usually due to a psychological rather than a physical problem and is not a cause for concern.

How common is the problem?

It is common and affects at least 1 in 20 males at 45 years and 1 in 3 males at 65 years.

What are the causes?

Most cases of erectile dysfunction (up to 75%) have a physical (organic) cause while the rest have a psychological (functional) cause.

Psychological causes
- stress and fatigue
- anxiety or depression
- marital disharmony
- negative thoughts about sex and sexual performance
- guilt feelings
- ignorance about sexuality
- situational stresses, such as presence of other people in the home (e.g. mother-in-law)

Physical causes
- alcohol excess
- chronic illness
- diabetes
- nervous system disorders (e.g. stroke)
- decreased circulation to penis
- drug reactions, for example:
  - marijuana, cocaine, narcotics
  - heavy smoking (4 times the risk by age 50)
  - sedatives, tranquillisers, antidepressants
  - blood pressure drugs
- hormone irregularities
- surgery (e.g. prostate surgery)

Sometimes we simply do not know what causes impotence. You can get an idea of whether you are functional by being aware of erections during sleep (which usually occur 3 to 5 times during the night and last for about 90 minutes) or morning erections or erections through masturbation.

What about getting old?

Although the risk of impotence increases with age, it is not inevitable. Most men keep the ability to get an erection, although more stimulation is usually required.

What tests need to be performed?

Tests will include blood tests and possibly special investigations for function of your penis. Special sleep studies on erections during sleep can be performed.

How can it be prevented?

- Careful treatment of any medical problem such as diabetes is important.
- Avoid drugs of addiction, including common 'social' drugs.
- Discuss the effects of any medicines with your doctor.
- Do not have more than 2 standard alcohol drinks a day.
- Cut down smoking.
- Promote sexual feelings:
  - Have good communication with your partner.
  - Talk over any concerns.
  - Choose a good atmosphere for lovemaking.

What is the treatment?

Lifestyle

All patients should be advised to reduce any high alcohol consumption and refrain from smoking (cigarette, cigar and pipe). Significant stress and overwork should be attended to.

Counselling for psychological causes

This will involve brief sexual counselling for which you may be referred to a specialist clinic. It is important to attend with your partner.

Hormone treatment

Hormones will only be given if blood tests find that you are lacking a certain hormone necessary for sexual function. This is very uncommon.

Injections

An important modern way to treat physical impotence is to give an injection of a special substance into the penis to achieve an erection. If a test dose works, you will be able to give yourself injections (up to a maximum of 3 a week) before you intend to have intercourse. The injection in common use is prostaglandin E_1 (Caverject).

Other methods

There are other ingenious ways to achieve intercourse should your impotence be permanent. These include:
- a vacuum device to make the penis erect
- surgery to implant a firm but flexible device
- surgery to implant an inflatable device

Remember

There is usually a way of achieving intercourse, whatever the cause.

John Murtagh, *Patient Education*, Second edition, McGraw-Hill Book Company

Prostate: your enlarged prostate

What causes 'trouble with the waterworks'?

This is usually caused by enlargement of the *prostate gland*. Nearly every man over 45 years of age has some degree of this enlargement, which is called *benign hypertrophy*. Some drugs cause trouble, especially when an enlarged prostate is present. These drugs include alcohol, some drugs used to treat depression, Parkinson's disease and irregular beats of the heart, and over-the-counter ephedrine-like compounds for coughs and colds.

How common is the problem?

Although enlargement of the prostate is common in men over 45, it rarely causes trouble before 50. By the age of 55 at least 50% of men will have 'waterworks trouble'. This increases to 80% of men over 80. Serious urinary trouble affects 2 in 10 elderly men.

What are the symptoms?

- frequency of urination
- an urge to urinate without much warning
- waking at night with this urge
- difficulty starting and sluggish stream, especially first thing in the morning
- a tendency to dribble after urinating, with wetting of pants
- a need to urinate a second time after only 20 minutes

The symptoms vary somewhat, but pain is a rare problem.

What is the prostate gland?

It is a brownish gland about the size of a walnut that surrounds the opening of the bladder and about the first 2.5 cm (1 inch) of the urethra (the tube passing from the bladder to the penis). It produces substances that make up a small part of the semen.

What are the risks?

Hypertrophy of the prostate is not dangerous, but it tends to squeeze the urethra and makes it difficult for the urine to pass through. This can cause the symptoms of dribbling and poor stream. More serious problems include:
- infection of urine
- sudden blockage (called *acute retention* of urine)
- slow blockage (called *chronic retention* of urine)

A catheter will usually be necessary to relieve a severe obstruction.

What will your doctor do?

Your doctor will perform a rectal examination with a gloved finger to feel the prostate and then may refer you to a urologist for special tests. Cancer of the prostate has to be excluded. A blood test called the PSA can test for cancer. The doctor will check what drugs you are taking to make sure these are not aggravating the problem.

What is the treatment?

Non-surgical
At least 1 in 3 mild cases will not require an operation. Although we cannot cure or shrink an enlarged prostate, you can learn to live with it for some time.
- Avoid or cut down alcohol, especially with and after an evening meal.
- Avoid fluids for at least 3 hours before retiring.
- Get up immediately at night when you wake up with the urge to go.
- Visit the toilet when you need to (do not hang on) and wait a while to make sure you empty your bladder completely.

Drugs
Fortunately there are now drugs that can improve the flow of urine in many patients. Your doctor will prescribe them if appropriate.

Surgical
This is eventually required for most prostate problems. About 1 in 10 men will need a prostatectomy. This usually is done through the penis, using an instrument about as wide as a pencil. The operation is called a *transurethral resection* (TUR).

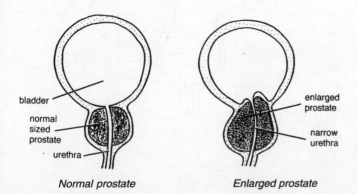

Normal prostate   Enlarged prostate

Prostate: your prostate operation

Why is the operation needed?

You have developed enlargement of your prostate, which cannot shrink by itself or with drugs. This enlarged tissue needs to be removed to allow your urine to flow normally from your bladder to your penis. If the obstruction continues, it can damage your bladder and possibly your kidneys. It may block off the urine completely and cause considerable pain. This emergency situation is called *acute retention*.

What will the operation do to your stream?

If successful, the operation will give you a good stream with full control, which you probably have not had for years. You will soon be able to pass urine normally without dribbling and will not have to get up more than once to urinate during the night.

How is the operation performed?

This is usually done through the penis. The urologist passes an instrument about as wide as a pencil through the urethra to cut away the enlarged prostate. This instrument (a *resectoscope*) has a loop of wire at its tip, which can cut tissue. It has a miniature telescope or camera and light to allow the surgeon to see clearly to slice and 'nibble' away pieces of the prostate from inside the urethra, thus making it nice and wide.

What anaesthetic will I have?

Usually a local anaesthetic is used—you will be made numb from the waist down for about 4 hours. This is done by giving a spinal injection. Sometimes a general anaesthetic may be necessary.

What happens after the operation?

A catheter is left in the urethra to drain the bladder for about 1–2 days. There is usually some blood loss for a few days. Taking the catheter out is simple and painless. You are in hospital for about 4–5 days. Although it tends to burn and be erratic at first, your urine stream will soon become strong and controlled.

What are the chances of becoming incontinent?

This is rare. Usually after 2 days of incontinence you begin to return to normal.

What about my sex life?

In most people the sexual desire and ability remains. Getting an erection soon returns and satisfactory intercourse is possible about 1–2 months later. You will have an orgasm, but you do not ejaculate fluid (semen) outwards. It goes back up into the bladder. This is quite harmless, and the fluid passes out later in the urine.

Can I become impotent?

This is most unusual—less than 1 in 10 men have a problem. If you have had a problem before the operation, it is unlikely to improve it.

What happens after I leave hospital?

Like after any operation, you make steady and good progress, with gradual improvement of your urination. Sometimes infection and bleeding can cause minor setbacks. You should take it very easy for 2–3 weeks, but should be well enough to return to work in about 4 weeks.

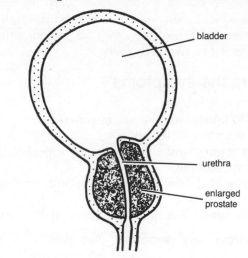

Before surgery

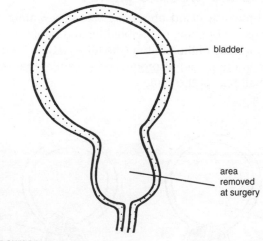

After surgery

John Murtagh, *Patient Education*, Second edition, McGraw-Hill Book Company

Testicular self-examination (TSE)

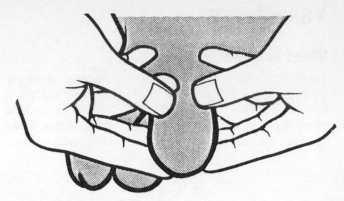

Why bother with TSE?

Although testicular cancer is rare, it is the commonest cancer in men between the ages of 15 and 34 years.

With early detection and recent advances in chemotherapy, testicular cancer is one of the most easily cured cancers. Some patients are only diagnosed after the tumour has well and truly spread into the body, but even these patients can respond well to modern treatment.

It is useful for young men to carry out TSE with the same regularity as women carry out breast self-examination. The examination is necessary for the early detection and for the successful treatment of cancer. Any delay in the diagnosis should be avoided. TSE might be a life-saving health habit.

TSE technique

What are the causes of testicular cancer?

They are not exactly known, but some factors that may lead to it are an undescended testicle, trauma (injury), heat exposure and heredity.

What are the symptoms?

The usual symptoms of testicular cancer include a lump on the testicle, painless swelling and a dull ache or heavy dragging sensation in the lower abdomen, groin or scrotum. The early symptoms are therefore mild and tend to be overlooked.

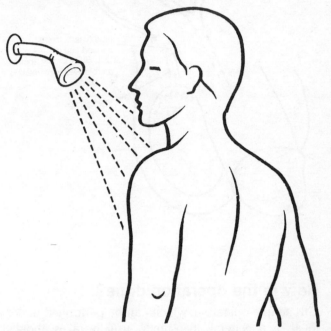

TSE is best performed after a warm bath or shower

How to do TSE

Testicular self-examination is a simple procedure that all young men should learn to do. Examination is best done using two hands, as illustrated.

- Explore each testicle individually.
- Using both hands, gently roll the testicle between the thumbs and fingers. If pain is experienced, too much pressure is being applied.

The examination should be done about once a month, preferably after a warm bath or shower, when the scrotal skin is most relaxed.

What to look for

A normal testicle is egg-shaped, fairly firm to touch and should be smooth and free of lumps. When you examine the testicles, you should feel for any changes in size, shape or consistency. If you do find something abnormal, most likely it will be an area of firmness or small lump on the front or on the side of the testicle.

Do not confuse the *epididymis* (the soft tube-like structure at the back of the testicle) with a tumour. If you do find something abnormal, you should see a doctor as soon as possible. However, remember that not all lumps are due to cancer.

Vasectomy

What is vasectomy?

Vasectomy, which is the commonest method of sterilisation in men, is an operation in which the two 'vas' tubes (the *vas deferens*) are cut and tied. This blocks the flow of sperm from the testicles into the penis, so that when the man ejaculates the semen does not contain sperm.

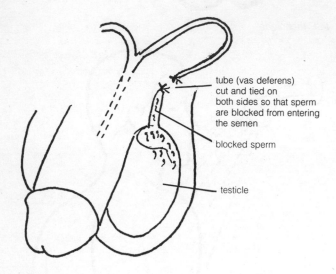

tube (vas deferens) cut and tied on both sides so that sperm are blocked from entering the semen

blocked sperm

testicle

How is the operation done?

This simple operation, which can be performed under a local or a general anaesthetic, usually takes about 30 minutes. It is done through two small cuts in each side of the scrotum (bag) or through one cut in the middle. The 'vas' tube, which lies just below the skin, is picked up and cut. About 1 cm of it is removed; the ends are tied off and then cauterised with a hot needle.

How effective is a vasectomy?

Vasectomy is reliable because every precaution is taken to separate the tubes so that they do not rejoin. Nevertheless, despite this, about 1 in 500 vasectomies fail because the tubes somehow manage to rejoin.

Is the man sterile immediately?

No. It takes about 12 to 15 ejaculations to clear all the sperm from the tubes above the cut. About 2 months after the operation it is necessary to have one or two (preferably two) sperm counts to make sure that the semen has no sperm. The semen has to be collected by masturbation and examined under a microscope.

Does vasectomy affect sexual function?

No. It makes no difference to a man's sex drive and performance. Some say that their sex life is improved because the worry about contraception is removed. Despite the absence of sperm in the semen, the fluid ejaculated seems normal because most of it is produced high in the tubes at the base of the penis.

Normal sexual activity can be started 4–5 days after vasectomy, but it is important to continue some form of birth control until the sperm count is zero.

What happens to the sperm?

Sperm are still produced in the testicles but lie around in the blocked tube for about 3 weeks before shrivelling up and being absorbed into the body in a similar way to blood after a bruise. Sperm only make up about 1% of the fluid ejaculated.

What are the side effects of vasectomy?

Bruising and swelling are common problems but settle after about 2 days. Bleeding and infection occur sometimes, but they settle quickly with treatment. A small lump caused by a build-up of sperm can develop at the operation site: these sperm *granulomas* usually settle themselves.

Can vasectomy be reversed?

The cut tubes can be rejoined by microsurgery, but there is no guarantee of regaining fertility. As a general rule about 40% of vasectomy reversals lead to successful pregnancy.

Vasectomy should be regarded as permanent and irreversible.

It is important to be definite about the decision to have the operation and not to have it under pressure.

7 The elderly

Arthritis in the elderly

Arthritis means inflamed joints, and there are many types of arthritis. The commonest type is *osteoarthritis*, which is a problem of wear and tear due to excessive use over the years and to old injuries in the affected joints. Most cases of arthritis are mild, and people cope with it. Arthritis does not necessarily get worse as you get older; sometimes it can get less painful (arthritis in the lumbar spine is a good example of this).

What are the symptoms of osteoarthritis?

- pain, swelling or stiffness in one or more joints
- pain or stiffness in the back or neck
- pain and stiffness after heavy activity such as gardening or housework or long walks and on getting up in the mornings; light activity might actually relieve some of the symptoms

Which joints are affected?

Osteoarthritis mostly affects the weight-bearing joints such as the spine, knees and hips. The base of the thumb, the ends of the fingers and the big toes are also common sites.

What is the treatment?

There is no cure, but there are many ways to make life more comfortable and keep you mobile and independent.

Diet

Keep your weight down to avoid unnecessary wear on the joints. No particular diet has been proved to cause, or improve, osteoarthritis.

Exercise

Keep a good balance of adequate rest with sensible exercise (such as walking, cycling and swimming), but *stop* any exercise or activity that increases the pain.

Heat

It is usual to feel more comfortable when the weather is warm. A hot-water bottle, warm bath or electric blanket can soothe the pain and stiffness. Avoid getting too cold.

Physiotherapy

This can be most helpful in improving muscle tone, reducing stiffness and keeping you mobile.

Walking aids

Shoe inserts, good footwear and a walking stick can help painful knees, hips and feet.

Medication

Aspirin and paracetamol are effective pain-killers. Your doctor may prescribe special antiarthritic medications, which should be taken with food. Inform your doctor if you have had a peptic ulcer or get indigestion.

Special equipment

It is possible to increase your independence at home. There is a wide range of inexpensive equipment and tools that can help with cooking, cleaning and other household chores. These can be discussed with your physiotherapist or occupational therapist.

Surgery

Modern surgery can give excellent results with relief of severe pain for most joints. The new techniques and artificial joints are improving all the time, and so there is no need to suffer with severe pain.

Osteoarthritis of the hip

Replacement of your worn-out joint with an artificial hip made of a combination of metal or plastic is a very common operation. More than 90% of these are most successful.

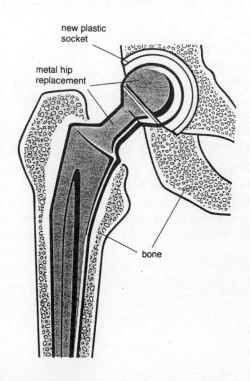

Total hip joint replacement

Osteoarthritis of the knee

Modern knee replacements are also giving excellent results, and if you have crippling knee pain this operation can give great relief.

Dementia

What is dementia?

Dementia is a disorder in which a previously normal brain does not function normally and the affected person becomes confused, forgetful and out of touch with the real world. It is rare in people under 65 years of age and appears more likely to develop with increasing age. It tends to progress slowly after it develops. The cause is not always known, but dementia can follow brain damage from physical abuse such as boxing, excessive alcohol and other drugs, and hardening of the arteries to the brain.

What is Alzheimer's disease?

This refers to a special type of dementia in which there is wasting of some brain cells, the cause of which is uncertain. It can occur at any age, but when it develops at a relatively young age (under 65) it is referred to as *presenile dementia*. It is commoner in people with Down syndrome.

What are the symptoms?

The main feature is *loss of memory* of things that have happened *recently*. You will notice that the person cannot remember what has happened a few hours (or even moments) earlier but can clearly remember events in the past. Other symptoms, which are slowly progressive, include:
- apathy
- confusion and restlessness
- a tendency to wander
- poor powers of reasoning and understanding
- loss of interest in previously enjoyable things
- sleeping problems
- personality changes, such as being suspicious, irritable, withdrawn, humourless, unco-operative or aggressive

The problem occasionally results in marked emotional and physical instability. It is sad and difficult for relatives to watch their loved ones develop aggressive and anti-social behaviour, such as poor table manners, poor personal cleanliness, rudeness and a lack of interest in others. Sometimes severe problems such as violent behaviour, sexual promiscuity and incontinence will eventuate.

How common is dementia?

The older the person, the more likely the problem. The incidence is probably 1 person in 10 over 65 years and 1 in 5 over 80 years.

What are the risks?

There is always the likelihood of accidents with household items such as fire, gas, kitchen knives and hot water. Accidents at the toilet, in the bath and when crossing roads may be a problem, especially if dementia is combined with failing sight and hearing. Such people should not drive motor vehicles.

Without proper supervision they are likely to eat poorly, neglect their bodies and develop medical problems such as skin ulcers and infections. They can also suffer from malnutrition and incontinence of urine or faeces.

What is the treatment?

If you suspect that a friend or relative has early dementia, take him or her to the doctor for assessment. There is no cure, but the best that can be offered is tender loving care.

Regular home visits by caring, sympathetic people are important. Such people include relatives, friends, general practitioners, district nurses, home help, ministers of religion and Meals-on-Wheels. The sufferers tend to manage much better in the familiar surroundings of their own home.

Special attention should be paid to organising memory aids such as lists, routines and medication, and to hygiene, diet and warmth. Adequate nutrition, including vitamin supplements if necessary, has been shown to help these people.

Support groups

It is important to contact an Alzheimer's support group in your state or locality. One such special support and advisory group is called ADARDS (the Alzheimer's Disease and Related Disorders Society).

John Murtagh, *Patient Education*, Second edition, McGraw-Hill Book Company

Eye problems in the aged

Many older folk have no problems at all with their eyes and vision, with most maintaining good eyesight into their 80s.

However, natural physical changes can cause some problems with age, and disorders such as *cataracts* and *glaucoma* are more likely to occur. Older people generally need brighter light for everyday tasks such as reading, cooking, mending and driving a car.

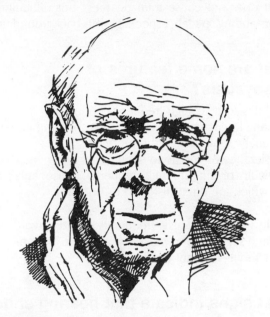

Common eye complaints

Presbyopia
This is a common disorder first noticed after the age of 40 (usually 45 years onwards) when a change in the eye muscles and lens caused by loss of elasticity makes reading more difficult. You can read only by holding the material at arm's length. This applies to small print as in telephone books and street directories. It is a focusing problem, which is easily corrected by having reading glasses with a convex lens.

Every few years you will need slightly stronger spectacles to allow for decreasing ability to focus. Bifocal lenses may be needed if you have another eye problem.

Floaters
A common complaint is of seeing tiny spots or specks that float across the eye, especially in bright light. They are normal and usually harmless but may be a warning of impending eye problems. If they become noticeable or cause flashes of light, report to your doctor.

Excessive tears
Excessive tears are usually a sign of increased sensitivity of the eyes to wind, light or temperature changes. This complaint is very common in a cold wind. It can be minimised by wearing glasses, especially sunglasses, in those conditions. However, it may indicate blocked tear ducts (*lacrimal ducts*) or an eye infection, and so an eye check is recommended.

Dry eyes
This is caused by a reduced production of tears by the tear glands. It can cause many problems, such as blurred vision, itching or burning. It is easily corrected by using artificial tears.

Common eye diseases

Glaucoma
Glaucoma is caused by too much fluid pressure in the eye, which can lead to blindness. It comes in two forms: the rarer *acute* form (which causes sudden pain and visual problems) and the common *chronic* form (which slowly develops without any early symptoms). It is important to have any unusual eye symptoms checked, and all elderly patients should have eye tests (including eyeball pressure) every 2–3 years. When detected, it can be treated and blindness prevented.

Cataracts
Normally the lens within the eye is clear and allows light to pass through it. A cataract is where the clear lens becomes cloudy or opaque and cuts down the light entering the back of the eye. Apart from deterioration of vision, there are no other symptoms. They can occur in anyone but are more common in diabetics and those taking cortisone tablets. Cataracts can also run in families. They are diagnosed during an eye examination. A modern lens implant (an artificial lens placed in the space left by the cataract lens) can give excellent results.

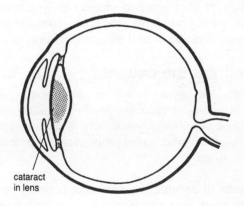

cataract in lens

Retinal disorders
Disorders of the *retina* (the photosensitive area of the eye) can lead to varying degrees of blindness. Diabetes and other diseases can cause retinal problems. Sometimes the retina can become detached and seriously affect your eyesight. Retinal detachment can be treated successfully if detected early.

> **Tips**
> - Light bulbs are better than fluorescent lights.
> - Have regular checks for blood pressure and diabetes.
> - Have an eye examination every 2–3 years.
> - Eye problems tend to run in families.

John Murtagh, *Patient Education*, Second edition, McGraw-Hill Book Company

Hearing impairment in the aged

Loss of hearing tends to gradually increase with advancing age. Every year after the age of 50 we lose some of our hearing ability. As many as 25% of people aged 60–70 report hearing impairment. The decline varies from person to person and, like greying of hair, occurs at different rates.

What are the symptoms?

The symptoms vary so that some barely notice a problem while others are severely disabled.

Common symptoms include:

- inability to hear speech and other sounds loudly enough
- inability to hear speech and music clearly, even when it is loud enough
- inability to understand speech, even when it is loud enough (a problem of language reception)

People with mild hearing loss notice only subtle differences and may have trouble hearing certain high frequency sounds such as *s*, *f* or *th*. They may also have trouble hearing in certain situations, such as at a party or in a crowd where there is a lot of background noise. Those with moderate hearing loss have trouble hearing in many situations.

In very old people, deafness can lead to unexpected behavioural problems such as confusion, agitation, anxiety, depression and paranoid delusions.

What are the causes?

Hearing loss takes two forms: *conduction loss*, where the sound waves are blocked in their passage to the inner ear, and *neurosensory loss*, where the inner ear cannot pick up the sound waves properly and thus transmit them to the brain.

Causes of conductive deafness (usually reversible)

- too much wax in the ears
- other debris in the ear canal (e.g. cotton bud tip)
- ear infection
- faulty vibrating bones (*otosclerosis*)

Causes of neurosensory deafness (usually not reversible)

- nerve damage
- exposure to loud noise, including sudden explosions

- certain drugs
- brain tumours
- presbycusis

What is presbycusis?

Presbycusis (pronounced 'prez-bee-ku-siss') is also known as 'old age' deafness and is the commonest type of hearing impairment in older people. It is caused by wear and tear in the very delicate workings of the inner ear. It does not cause total deafness but difficulties in understanding speech, especially with background noise.

What are some features of presbycusis?

- inability to hear high frequency sounds
- usually an association with tinnitus (ringing in ears)
- a genetic tendency to the problem
- intolerance of very loud sounds
- difficulty picking up high frequency consonants (e.g. *f*, *s*), which are often distorted or unheard

People with presbycusis frequently confuse words such as *fit* and *sit*, *math* and *mass*, *fun* and *sun*. They often say 'Don't shout—I'm not deaf'.

What signs indicate that hearing should be tested?

- speaking too loudly
- difficulty understanding speech
- social withdrawal
- lack of interest in attending parties and other functions
- complaints about people mumbling
- requests to have speech repeated
- complaints of tinnitus
- setting television and radio on high volume

Patients are usually referred to an audiologist after a medical check.

What can be done?

If medical problems such as fluid or wax in the ear are not present and 'old age' deafness is proved on testing, a hearing aid is usually fitted. There is no cure for the problem and hearing aids are not the perfect answer. However, modern hearing aids can be tailor-made for the individual person and are usually quite effective.

John Murtagh, *Patient Education*, Second edition, McGraw-Hill Book Company

Leg ulcers

What are leg ulcers?

Leg ulcers are abnormal 'holes' that occur in breaks in the skin in the lower leg. Ulcers can occur in any person, but the elderly who have poor circulation are most likely to develop ulcers. They usually occur in the area known as the *gaiter* area of the leg. Twice as many women as men are affected.

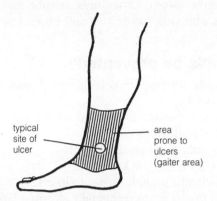

typical site of ulcer

area prone to ulcers (gaiter area)

What is the cause?

Ulcers are usually caused by a combination of two problems: rather sluggish circulation to the leg and poor drainage due to varicose veins. The further the distance is from the pump (the heart), the more likely the area is to be affected by poor circulation, so that the ankle area is the most vulnerable. The skin becomes thin, and because injuries such as from knocks or scratches are common here the skin tends to break down and heal poorly. The small crack in the skin may enlarge and gradually become an ulcer.

What are the symptoms?

The ulcer has dead tissue in it and usually weeps. The commonest site is the skin on the inside of the leg just above the ankle. The skin around the ulcer usually becomes red, itchy, flaky and discoloured. Many are not painful, just uncomfortable, but those due to very poor circulation can be quite painful, especially if on the foot.

What are the problems?

Slow healing is the main problem. This is usually not a serious problem, but an ulcer can take months or years to heal in an older person. Ulcers in younger persons usually heal in a few weeks. Those with diabetes or peripheral vascular disease (clogged arteries) heal slowly. Rarely the ulcer is due to an infection or can develop skin cancer and therefore needs careful medical attention.

What is the treatment?

Self-help

The key to healing is to keep the leg elevated as much as possible and also to keep fluid out of the leg, which is helped by a firm bandage. Raising the legs above the level of the heart reduces swelling and quickens healing. Avoid standing for long periods, but undertake moderate walking exercise. Avoid smoking and have a nutritious diet. Be extremely careful not to injure the leg, as the skin of the legs is fragile. Do not scratch, watch out for sharp stakes in the garden and be careful of hot-water bottles.

Keep ulcers covered and sterile (ulcers require moisture to heal).

Medical help

The ulcer will require regular dressings to keep it clean and free from infection. Special substances may be added to clean out the debris in the ulcer. A nurse may be able to call regularly to dress the ulcer. It is usually better to keep the dressing on for a few days. You will be provided with a knee-high elastic bandage or a thick elastic stocking to wear during the day. It may be necessary to apply a skin graft to promote the healing.

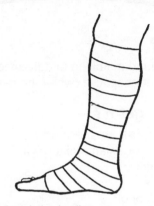

An elastic bandage helps healing

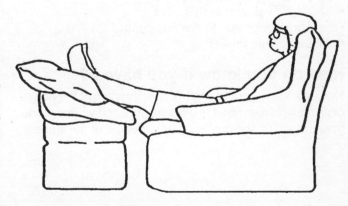

Rest and elevate the legs as much as possible

Remember

- Keep your leg elevated as often as possible.
- Keep the leg compressed with a firm bandage, tights or support stockings.
- Avoid further knocks and other injury.

Osteoporosis

What is it?

Osteoporosis is a condition leading to thinning of bones so that they become weak and brittle.

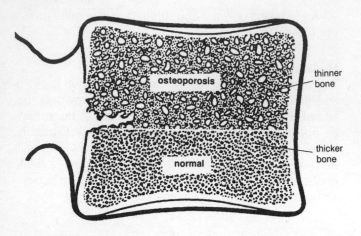

Who gets it?

Osteoporosis is found mainly in middle-aged and elderly women, after the menopause (when the periods cease).

Why do they get it?

Women at greatest risk are those who:
- are of Caucasian or Asian racial origin
- are thin and slight
- smoke cigarettes
- drink a lot of alcohol
- drink a lot of coffee
- get little exercise
- have little calcium in their diet
- lack hormones due to the menopause
- take cortisone tablets

How do you know if you have it?

Most women do not know, because thinning of the bones occurs unobtrusively. It is often first noticed when a bone breaks, usually the hip, wrist or vertebrae of the spine.

What can you do about it?

- Take regular weight-bearing exercise such as walking (e.g. brisk walking for 30 minutes 4 times a week).
- Stop smoking.
- Cut down on alcohol and caffeine.
- Have adequate calcium in your diet: 1000–1500 mg per day (1500 mg if postmenopausal). Eat calcium-rich foods such as low-fat calcium-enriched milk (500 mL contains 1000 mg), other low-fat dairy products (e.g. yoghurt or cheese), fish (including tinned fish such as salmon, with the bone), citrus fruits, sesame and sunflower seeds, almonds, brazil nuts and hazelnuts.

How can falls be prevented?

Falls tend to cause fractures in osteoporotic bones. They can be prevented by:
- removing loose or worn carpets and scatter rugs
- wearing low-heeled shoes
- holding onto railings when using stairs
- installing safety bars in the bathroom
- using night lights to provide better visibility
- being careful taking drugs, especially sleeping tablets
- having good eyesight: regular checks are advised

What can your doctor do?

Your doctor may:
- discuss your diet
- suggest hormone tablets and calcium supplements
- review your 'risks' for osteoporosis, and if you are at high risk suggest further tests such as bone density measurement

---

Key points

- Osteoporosis is a common condition.
- It starts from a young age but develops faster in middle and older age.
- The main aim is to *prevent* it from occurring.

John Murtagh, *Patient Education*, Second edition, McGraw-Hill Book Company

Parkinson's disease

What is Parkinson's disease?

Also known as *shaking palsy* or *paralysis agitans*, Parkinson's disease is due to an imbalance of chemicals in the nerve cells in the brain that regulate movement. Because these cells do not 'fire' smoothly, various body movements are affected.

How common is the problem?

About 1 person in 1000 develops Parkinson's disease, and these are mainly elderly or in late middle age. It can be caused by some drugs and toxic fumes or substances such as carbon monoxide and lead.

What are the symptoms?

The symptoms are:
- stiff and slow movements, causing difficulty starting a movement
- a shuffled walk
- an expressionless face
- slow and flat speech
- difficulty writing
- a tremor, especially on the hands and arms, with a rubbing together of the thumb and forefinger; the tremor is worse at rest and tends to go away when an action such as picking up a pen or other object is performed

There is no pain, numbness or pins and needles. Later on falls may be a problem.

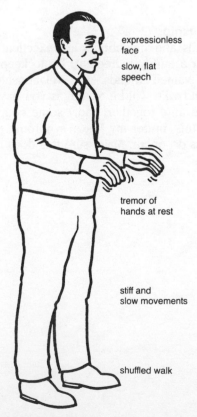

Symptoms of Parkinson's disease

expressionless face

slow, flat speech

tremor of hands at rest

stiff and slow movements

shuffled walk

What causes the symptoms?

The problem is caused by the lack of a special chemical in the brain called *dopamine*, which the nerve cells need to 'fire'. It is rather like the chemical in a battery gradually running out so that the battery becomes flat.

It is not caused by a brain tumour or a stroke, but in some cases poor circulation to that part of the brain can be responsible for the problem.

What is the outlook?

There are many different grades of severity but many people have a mild problem and are able to cope, even without the need for dopamine-producing drugs. If the disease gets worse, it is usually only a very slow process; it is rare that a person gets severely disabled and confined to a wheelchair. If you develop Parkinson's disease after the age of 60, you may expect to live out your normal life expectancy.

What are the risks?

The disease is not life-threatening because it does not affect nerves that supply the heart or other vital organs.

Two common risks are falls and mental depression.

What is the treatment?

Self-help

An important part of managing at home is to keep as active as possible with the help of a caring family, friends and other people. Your mobility can be assisted, for example, by bath rail supports, special banisters where you normally walk and chairs with high seats and arms.

It is important to have regular exercise and to stick to your everyday routine as actively as possible. Your doctor should see you regularly to assess your progress.

Medication

No drug will cure the problem, but there are modern drugs that can do much to relieve symptoms, particularly stiffness and poor mobility. Drugs that lead to higher levels of dopamine in the brain can be prescribed and it is better to prescribe them early rather than wait until the symptoms are more severe.

The drugs can have side effects such as feeling sick in the stomach (nausea) and a dry mouth, and so your doctor will have to juggle them according to the progress you are making.

Retirement planning

Retirement can be a most enjoyable period of the life cycle, one of productivity and self-realisation. However, for many people it can bring considerable unforeseen sadness and stress. This is mainly brought about by inadequate planning and changes of relationships. Studies show that very few people plan for it until just before the time.

What are the main problems?

Common problems in retirement are:
- loneliness
- boredom
- financial worries

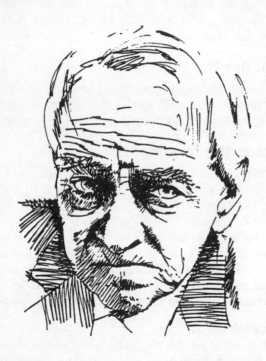

Loneliness

Loneliness is a terrible problem; it can lead to depression and a feeling of worthlessness. A common mistake is to sell the family home and move to another location, usually in a small unit. This separation from old friends, neighbours and family can cause much heartache. It often happens to country people who move to the city. You need your family around you, especially if your spouse dies. You should give consideration to keeping your family home, because it encourages your family to visit you. Children often interpret a move to a small unit as 'don't come and stay with us', although this may not be the intention.

Financial security

You really need sound advice for a secure financial future, including investments. Try to work out your finances 5 years in advance and allow for inflation and home maintenance. If you own your home and car, you have a good basis.

Health

You need good health to enjoy your deserved retirement. Take care not to get into bad eating and exercise habits. Plan a sensible, healthy, balanced diet. Avoid smoking and excessive drinking. Regular and effective exercise is important. Appropriate exercises are walking for 20–30 minutes each day, swimming, cycling and golf.

Activities

Retirement gives you the opportunity to devote more time to those interests and hobbies that you already enjoy. It will also give you the chance to pursue new ones. There are many agencies that will provide information on programs for the retired, adult education courses (especially in the arts and crafts) and community work. If your hobby can supplement your income, that is a bonus.

Useful activities include sports such as bowls, golf and tennis, travel, nature walking, voluntary or part-time work. Many retired people get considerable pleasure out of carpentry and woodwork.

Housing

Keep your family home if you can. Carefully weigh up the pros and cons of moving—it can bring much stress, worry and financial problems. As you get older it is most important to have transport, shopping and medical facilities nearby.

Companionship

Good friends and neighbours are excellent 'insurance policies' for a happy retirement. Try to keep in contact with your valued friends. The relationship between husband and wife will be tested, as you have to spend much more time together. Sadly some couples cannot cope with this 'under my heels' syndrome and marital breakdowns do occur. Make sure this does not happen to you.

John Murtagh, *Patient Education*, Second edition, McGraw-Hill Book Company

Stroke

What is a stroke?

A *stroke* occurs when an area of the brain is damaged following interruption to its blood supply. This results in deterioration of the mental and physical functions controlled by that particular area.

What is the cause?

There are three main causes:
- *thrombosis*: a clot forming in the artery to the area
- *embolus*: a small clot from elsewhere blocking the artery
- *haemorrhage*: bleeding into the brain (unlike the others, where the artery is blocked)

Some common underlying causes are high blood pressure and hardening of the arteries (*atherosclerosis*).

What are the symptoms?

The symptoms depend on the area of the brain affected and the cause. A haemorrhage usually has a sudden onset and a less favourable outlook. Sometimes a stroke is mild and the effects pass off in a day or so.
   Symptoms include:
- unconsciousness
- confusion
- loss of power of speech
- loss of movement of part of the body (e.g. on one side of the body)
- double or blurred vision
- difficulty understanding questions
- dizziness
- difficulty walking or using arms
- numbness on one side of the body

What is a transient ischaemic attack?

This is a transient loss of function due to a temporary blockage in the artery. It is usually caused by a small embolus and the patient recovers in a period ranging from a few minutes to 24 hours (average time 5 minutes). It can be a warning of an impending stroke, and so it needs urgent medical attention.

How common are strokes?

They are very common, especially in people over 65 years and more so in males. In Western countries they are the third commonest cause of death and after heart attacks the second commonest cause of sudden death. Those at special risk are those with high blood pressure, diabetes or high blood cholesterol and heavy smokers.

What is the outcome?

About one-third recover almost completely one-third have some permanent disability and one-third will die.

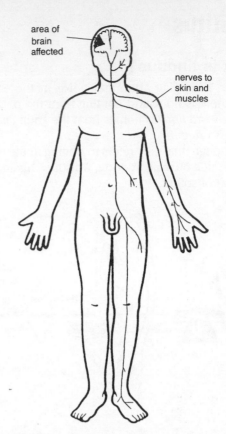

area of brain affected

nerves to skin and muscles

Stroke: an accident to one side of the brain will lead to paralysis of the opposite side of the body

How can strokes be prevented?

The risk factors need to be checked, especially high blood pressure, which must be kept under control. Other things to do are avoid smoking, avoid excessive alcohol intake, eat a low-fat healthy diet, keep to ideal weight and have regular exercise.
   If you have been found to have hardening of the arteries to the brain, you may be advised to have tablets to prevent blood clots (thrombosis) forming. Aspirin can do this, and only a small dose is needed. Garlic tablets are reported to help prevent clots, and special blood-thinning tablets called *anticoagulants* (commonly warfarin) can be prescribed.

Surgery

If a person has partially clogged arteries to the brain (the *carotids*), it may be possible to clean them out rather like a brush cleaning out a chimney. This is a good option in some patients, especially in those who have had transient ischaemic attacks.

What is the treatment for stroke?

Once the stroke has occurred, the brain tissue will not heal normally. Even though the person has survived, it is important to still attend to the risk factors, especially checking the blood pressure. Intense rehabilitation to get limbs and speech working again will begin. This involves a team approach with the physiotherapist being the key person. The results are usually a pleasant surprise to all concerned, with a gradual improvement occurring over 2 years (at least).

Tinnitus

What is tinnitus?

Tinnitus is hearing abnormal noise in the ear or head when there is no sound coming from the outside.

The word *tinnitus* comes from the Latin *tinnire*, which means 'to ring'.

Although it usually refers to ringing in the ear, tinnitus may include buzzing, roaring, whistling, hissing or a combination of sounds.

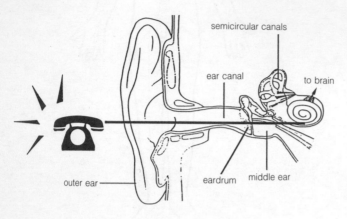

How common is tinnitus?

Although most of us experience tinnitus at some time, especially with a lot of wax blocking an ear, it is only a temporary problem. About 1 in 4 people are bothered by it, but it is a severe problem for 2% of the population.

What causes or aggravates it?

- ear disorders such as infection
- excessive noise exposure for a long time
- wear and tear of the ear with ageing
- some prescribed drugs
- stress and fatigue
- excessive alcohol
- smoking
- social drugs, including caffeine and marijuana
- head injury

How serious is tinnitus?

Tinnitus in itself is not a serious condition, does not cause pain or deafness but can be frustrating. Most people with tinnitus have a hearing loss, but there are also many people with normal hearing who have tinnitus. Many people with tinnitus worry that it is a symptom of a brain tumour, a stroke, a nervous disorder or some other serious head problem. However, this is rarely the case.

What are its effects?

The main problem is the psychological effect, as the noise tends to affect one's concentration, ability to think and peace of mind. Stress can aggravate the problem.

It can also be a problem at night, when it is more noticeable and affects the ability to sleep.

What can be done for tinnitus?

Tinnitus is less noticeable when there is background noise, and therefore it is important to 'switch off' from the ear ringing as much as possible and focus on other noise.

The following methods can help one cope with tinnitus:

Stress management and relaxation techniques

Since tinnitus is more noticeable when you are stressed, tired or emotionally upset, learning relaxation or meditation techniques to focus your attention outwards may be helpful. Some patients are helped by hypnosis. Your doctor will advise on these methods.

Background sound treatment

A useful treatment, especially for those having trouble getting to sleep, is to have background music playing when retiring at night. Other sounds that are sometimes used include FM static produced by a radio set off the station and environmental sound masking tapes.

Tinnitus maskers

Some people are helped by wearing a tinnitus masker, which is a device like a hearing aid worn behind the ear. It produces a type of hissing noise that tends to counter-balance the tinnitus noise.

Hearing aids

If a hearing loss accompanies the tinnitus, the use of a hearing aid can mask the tinnitus with amplified sound. This makes it easier to focus on outside sound.

Distracting activities

Some people can cope by diverting their attention away from their tinnitus by keeping themselves busy and undertaking interesting activities that focus their mind elsewhere. Examples include gardening, power walking, music, television, handicrafts, jigsaw puzzles, card playing and discussion groups.

Counselling and support

Most cities have a counselling service for tinnitus sufferers. Ask your doctor about the Australian Tinnitus Association.

John Murtagh, *Patient Education*, Second edition, McGraw-Hill Book Company

PART II

General health—various ages

8 Prevention

Cholesterol: how to lower cholesterol

Why bother?

Heart disease is the number one killer in Australia. It is mainly caused by clogging up of the arteries by a fatty substance known as *atheroma*, which comes from having too much 'fat' in the blood. This serious process is called *atherosclerosis*—the condition that can lead to heart attack or stroke. There are two types of fat that cause damage if their levels are too high—*cholesterol* and *triglyceride*. A special blood test taken after fasting for at least 12 hours can tell if one or both of these fats are too high.

Triglyceride

If your triglyceride level is too high, fixing the problem is usually quite straightforward because it is mainly due to being overweight. It is caused by having too many calories in the diet, especially from sugar and other carbohydrates and high-calorie drinks (e.g. soft drinks and alcohol, in particular beer). The aim is to get your weight down to an ideal level.

Cholesterol

High cholesterol is a bigger problem, and if your level is too high it is important to reduce it. Cholesterol is a white fatty substance made mainly in the liver by animals, including humans. We get high levels mainly through our diet, by eating animal foods. (Therefore it is a rare problem in vegetarians.) Most people can lower the level through changing their diet. Occasionally the level is so high in some people that in addition to the diet special medicine is necessary to reduce it to the right level.

Note: Although cholesterol is present in animal food, it has been shown that it is necessary to reduce the amount of *all* the saturated fats (plant and animal) in our diet and to lose excess weight in order to get our cholesterol down. Foods rich in starch (such as bread, rice and pasta) and fibre also help.

Golden rules

- Keep to your ideal weight.
- Take a high-fibre diet.
- Eat fish at least twice a week.
- Beware of 'fast' foods.
- Avoid deep-fried foods.
- Take regular exercise.
- Always trim fat off meat.
- Avoid biscuits between meals.
- Drink more water.
- Do not smoke.

The low cholesterol diet

	Foods to avoid	Suitable foods
Eggs	whole eggs, egg yolks	egg whites
Milk	whole milk and its products—butter, cream, cheese, ice-cream, yoghurt, condensed milk	low-fat milk, skim milk and its products—cottage and ricotta cheese, buttermilk, non-fat yoghurt
Organ meats	brains, liver, pâté, liverwurst, kidney, sweetbread	—
Seafood	prawns, squid (calamari), fish roe, caviar, fish 'fingers', canned fish in oil (e.g. sardines)	fresh fish, scallops, oysters, canned fish in water, lobster and crab (small amounts)
Meat	fatty meats—bacon, ham, sausages, salami, canned meats, pressed meats, meat pastes, hamburger mince	rabbit, veal (without fat), lean cuts of beef, lamb and pork (in moderation)
Poultry	duck, goose, skin of chicken and turkey, pressed chicken	chicken, turkey (lean and without skin), preferably free-range
Bakery food	pies, pasties, pastries, cakes, doughnuts, biscuits	bread, crumpets, crispbreads, water-biscuits, homemade items (pies, etc.) if proper ingredients used
Fast food	fried chicken, chips, fish, dim sims, spring rolls, etc., hot-dogs, pizzas, fried rice	—
Nuts	cashews, macadamia nuts, coconut, roasted nuts, brazil nuts, peanuts, peanut butter (can have in very small amounts)	pecan nuts, hazelnuts, walnuts, almonds, seeds (in moderation)
Fruit and vegetables	—	all types (very important)
Miscellaneous	gravies, potato crisps, caramel, chocolate (including carob), butterscotch, 'health food' bars, fudge coffee whitener and other cream substitutes, toasted breakfast cereals (especially with coconut)	rice, pasta, cereals, jelly, herbs, spices, canned spaghetti, Vegemite, tea, coffee, honey, jam, alcohol (small amounts)
Oils and fats	saturated fats—lard, dripping, suet, copha, cooking (hard) margarine, coconut and palm oils, mayonnaise	polyunsaturated fats—margarines, salad dressings; vegetable oils—olive, walnut, corn, soya bean, sunflower, safflower, cottonseed (all in moderation)
Cooking methods	frying, roasting in fat	using vegetable oils (as above), baking, boiling, grilling, stewing

---

Coronary risk factors

The problem of coronary heart disease

The number one cause of death in modern Western society is coronary heart disease (CHD), whether it be from sudden fatal heart attacks or blocked coronary arteries causing angina and heart failure. CHD is responsible for 1 in 3 deaths in Australia. However, there has been a very pleasing reduction in deaths from coronary heart disease and stroke in the past 20 years because people have made the effort to reduce their risk factors. In spite of this, it is still a major cause of preventable death and we still need to work hard at reducing the risk.

What are the risk factors?

- hypertension (high blood pressure)
- smoking
- high cholesterol
- diabetes
- obesity
- lack of exercise
- stress
- alcohol excess
- family history

These risk factors increase the likelihood of development of hardening of the arteries (or *atherosclerosis*); the benefit of reducing them is obvious. The factors are inter-related; for example, excessive intake of alcohol will lead to hypertension.

Hypertension

The higher the blood pressure, the greater the risk. Regular checks, say yearly for people over 40 years, are advisable. Doctors recommend that you have the *diastolic level* (lower level) of blood pressure kept at 90 mm Hg or below.

Smoking

Cigarette smoking has been clearly shown to increase the risk of heart disease. The death rate from coronary heart disease is about 70% higher for smokers than for non-smokers and for very heavy smokers the risk is almost 200% higher. The more one smokes, the greater the risk.

It has also been proved that the incidence of heart disease falls in those who have given up smoking.

High cholesterol

It has been proved that high blood cholesterol is related to heart attacks. High cholesterol is caused by a diet high in *saturated* fats, as compared with *polyunsaturated* fats. It is recommended that every effort should be made to keep the blood cholesterol level as low as possible and preferably below 5.5 mmol/L in adults. This acceptable level can usually be achieved through dieting. Saturated fats are found in regular milk and its products (e.g. cream, butter, cheese); fatty meats; pies and pastries, cakes, biscuits and croissants; cooking fats; most fast foods and potato crisps.

Stress and heart attacks

The stress of our modern lifestyle is regarded as a risk factor. Evidence for this is supported by the increased incidence of heart attacks in Asians (who have a low incidence) when they move into Western societies or become business executives in their own environment. Consider ways to modify your stress factors and seek relaxation programs such as meditation.

The significance of risk factors

Most of the risk factors are interdependent, and if two or more are present they have a multiplication effect. If only one risk factor is present, the patient does not have so much cause for concern. Your doctor is the best person to assess the combined risk.

Rules for living

- Do not smoke.
- Drink alcohol in only very small amounts or not at all.
- Keep to an ideal weight.
- Avoid saturated fats.
- Take regular exercise.
- Practise relaxation.

Note: The risk factors for coronary heart disease apply also to other cardiovascular disease, such as cerebral artery disease and hardening of the arteries of the legs.

John Murtagh, *Patient Education*, Second edition, McGraw-Hill Book Company

Diet guidelines for good health

At times we get confused about what we should or should not eat. The following recommendations come from authorities on nutrition, such as government Health Departments. These guidelines ensure an adequate intake and balance of all important nutrients—carbohydrates, proteins, fats, fibre, vitamins and minerals.

1. Choose a nutritious diet

Choose from a wide variety of foods to provide meals that are healthier, cheaper, tastier and easier to prepare.

2. Control your weight

Prevent obesity by cutting back fats, sugar and alcohol. Reduce the size of servings (say 'no' to seconds) and increase physical activity.

3. Eat less fat

Select fish, poultry and lean meats; trim excess fat from meat and the skin from poultry. Limit the amount of butter or margarine on vegetables and bread. Use the minimum of cooking fats. Limit the intake of full-cream products, fried foods, fatty takeaway and snack foods.

4. Eat less sugar

Avoid or reduce sweet foods such as lollies, sugar, soft drinks, syrups, biscuits and cakes. Reduce the sugar in recipes. Use fresh fruit instead of canned fruit.

Instead, increase your intake of complex carbohydrates that contain starch and fibre. Eat more wholegrain breads and potatoes prepared without added fat.

5. Eat more breads and cereals, fruit and vegetables

Eat more fruit and vegetables, including dark-green vegetables, potatoes and corn. Choose wholegrain products—cereals, bread, bran, rice and oatmeal.

6. Drink less alcohol

Limit alcohol to no more than two drinks a day. Drink with smaller sips each time. Reserve alcohol for special occasions and to only one occasion in the day.

7. Use less salt

High sodium intake may raise your blood pressure. Use few salty processed foods, including canned vegetables, meats, chips, crackers, sauces and meat pastes. Read labels on canned and packaged foods for their sodium content. Use little salt for cooking and at the table.

8. Encourage breastfeeding

Breastfeeding gives the best nutritional start to life.

9. Drink more water

Use water in preference to soft drinks, coffee and tea, cordials and alcohol. Use water filters and purifiers if your water supply is not pure.

Extra tips on diet

- Do not eat animal meat every day, and then eat small portions.
- Limit tea and coffee intake.
- Eliminate or reduce takeaway foods (high in salt and fat).
- Eat fish at least twice a week.
- Plant food is good for you—have it as part of breakfast.
- What you *usually* eat matters most, not what you *occasionally* eat.

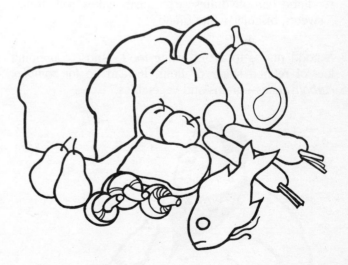

Obesity: how to lose weight wisely

Why bother to lose weight?

Those who are overweight, whether mildly obese or unattractively fat, have much to gain. You will look and feel so much better—your self-esteem will return. It will reduce your risks of heart disease, stroke, diabetes, cancer, gall bladder trouble, hiatus hernia, high blood pressure and arthritis, especially of the hips and the knees. Taking your obesity into old age creates many uncomfortable problems.

The two keys to success

- Eat less fattening food (especially fats and alcohol).
- Burn off the calories with exercise.

If we eat more fuel (joules) than we burn, we get fat.

Fattening foods

It is essential to cut down on high-calorie foods. These include:
- fats (e.g. oils, butter, margarine, peanut butter, some nuts)
- alcohol
- refined carbohydrates (e.g. sugar, cakes, soft drinks, sweets, biscuits, white bread)

A good rule is to avoid 'white food'—those containing lots of refined sugar or flour. Instead go for *complex carbohydrates*—grains and vegetables.

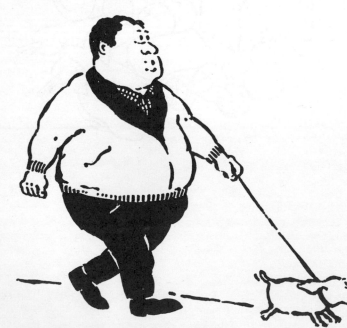

Losing weight wisely includes regular exercise

Physical activity

- A brisk walk for 20–30 minutes each day is the most practical exercise.
- Other activities, such as tennis, swimming, golf and cycling, are a bonus.

A plan that works!

Breakfast

- oatmeal (soaked overnight in water); after cooking, add fresh or dried fruit; serve with fat-reduced milk or yoghurt

or

- muesli (homemade or from a health-food store)—medium serve with fat-reduced milk; perhaps add extra fruit (fresh or dried)
- slice of wholemeal toast with a thin scraping of margarine, spread with Vegemite, Marmite or sugar-free marmalade
- fresh orange juice or herbal tea or black tea/coffee

Morning and afternoon tea

- piece of fruit or vegetable (e.g. carrot or celery)
- freshly squeezed juice or chilled water with fresh lemon

Midday meal

- salad sandwich with wholemeal or multigrained bread and a thin scraping of margarine. (For variety use egg, salmon, chicken or cheese fillings.)
- drink as for breakfast

Evening meal

- *Summer* (*cold*): lean meat cuts (grilled, hot or cold), poultry (skin removed) or fish; fresh garden salad; slices of fresh fruit
- *Winter* (*hot*): lean meat cuts (grilled), poultry (skin removed) or fish; plenty of green, red and yellow vegetables and small potato; fruit for sweets

Weight-losing tips

- Have sensible goals: do not 'crash' diet, but have a 3–6 month plan to achieve your ideal weight.
- Go for natural foods; avoid junk foods.
- Avoid alcohol, sugary soft drinks and high-calorie fruit juices.
- Strict dieting without exercise fails.
- If you are mildly overweight, eat one-third less than you usually do (only).
- Do not eat biscuits, cakes, buns, etc. between meals (preferably at no time).
- Use high-fibre foods to munch on.
- A small treat once a week may add variety.
- Avoid seconds and do not eat leftovers.
- Eat slowly—spin out your meal.
- Avoid medicines that claim to remove weight.

John Murtagh, *Patient Education*, Second edition, McGraw-Hill Book Company

Smoking—quitting

What are the facts on smoking?

Each year over 20 000 Australians die from diseases caused by smoking. Out of every 5 people who smoke 20 or more cigarettes a day, 2 die before the age of 65.
- *Cancer*: Smoking is the major cause of death from cancer, especially lung cancer (86% caused by smoking).
- *Other lung disease*: Smoking causes chronic bronchitis (smokers' cough) and emphysema.
- *Hardening of the arteries*: Smoking can cause hardening of the arteries of the heart (angina and coronary attacks), brain (strokes) and legs.

Women smokers have problems with pregnancy (including smaller babies), increased chance of infertility, an earlier menopause and an increased risk of osteoporosis.

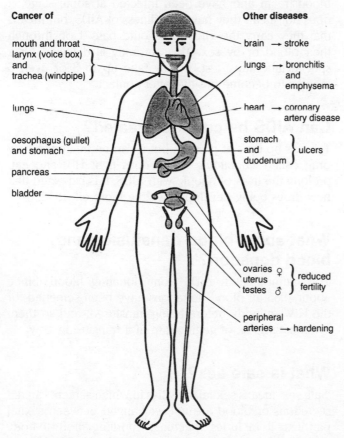

Cancer of
- mouth and throat larynx (voice box) and trachea (windpipe)
- lungs
- oesophagus (gullet) and stomach
- pancreas
- bladder

Other diseases
- brain → stroke
- lungs → bronchitis and emphysema
- heart → coronary artery disease
- stomach and duodenum } ulcers
- ovaries ♀ uterus testes ♂ } reduced fertility
- peripheral arteries → hardening

Harmful effects of smoking

What is in a cigarette?

The most harmful chemicals in cigarettes are tar, nicotine and carbon monoxide. Nicotine causes the addictive effect.

How will it help me if I quit?

The risk of death from heart attacks, lung cancer and other lung diseases will drop dramatically. Many of the bad effects of smoking can be reversed after quitting.

Other reported good effects are increased 'wind' on exercise, better senses of taste and smell, improved sexual pleasure and much more pocket-money. It is unnatural to smoke.

How should I quit?

The best way is to stop completely, going 'cold turkey'. It may help to use nicotine gum or skin patches, because nicotine is very addictive. Changing to pipes or cigars is not as good as completely stopping. Gradual reduction (e.g. by 3 or 4 a day) is a reasonable method, but it is best if you can stop completely within 2 weeks.

What are the unpleasant effects of quitting?

For the first few days it is normal to have the withdrawal effects of feeling restless, irritable, tense, tired and sweaty. You will crave for a cigarette, but these feelings are signs of recovery from the addictive effects of nicotine as your body adjusts itself for a return to normal health. After about 10 days, most of these uncomfortable feelings will have disappeared and you will start feeling absolutely marvellous. Ask a smoker who has quit.

What are some good tips for quitting?

- Make a definite date to stop (e.g. during a holiday).

After quitting:
- Eat more fruit and vegetables (e.g. munch carrots, celery and dried fruit).
- Foods such as citrus fruit can reduce cravings.
- Chew low-calorie gum and suck lozenges.
- Increase your activity (e.g. take regular walks instead of watching TV).
- Avoid smoking situations and seek the company of non-smokers.
- Drink more water and avoid substituting alcohol for cigarettes.
- Be single-minded about not smoking—be determined and strong.
- Take up hobbies that make you forget smoking (e.g. water sports).
- Put aside the money you save and have a special treat. You deserve it!

Where can I get more help?

There are many quitting programs and community groups to help smokers. Many excellent tapes and booklets are also available. Chewing nicotine gum or using nicotine skin patches, which are available only by prescription from your doctor, can help. However, these are only temporary measures and are generally not used for longer than 6 months.

A final word!

Ask your general practitioner for help ASAP—do not put it off—ask for help now. It is unnatural to keep smoking. Choose the good, healthy life.

John Murtagh, *Patient Education*, Second edition, McGraw-Hill Book Company

9 Infections

AIDS and HIV infection

What is AIDS?

Acquired—not inherited
Immune—body's defence system
Deficiency—not working properly
Syndrome—a collection of signs and symptoms

What is the cause of AIDS?

AIDS is caused by a virus called the *human immuno-deficiency virus* (HIV). It may start as an acute glandular fever or flu-like illness that soon settles. However, the incubation period is thought to be about 5–7 years, after which about 30% of people infected with HIV will develop full-blown AIDS, 40% may develop milder AIDS-related conditions (ARC) and 30% appear to remain healthy although carrying the virus. These fit people are called *antibody positive*, and although they are healthy they can pass the virus on to others. However, usual non-sexual contact is safe and an HIV positive person is otherwise not a risk to the general population.

How do you catch AIDS?

HIV is transmitted in semen, blood and vaginal fluids through:
- unprotected sexual intercourse (anal or vaginal) with an infected person
- infected blood entering the body (through blood transfusion or by IV drug users sharing needles/syringes)
- artificial insemination
- infected mothers (to babies during pregnancy, at birth or in breast milk)

It is not 'easy to catch' other than by these means. There is no evidence anywhere that it is spread from public places (e.g. toilets, swimming pools), shaking hands or kissing, eating utensils and so on.

Infection with HIV can occur via the vagina, rectum or open cuts and sores, including any on the lips or in the mouth.

What are the symptoms?

Most patients with HIV infection have no symptoms, but when AIDS develops any one or a combination of the following may be present:

- constant tiredness
- unexplained weight loss
- recurrent fever or night sweats
- decreased appetite
- persistent diarrhoea
- persistent cough
- swollen lumps (glands) in the neck, groin or armpit
- unusual skin lumps or marks
- recurrent thrush in the mouth
- mouth sores

What does 'antibody positive' mean?

It means that people have antibodies to HIV in their bloodstream and have been infected at some stage. It does not mean they have the illness of AIDS, but means that they carry the virus and could pass it on through their blood or by sex. This antibody is detected by a special laboratory test. It may take up to 3 or even 6 months to become positive after contact.

Can AIDS be cured or treated?

There is no cure at present, but it can be treated. A new drug called *zidovudine* (AZT) does fight HIV and can prolong the lives of people with AIDS. It is expected that new drugs being developed will be more effective.

What about blood transfusion and blood donation?

You cannot catch AIDS from donating blood. Since about 1985 all blood donations have been screened for the HIV antibody before being transfused, and so there is almost no risk of getting it from a transfusion now.

What is safe sex?

'Safe sex' means sexual activities in which semen, vaginal secretions or blood are not exchanged between sexual partners. It includes touching, cuddling, body-to-body rubbing and mutual masturbation. The proper use of condoms during vaginal, anal or oral intercourse will reduce the risk of transmitting HIV. A water-based lubricant such as KY jelly or Lubafax should be used: oil-based lubricants such as Vaseline weaken condoms.

John Murtagh, *Patient Education*, Second edition, McGraw-Hill Book Company

Chronic bronchitis

What is chronic bronchitis?

It is a persisting inflammation of the bronchial tree (air passages) of the lungs. It is a potentially dangerous problem because it starts so quietly that many people do not realise that they have it. Repeated irritation thickens and damages the delicate lining of these important tubes. This leads to lots of mucus and thus narrowing of the tubes.

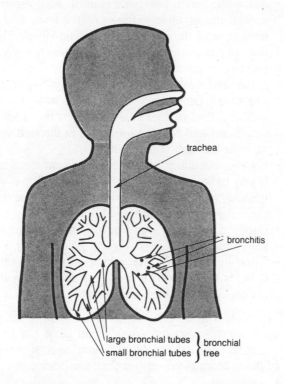

trachea

bronchitis

large bronchial tubes } bronchial
small bronchial tubes } tree

What are the symptoms?

The main symptom is a morning cough with sputum (phlegm). Smokers may consider this to be a normal smoker's cough, but there is nothing normal about it. As time goes by, this productive cough increases.

Later on, wheezing and breathlessness become a problem. If you are breathless when you exert yourself, you probably have significant lung damage.

What are the causes?

Smoking is the main cause.

People who work in dusty atmospheres are also at risk. Air pollution is a minor factor.

At first the bronchitis gets worse with bad colds or influenza, but eventually even a mild cold can bring on a nasty flare-up. Colds or other infections can cause deterioration, especially in winter. However, chronic bronchitis is not caused by chronic infection. It is usually caused by chronic irritation from smoke.

What are the risks?

Once bronchitis is chronic, a vicious cycle is established so that increasing infections and lung damage occur.

The end result is severe permanent lung damage and then heart failure.

How common is the problem?

In Australia about 4500 people die of chronic bronchitis each year.

What is the treatment?

Self-help

If you smoke, you should stop. This is the vital first step—it will stop further damage. The lungs may return to normal. Avoid smoke-filled rooms.

If you work in a polluted or dusty atmosphere, it would be wise to change your job. A warm, dry climate is preferable to a cold, damp place: it may make you feel more comfortable and may make you less susceptible to winter colds and 'flu'.

Avoid close contact with people with colds, since any viral respiratory infection is a problem to your lungs.

Medical help

Prevention of more infections is important. This may be achieved by giving high doses of vitamin C, anti-influenza injections and antibiotics. Your doctor may prescribe small doses of antibiotics throughout the winter months or may advise you to take a full dose at the first sign of a flare-up. The reason for this is that bacterial infection soon complicates the viral infection.

See your doctor as soon as possible if you notice your sputum changing to a yellow or green colour.

If you have wheezing and breathlessness, an aerosol inhaler will be prescribed if tests show that your breathing capacity is reduced.

Your doctor can help you with techniques to stop smoking.

Physiotherapy can help if you have difficulty coughing up sputum.

Common cold

What is the common cold?

The common cold is an infection of the upper respiratory passages, especially the nose and throat. It is caused by any of several types of viruses. It is quite different from influenza (the flu), which is caused by more intense viruses.

What are the symptoms?

The usual symptoms are:
- runny nose
- sore throat
- coughing
- sneezing
- sore eyes
- feeling generally unwell

Other possible symptoms are:
- headaches
- hoarseness
- fever, with general aches and pains

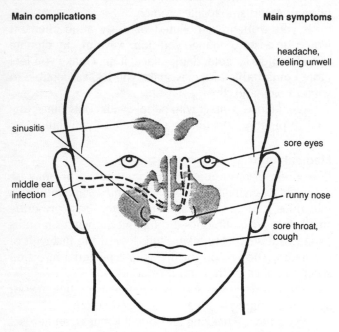

Main complications

sinusitis

middle ear infection

Main symptoms

headache, feeling unwell

sore eyes

runny nose

sore throat, cough

The main symptoms and complications of the common cold

How is it caught?

If you have a cold, you must have breathed in the virus, which is carried in the air after being coughed or sneezed out by another person with a cold.

What is the treatment?

There is no cure for the common cold. Antibiotics are of no use for viral infections and are only useful for certain complications. Fortunately, the body's immune system eventually is able to fight the virus by making antibodies. This takes several days. There are several things you can do to feel more comfortable, and to help your body's immune system:
- Rest. It is important to have plenty of sleep and rest when you have a cold. Physical activity puts extra demands on the immune system.
- Analgesics such as paracetamol and aspirin have several useful effects: they control fever and inflammation, and they are effective pain-killers. The adult dose of paracetamol or aspirin is 2 tablets every 4 hours (up to a *maximum* of 8 per day).
- A blocked nose can be considerably helped by inhaling steam. One way is to put boiled water into a basin with menthol or friar's balsam, then put a towel over your head and breathe the steam in through your nose and out through your mouth.
- Usually, coughing is to clear away unwanted material. If you have a dry cough, however, and it is very distressing, you may suppress it with a cough mixture. Ask your pharmacist or doctor about this.
- Gargling aspirin in water or lemon juice can soothe a sore throat.
- Some people claim that taking large doses of vitamin C helps them recover more quickly from a cold. An average dose is 1–2 grams a day.

Your cold can be cleared up in a few days, but can last up to 10 days. Sometimes you can get a bacterial complication, which may require antibiotics. If you get any of the following, you should see the doctor:
- a sore ear
- chest pain or difficulty in breathing
- a lot of green mucus from your chest or nose
- a sore throat without other symptoms

How can it be prevented?

It is important to consider whether you have a reason for this cold. Regular exercise, a balanced diet and adequate sleep are important to keep your immune system in tiptop shape.

John Murtagh, *Patient Education*, Second edition, McGraw-Hill Book Company

Conjunctivitis

What is conjunctivitis?

It is an inflammation of the *conjunctiva*, which is a thin, clear tissue that lines the eyelids and the eyeball, except the cornea. It is very common, but not a serious problem except in newborn infants.

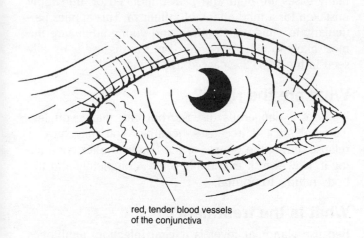

red, tender blood vessels of the conjunctiva

What causes conjunctivitis?

- bacterial infection
- viral infection
- allergies such as hay fever

Bacterial infections are common; the bugs are usually picked up from contaminated fingers, face cloths and towels. They are more likely to occur when you are run down, such as with a heavy cold, and when the tear ducts are blocked with a respiratory infection.

What are the symptoms?

Bacterial infection (usually both eyes)

- whites of the eyes red and sore
- yellow pus discharging from the eyes, making them sticky
- during sleep, this matter causing the eyelids to stick together so that they have to be prised open upon waking

Viral infection

- a painful red eye
- slight discharge only

Allergic conjunctivitis

- itchiness and redness of the whites of the eyes
- a gritty feeling in the eyes
- no discharge

A feeling of irritation and watering may be found with all these types.

What is the treatment?

It is important to visit your doctor for care. Sometimes the cause is a foreign body, such as a piece of metal or a piece of an insect or another speck that has entered your eye without your being aware of it.

Your doctor may prescribe antibiotic or antiallergy drops or ointment, which you place in the eye as directed. The infection usually responds rapidly to treatment within 48 hours. If not, inform your doctor.

Other points

- Avoid touching your eyes directly.
- Wash your hands regularly.
- Do not use make-up.
- Gently wipe any discharge with disposable tissues.

Eye bathing with salt water

Antibiotics will not work if there is discharge still in your eyes, and so it is vital to wash away this debris with a weak, salty solution. It is preferable to have this warm. The solution can be made by dissolving 1 teaspoon of salt in half a litre (500 mL) of boiled water. Use this solution before instilling eye drops.

Another method is to add a pinch of salt to an eyebath of lukewarm water. Apply the eyebath closely to the rim of the eye, look upwards and blink the eye, which will then be irrigated by the solution.

Glandular fever

What is glandular fever?

Glandular fever (properly known as *Epstein–Barr mononucleosis*) is a viral infection that causes an illness similar to influenza. It is sometimes called 'the kissing disease' because it was observed to be passed from one person to another through the mouth. It is also transmitted by coughing and sharing food. The virus spreads through the bloodstream and the lymphatic system, causing the spleen, liver and lymph glands to swell as well as causing a fever (hence the term 'glandular fever').

What are the symptoms?

The symptoms are similar to those of the flu: fever, headache, blocked nose, nausea, mouth breathing, sore throat (you may have tonsillitis) and a general sense of feeling 'out of sorts'. The patient may be aware of having swollen, tender glands (lymph nodes) in the neck, armpits and groin. Less common symptoms include a rash and jaundice.

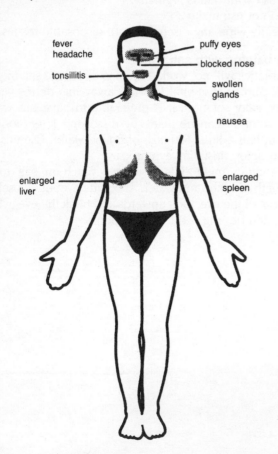

fever
headache

puffy eyes

blocked nose

tonsillitis

swollen glands

nausea

enlarged liver

enlarged spleen

Symptoms of glandular fever

How is it diagnosed?

The best way to diagnose the illness is for a blood test to be done. The blood shows abnormal cells (called *monocytes*) under the microscope, hence the name *mononucleosis*.

How long does it last?

The major symptoms usually disappear within 2 or 3 weeks, but for a further period of at least 2 weeks you may feel weak, lacking in energy and depressed. Occasionally the lethargy can last for months.

How common is the problem?

It is probably more common than realised, because many cases are mild and pass unnoticed or are simply mistaken for a mild attack of influenza. This applies particularly to children. Children and young adults are the most likely to catch the virus, but the disease is usually seen in the 15 to 25-year-old age group.

What are the risks?

It is not a dangerous disease, but can make you feel extremely sick if it causes hepatitis. You may have a relapse during the course of the first year after contracting it. However, it eventually settles completely and the body returns to normal.

What is the treatment?

Because glandular fever is a viral infection, antibiotics will not help. The illness must simply run its course.

Advice

Do:
- Take paracetamol (in modest doses) to relieve discomfort or pain.
- Rest (the best treatment), preferably at home and indoors.
- Drink plenty of fluids such as water and fruit juices.
- Gargle soluble aspirin or 30% glucose to soothe the throat.

Do not:
- Drink alcohol or eat fatty foods.
- Push yourself to perform tasks.
- Attempt to return to your normal daily routine until advised to do so by your doctor (about 4 weeks after the illness starts).
- Participate in contact sports until at least 4 weeks after complete recovery.

Finally, it is common to feel depressed during the illness and in the recovery phase because you may feel tired and lethargic. Report any such problems to your doctor.

John Murtagh, *Patient Education*, Second edition, McGraw-Hill Book Company

Gonorrhoea

What is gonorrhoea?

Gonorrhoea (also known as 'the clap') is a sexually transmitted disease (STD) caused by the bacterium *Neisseria gonorrhoeae*. It commonly affects the urethra, especially in men, and other genital areas but may also develop in the anus or throat, depending on the sexual activity.

What are the symptoms?

The symptoms usually appear about 2–10 days after vaginal, anal or oral sex, but the incubation period can be as long as 3 weeks.

In men

The main symptoms (due to urethritis) are:
- a burning sensation on passing urine
- a pus-like (white or yellow) discharge or leak

The first noticeable symptom is a slight discomfort on passing urine, which can later become very painful 'like passing razor blades' if it is not treated. A discharge of creamy pus from the tip of the penis follows. Sometimes there is no discharge, just pain, and sometimes there are no symptoms at all.

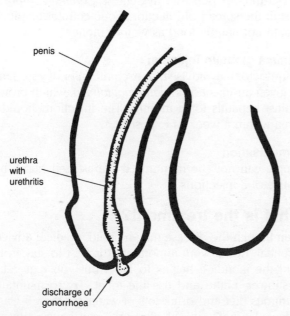

penis

urethra with urethritis

discharge of gonorrhoea

Gonorrhoea in men

In women

In women gonorrhoea often causes no symptoms but can produce vaginal discharge or pain on passing urine. If it produces pelvic inflammatory disease (PID) it can cause:
- pain and tenderness deep in the pelvis
- lower abdominal pain and tenderness
- fever, an unwell feeling and painful periods
- pain on intercourse

In both sexes

Gonorrhoea of the anus and throat may have no symptoms or soreness. There may be a discharge (a feeling of dampness) around the anus.

Gonorrhoea is diagnosed by taking special swabs from the infected areas.

How is gonorrhoea spread?

It is spread through vaginal and anal intercourse and oral sex, whether homosexual or heterosexual, where one partner is already infected.

What are the risks?

- It can cause PID in women, sometimes leading to infertility.
- It can cause infection in the joints.
- In men it can infect the testicles and also may cause a urethral stricture (narrowing of the urethra).

What is the treatment?

You must see your doctor or go to an STD clinic. Gonorrhoea is treated with a course of antibiotics (by tablets, capsules or injection, depending on where you picked up the infection and on the test results). It is cured in about 2 weeks.

Sexual partners should be tested, even if they have no symptoms, and even if a checkup has failed to detect the infection.

Sexual intercourse must be avoided until the infection has cleared up (both you and your partner).

How is gonorrhoea prevented?

Using condoms for vaginal, anal and oral sex provides good protection. Sexually active men and women (especially those at risk, e.g. those with multiple partners) should have regular checks (at least annually).

Important points

- Gonorrhoea may cause no symptoms, especially in women.
- It can cause infertility in women (and less commonly in men).
- It is readily treated by antibiotics.
- All sexual partners need to be treated.
- Sexual intercourse should be avoided until the infection is cleared.
- Condoms provide protection.

Hepatitis A

What is hepatitis A?

Hepatitis A, also known as *infectious hepatitis* and *yellow jaundice*, is a viral infection of the liver. *Hepatitis* means inflammation of the liver. Unlike most other types of hepatitis, hepatitis A invades the liver after it enters the body from the bowel by taking in infected food or water.

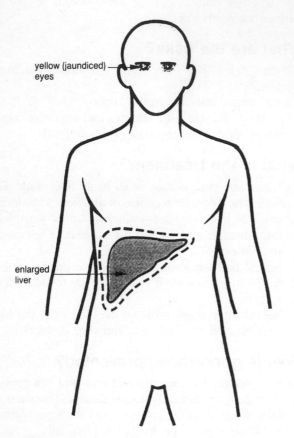

yellow (jaundiced) eyes

enlarged liver

Signs of hepatitis A

What are the symptoms?

The main sign is yellow skin (jaundice) due to a building up of the waste pigment *bilirubin* in the body. Another is darkening of the urine. A flu-like illness may be noticed before the jaundice, including loss of appetite, nausea, fever, muscle aches and pains. Some people may never have symptoms. It is diagnosed by a simple blood test.

How serious is it?

Hepatitis A is usually a mild disease, especially in children, although some cases can be severe. Complete recovery is usual, but some people can be left with chronic hepatitis and liver damage.

How is it spread?

The virus is present in the bowel and is spread from person to person through close contact such as infected hands, towels and food. That is, it gets from the faeces of the infected person to the mouth of another. It may take 15–50 days after picking up the virus before the disease becomes evident, with 28 days being the average time.

The patient is most infectious 2 weeks before and 1 week after the onset of jaundice.

Hepatitis A is more likely to be contracted overseas in a Third World country with poor hygiene.

How is the spread prevented?

A few simple measures can stop the disease spreading to close contacts and family members. These are:
- Wash your hands carefully after using the toilet and disinfect them with antiseptic. Also disinfect the bathroom doorknob.
- Do not handle food with your fingers.
- Do not share crockery and cutlery during meals.
- Protect food from flies.
- Do not use tea-towels to dry dishes.
- *All* family members should wash their hands often and carefully.

Note: Normal dishwashing and hot-water laundering is sufficient to sterilise your crockery, cutlery, clothing and bed linen.

Scrupulous personal hygiene is *extremely* important to stop the spread of infection. Food-counter employees should not handle food as well as money.

Gamma globulin injection

Your doctor may advise that each member of your family be given an injection of *immunoglobulin*, which protects against hepatitis for 3 months. The injection should be given within a week of exposure.

Immunisation

People can now be immunised against hepatitis A by a course of 3 injections.

What is the treatment?

Even though the disease may be mild, medical advice is essential. Rest is very important. It is best to stay in bed until the jaundice begins to fade, but you can get up to shower, bathe and use the toilet. Try to maintain a nutritious diet and drink lots of water (at least 8 glasses a day). Do not drink alcohol until you have recovered. If fatty foods upset your stomach, avoid them until you feel better. Your doctor may recommend that you stop taking certain medications (e.g. the contraceptive pill).

John Murtagh, *Patient Education*, Second edition, McGraw-Hill Book Company

Hepatitis B

What is hepatitis B?

Hepatitis B is a virus that infects the liver. It is very infectious, more so than the AIDS virus.

How serious is the problem?

It is very epidemic in some parts of the world and is now on the increase in the world.

Most people with hepatitis B recover, although some have a long and serious illness. It may be fatal in people who get cirrhosis or cancer of the liver from it. 5–10% of sufferers become carriers.

What is a carrier?

A *carrier* is a person who has not been able to get rid of the virus from his or her body. Carriers are a risk to other people and have a responsibility to tell dentists, doctors and other people about this. The doctor will advise on how to cope.

What are the symptoms?

This depends on whether the attack of hepatitis is *acute* or *chronic*. The acute attack produces a flu-like illness and yellow skin (jaundice). The chronic form comes on slowly and is more serious. It may take months from the time you get the virus until the illness develops.

Some people may never have symptoms.

How is it spread?

The virus is carried in all body fluids: blood, saliva, semen and vaginal secretions, breast milk, tears and perspiration. It is usually picked up by absorption of infected blood through cuts and sores in the skin, by sexual intercourse or by sharing infected items such as razor blades, toothbrushes, needles and syringes. Procedures such as ear piercing and tattooing can also spread it. The commonest ways are through intravenous drug use and sexual intercourse with carriers.

Who are at highest risk?

- intravenous drug users
- male homosexuals
- heterosexuals and bisexuals with multiple sex partners
- prostitutes
- prisoners and other institutionalised people
- certain ethnic groups
- health-care workers (e.g. doctors, dentists, nurses)
- babies born to carrier mothers
- children in kindergartens and schools, especially where exposed to a variety of people

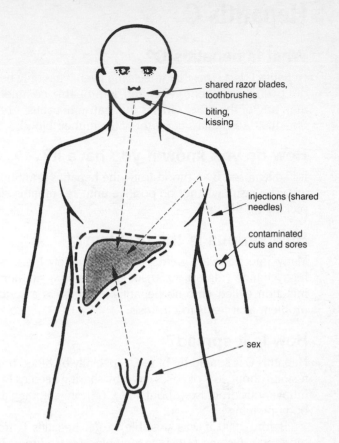

Transmission of hepatitis B

Labels: shared razor blades, toothbrushes; biting, kissing; injections (shared needles); contaminated cuts and sores; sex

Is there a cure?

- There is no cure, but it can be prevented.
- Prevention is the only cure.
- This is done by good hygiene and vaccination.

Good hygiene

- Do not share personal items (e.g. razors, toothbrushes).
- Use a condom for sex.
- Be careful not to get another's blood on cuts or wounds.
- Do not share needles.

Vaccination

This involves a course of 3 injections.

What is the treatment?

Carriers should follow the 'good hygiene' guidelines. They should eat a normal healthy diet and reduce any alcohol to no more than one standard drink per day.

If there is liver damage, interferon may be prescribed.

> **Remember**
> - A blood test can tell whether you have immunity or are a carrier.
> - Talk to your doctor about the prevention of hepatitis B.

Hepatitis C

What is hepatitis C?

Hepatitis C is a virus that infects the liver. It has only been discovered in recent years and is probably commoner than any of the other viruses that cause hepatitis. About 3 in 1000 Australians carry the virus in their blood.

How do you know if you have it?

It is diagnosed by a blood test—the hepatitis C antibody test. The result will not be positive until 2–3 months after picking up the virus.

How serious is the problem?

Many infections are mild, but unfortunately there is a high chance (almost 50:50) of developing a simmering infection called chronic hepatitis C, which is a serious problem as it leads to cirrhosis.

How is it spread?

Hepatitis C is spread by blood, especially by blood transfusion (about 40% of cases) and by sharing needles from intravenous drug use (about 40%), or from tattooing and body piercing.

Before 1990 it was possible to get hepatitis C from blood transfusions, but since then blood from donors has been tested for hepatitis C. There appears to be a small risk of spread during homosexual or heterosexual intercourse. It also does not spread easily through normal family or household contact.

What are the symptoms?

The symptoms vary from person to person and in many cases the infection may not cause any symptoms. Symptoms may take from 15 to 180 days to appear from the time of infection. The acute attack produces a flu-like illness with tiredness and yellow skin (jaundice). The serious chronic form comes on slowly, even after several years.

What happens with chronic hepatitis C?

Chronic hepatitis is more likely to occur with hepatitis C than with any of the other hepatitis viruses. This gradually causes damage to the healthy liver cells, causing hardening of the liver. This is called *cirrhosis*, which makes the liver fail and sometimes leads to cancer of the liver.

Who is at highest risk?

- intravenous drug users
- male homosexuals
- prostitutes
- renal dialysis patients
- people who received blood transfusions before testing was available (February 1990)

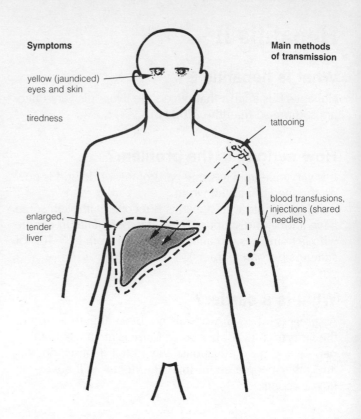

Symptoms

yellow (jaundiced) eyes and skin

tiredness

enlarged, tender liver

Main methods of transmission

tattooing

blood transfusions, injections (shared needles)

How can the spread of hepatitis C be stopped?

If you have a positive hepatitis C test:
- Do not donate blood.
- Do not share needles.
- Advise health-care workers, including your dentist, about your hepatitis C.
- Do not share personal items (e.g. razors, toothbrushes).
- Wipe up blood spills with household bleach.
- Cover cuts and wounds with a firm dressing.
- Safely dispose of blood-stained tissues, tampons and the like.
- Practise 'safe' sex.

Hepatitis C does not seem to spread easily from mother to baby.

Is there a cure?

There is no cure, although there are new drugs to treat chronic hepatitis. Prevention is really the only 'cure'. There is no vaccine available.

What is the treatment?

- Rest if you feel unwell.
- Maintain a nutritious diet: well balanced and low fat.
- Avoid alcohol or have only small amounts upon recovery.
- Keep in touch with your doctor.
- Chronic hepatitis C may be treated with interferon.

John Murtagh, *Patient Education*, Second edition, McGraw-Hill Book Company

Herpes: genital herpes

What is genital herpes?

It is a form of sexually transmitted disease (STD) caused by the *herpes simplex* virus. It produces painful ulcers on and around the genitals of both sexes.

How is it caught?

It can be caught by direct contact through vaginal, anal or oral sex. Rarely is it transferred to the genitals from other areas of the body by the fingers, and it has never been proved that it can be transferred from places or objects such as toilet seats, towels, spas or swimming pools.

Contact is from person to person.

What are the symptoms?

With the first attack there is a tingling or burning feeling in the genital area. A crop of small blisters then appears; these burst after 24 hours to leave small, red, painful ulcers. The ulcers form scabs and heal after a few days. The glands in the groin can become swollen and tender, and the patient might feel unwell and have a fever.

The first attack lasts about 2 weeks.

Males

The virus usually affects the shaft of the penis, but can involve the glans and coronal sulcus, and the anus.

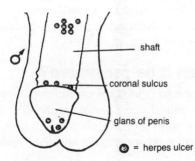

shaft

coronal sulcus

glans of penis

= herpes ulcer

Usual sites of blisters in males

Females

Blisters develop around the opening of, and just inside, the vagina and sometimes on the cervix and anus. Passing urine might be difficult, and there can be a vaginal discharge.

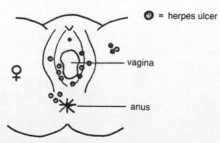

= herpes ulcer

vagina

anus

Usual sites of blisters in females

In both sexes, it can affect the buttocks and thighs. A serious but uncommon complication, especially in females, is the inability to pass urine.

Does it recur?

After the first infection, the herpes virus remains deep in the nerves that supply the affected area of the skin. Half of those who have the first episode have recurrent attacks; the others have no recurrences.

Fortunately attacks gradually become milder, less frequent and usually stop eventually. Recurrences after many months or years can be precipitated by menstruation, sexual intercourse, masturbation, skin irritation or emotional stress.

What should you do?

If you think you have herpes, see your doctor or attend a clinic specialising in STD. You should not have intercourse during an attack, because you are likely to transmit the infection to your partner.

What is the treatment?

- Rest and relax as much as possible. Warm salt baths can be soothing.
- Antiviral ointments can help if they are used as soon as symptoms start. Other agents that help are Betadine lotion or 10% silver nitrate solution.
- Icepacks or hot compresses can help.
- Pain-killers such as aspirin or paracetamol give some relief.
- If urination is painful, pass urine under water in a warm bath.
- Keep the sores dry; dabbing with alcohol or using warm air from a hairdryer can help.
- Leave the rash alone after cleaning and drying; do not poke or prod the sores.
- Wear loose clothes and cotton underwear. Avoid tight jeans.
- Your doctor can prescribe a special antiviral drug (*acyclovir*) for a severe infection.

How can it be prevented?

Spread of the disease can be prevented only by avoiding sexual contact during an attack. If you are not sure whether you are infective or not, use a condom (however, this is not absolutely protective) and wash your genitals with soap and water immediately after sex. Condoms should always be used where a partner has a history of infection.

Can herpes cause cancer in women?

There may be a connection between genital herpes and cancer of the cervix, but that cancer is treatable if diagnosed early—'a smear a year' is the rule.

Herpes simplex (cold sores)

What is herpes simplex?

Herpes simplex (cold sores) is a viral infection of the skin that causes two types of infection:

1. the classical cold sores on the lips and around the mouth

2. genital cold sores, which are spread by sexual contact

This pamphlet will consider cold sores on the face.

What are the symptoms?

This common infection is known also as 'fever blisters'. The first symptom is itchiness and tingling at the site of the developing infection, usually on the edge of the lips. Blisters soon appear and later burst to become crusted sores. The person usually feels unwell. The infection occurs only occasionally in some people but frequently in others.

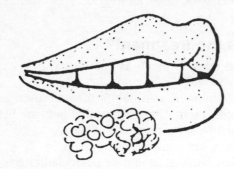

Herpes simplex

How does herpes simplex develop?

It usually begins in childhood as a mouth infection. The virus then lives in the nerves supplying the skin or eyes, waiting for an opportunity to become active. It may erupt on any area of the body's skin or in the eyes. The following may precipitate eruptions:

- overexposure to sunlight
- overexposure to wind
- colds, influenza and similar infections
- heavy alcohol use
- fever from any cause
- the menstrual period
- physical stress
- emotional stress

Does it spread?

Herpes simplex is contagious. It is present in saliva of affected persons and can be spread in a family by the sharing of drinking and eating utensils and toothbrushes or by kissing.

It is most important not to kiss an infant if you have an active cold sore.

Is herpes simplex dangerous?

It usually presents no serious risk, but it can be very unpleasant for patients who have eczema. It also can infect the eyes, and can cause a serious ulcer on the cornea.

What is the treatment?

There is no special treatment; most sores heal and clear in a few days. They should be kept dry: dabbing them with plain alcohol or, better still, a solution of menthol in SVR alcohol, will relieve itching and help keep them clean and dry.

When you feel them developing, the application of an ice-cube to the site for up to 5 minutes every hour for the first 12 hours is soothing. Also, an antiviral ointment may help, but it must be applied early to be effective.

Notify your doctor if you have a persistent fever, pus in the sores or irritation of an eye.

How can it be prevented?

Those prone to cold sores should avoid overexposure to sun and wind. If you cannot, apply 15+ sun protection lip balm or zinc oxide ointment around the lips and other areas where cold sores have erupted previously.

John Murtagh, *Patient Education*, Second edition, McGraw-Hill Book Company

Herpes zoster (shingles)

What is herpes zoster?

It is an infection in a nerve by the virus that causes chickenpox. The term comes from the Greek *herpes* (to creep) and *zoster* (a belt or girdle). *Shingles* is from the Latin *cingere* (to gird) or *cingulum* (a belt).

How does it occur?

Contact with someone with chickenpox may cause it, but usually it is a reactivation of the chickenpox virus lying dormant (often for many years) in the root of a nerve in the brain or spinal cord. The dormant virus can be stirred into activity by stress or by the loss of natural immunity as we get older. The virus multiplies and spreads, causing pain in the nerve in which it resides.

Where does it occur?

Almost any part of the body can be involved, but common sites are the right or left side of the chest or abdomen and the face.

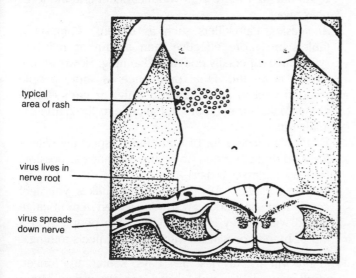

typical
area of rash

virus lives in
nerve root

virus spreads
down nerve

Herpes zoster

What are the symptoms?

Apart from feeling unwell, sometimes with a fever, the main symptoms are pain and a rash.

Pain
- This can vary from mild to severe.
- It is burning in nature, but can be knife-like.
- It precedes the rash and lasts for 1–4 weeks after the blisters disappear; it can persist for several weeks.
- It always improves in time.

Rash
Groups of blisters appear in the skin that is supplied by the nerve. They itch and become crusted. The rash disappears after about 7 days but will leave scars or discoloured skin.

Who gets herpes zoster?

This relatively common disease is unpredictable and a person of any age can be affected. It is seen more often in people over the age of 50; sometimes children will get it during a chickenpox epidemic.

Is it contagious?

Yes, but only mildly. Rarely, children might acquire chickenpox after contact with someone who has herpes zoster, but it would be very unusual to 'catch' herpes zoster from another person.

Can the problem recur?

It is possible but most unlikely. One attack generally protects you from a second attack and gives lifelong immunity.

Old wives' tales

It is not true that it is a dangerous disease or that the patient will go insane. Another myth is that a person will die if the rash spreads from both sides and meets in the middle: this is nonsense.

For the majority, herpes zoster is a mild disease and an excellent recovery can be expected.

What is the treatment?

There is no cure for this viral infection, but you should see a doctor without delay because proper treatment may reduce the likelihood of pain after the sores have healed. You should:
- Rest as much as possible.
- Take simple pain-killers, such as aspirin or paracetamol, regularly.
- Avoid overtreating the rash, which may get infected. Calamine lotion may be soothing, but removal of the calamine crust can be painful. A drying lotion such as menthol in flexible collodion is better.
- New drugs that help relieve severe infections are *acyclovir* for the acute illness and *capsaicin* cream for painful skin.

Influenza

What is it?

Influenza, usually called *flu*, is a respiratory infection caused by a virus, which is a tiny germ that cannot be seen even under an ordinary microscope. There are several kinds of influenza virus, and they seem to keep changing just when we seem to be immune to them. However, they all produce a similar illness.

What are the symptoms?

The main symptoms are:
• fever
• headache
• muscle aches and pains

These may be followed by a sore throat, a cough and a runny nose.

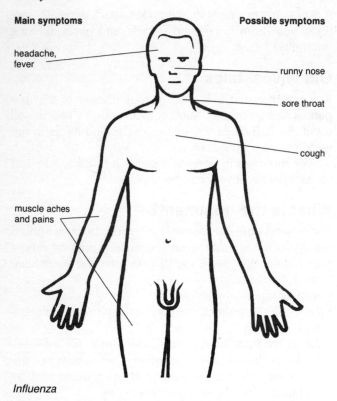

Main symptoms

headache, fever

Possible symptoms

runny nose

sore throat

cough

muscle aches and pains

Influenza

How is it caught?

Influenza usually comes in epidemics, when it spreads from one person to another in the spray from coughs and sneezes (called *droplet infection*). The virus enters the nose or throat and may spread to the lungs. It is extremely infectious.

How is it different from the common cold?

Many people refer to the common cold (which is more common) as 'the flu', but influenza is a more serious respiratory infection that usually makes the victim sick enough to go to bed. Flu tends to go to the chest and makes the whole body ache; the common cold usually only affects the upper respiratory passages, causing a runny nose, sneezing and a sore throat.

What are the risks?

The main risk of influenza is that the infection may spread to the lungs, causing bronchitis or, worse still, pneumonia. Such complications are rare, and are more likely to occur in people with poor health (especially those with a chest complaint), in the elderly and in heavy smokers.

Although influenza makes people quite ill, it is usually not dangerous. Feeling depressed after the flu is a common problem.

What is the treatment?

Like any viral infection, influenza must run its course. Symptoms can be eased and complications prevented by proper care and common sense.

Self-help

• *Rest*. Just as a broken leg needs rest, so does the body overcome by flu. Go to bed as soon as the symptoms begin and stay there until you feel better and the fever goes away.
• *Analgesics*. Pain-killers such as codeine compound tablets are more effective than aspirin at relieving symptoms, especially cough and aching. However, the choice is an individual preference as some people respond well to aspirin (adults only) or paracetamol alone. Make sure you are not allergic to the particular analgesic.
• *Fluids*. You lose a lot of body fluid, especially with a fever, so drink as much water and fruit juice as possible (at least 8 glasses a day).
• *Special remedies*. Any remedy that makes you feel comfortable is good. Freshly squeezed lemon juice mixed with honey is very good. Some people find a nip of brandy or whisky with the fruit juice soothing.

The flu will usually last 3–4 days, sometimes longer. Consult your doctor only if you are concerned about complications. There is no specific treatment for flu, and routine antibiotics are not helpful. They are reserved for complications. Some people find that taking 1–2 grams of vitamin C each day helps recovery.

What about prevention?

The influenza vaccine appears to help some people, but vaccination cannot guarantee total immunity as the strain that sets off the epidemic may be new. Vaccination is worthwhile for patients at risk: diabetics, those with chronic lung disease and heart disease, those over 65 years, and those whose occupation (working with crowds or sick patients) puts them at risk in an epidemic.

John Murtagh, *Patient Education*, Second edition, McGraw-Hill Book Company

Lice: head lice

What is the cause?

Pediculus humanus capitis is the head louse. This small insect, which lives on human hair, sucks blood from the skin of the scalp. The female louse lays eggs (or 'nits'), which are glued to the hairs and hatch within 6 days, mature into adults in about 10 days and live for about a month.

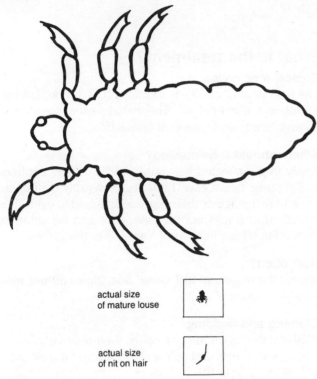

actual size
of mature louse

actual size
of nit on hair

An adult head louse

How is it spread?

Head lice spread from person to person by direct contact, such as sitting and working very close to each other. They can spread by sharing combs, brushes and headwear, especially within the family. Children are the ones usually affected, but people of all ages and from all walks of life can be infested. It is more common in overcrowded living conditions.

What are the symptoms?

Head lice may cause itching of the scalp, but often there are no symptoms. The white spots can be mistaken for dandruff.

How is it diagnosed?

The finding of lice or nits on the head is the only way to diagnose infestation. The nits are seen as small, whitish flecks securely attached to the base of the hairs, especially behind the ears and on the forehead. Unlike dandruff, they cannot be brushed off.

What is the treatment?

Topical medication

The best treatment is *pyrethrin/piperonyl butoxide* (*Lyban*) foam or shampoo, which is effective in killing both the lice and eggs. *Malathion* or *permethrin* is also useful, but *lindane* is less effective and does not kill the eggs. Follow the instructions on the bottle carefully. The hair does not have to be cut short if the medication is properly and thoroughly applied.

Where should it be applied?

Apply to the hair of the head only.

How often?

Apply once a week for 2 weeks. Two applications of Lyban should be sufficient to clear the lice.

Combing

The eggs can be removed after treatment by combing with a fine-tooth metal comb while the hair is wet.

Note

- Head lice are *not* associated with lack of cleanliness.
- Ordinary hair washing cannot prevent or cure it.
- If one member of the family has it, *all* members must be treated whether or not lice or nits can be detected.
- The source of head lice is the home, not the school.
- Wash clothing and bedclothes after a treatment using a normal machine wash.
- Although regulations vary from state to state, exclusion from school should *not* be necessary after proper treatment.
- All antilouse preparations are toxic, but they are safe if the special head louse lotions are used according to the directions. Keep all preparations out of the eyes and out of the reach of children.

Under no circumstances should garden formulations of the malathion insecticide be used.

Lice: pubic lice

What is the cause?
Pubic lice or 'crabs' is caused by the pubic louse (or *crablouse*), *Pthirus pubis*. These insects are usually found tightly attached to the hairs of the pubic region, less commonly to the hairs of the legs, the underarms or the beard. In young children the lice can occasionally be found on the eyelashes or on the hair of the forehead. Eggs are attached to the hair shaft after being laid. The lice live for about 3 weeks.

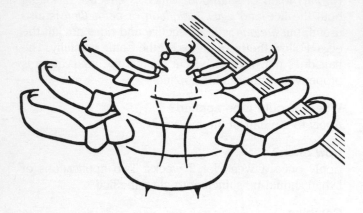

A crablouse attached to a hair shaft (actual size is 1–2 mm)

How is it spread?
Crablice are transmitted by close personal contact, especially during sexual intercourse. They may rarely be transmitted to young children by contact with heavily infested parents.

What are the symptoms?
There may be no symptoms, but the infestation or itching may be the main complaint. The pubic area may have a musty smell.

How is it diagnosed?
Diagnosis is made by finding eggs or lice tightly applied to the hair shaft. The lice may be seen to move like crabs, but usually are seen as rust-coloured specks in the pubic hair.

What is the treatment?
Topical medication
The treatment of choice is *maldison* 0.5% lotion. *Lindane* 1% lotion is also effective. The sexual partner should also receive treatment to prevent reinfection.

Where should it be applied?
Apply to the affected hair only. This is usually confined to the pubic hair. Leave 12 hours, preferably overnight.

Where the lice or their eggs are attached to eyelashes, insecticides should not be used; cure can be achieved by the liberal application of Vaseline to the lashes.

How often?
Repeat the treatment in 1 week. Sometimes a third treatment is necessary.

Clothing and bedding
Wash off the lotion after 12 hours, then remove pyjamas, underwear, sheets and pillow slips for normal washing in hot water. Repeat this in 1 week.

John Murtagh, *Patient Education*, Second edition, McGraw-Hill Book Company

Non-specific urethritis (NSU)

What is NSU?

NSU is a sexually transmitted disease (STD) and refers to any infection of the urethra except those caused by gonorrhoea. It is also called *non-gonococcal urethritis* and is probably the commonest STD. It is 3 times more common than gonorrhoea.

What causes NSU?

NSU is caused by a number of organisms, some of which are as yet undetected. About 50% of cases are caused by the organism *Chlamydia trachomatis* and 5% by *Trichomonas vaginalis*.

What are the symptoms?

The symptoms appear about 2–4 weeks after intercourse, although the incubation period can be as long as 12 weeks and as short as 7–10 days.

In men

The main symptoms (if present) are:
- a burning sensation when passing urine
- a discharge (clear, white or yellow) from the penis

Sometimes there is no discharge, just pain. Most often the symptoms are trivial.

The first noticeable symptom is a slight tingling or burning at the tip of the penis, usually first thing in the morning. The pain sometimes becomes quite severe. The discharge soon follows. It is usually clear at first, but if untreated can become heavier and yellowish. The infection can spread to the prostate gland and testicles.

In some, the only symptoms are spots on the underpants or dampness under the foreskin.

In women

In women, NSU usually causes no symptoms at all but may cause vaginal discharge. Some may notice burning on urination.

If untreated, as is often the case, it can infect the Fallopian tubes. This is the commonest form of pelvic inflammatory disease, which can result in infertility.

NSU is diagnosed by taking special swabs from the affected areas.

How is NSU caught and spread?

It is transmitted from one person to another during sexual intercourse. Men can pick it up through vaginal sex (often the woman carries the infection without knowing) or, less commonly, through anal or oral sex with either sex.

How is NSU treated?

NSU is treated with a 10–21 day course of antibiotics such as *tetracycline* or *doxycycline*. It usually responds very well to treatment, but can be slow to respond in some people and may recur in some others. About 1 in 5 patients will need more than 1 course.

It is the male who usually notices symptoms and comes for treatment. However, it is important that the sexual partner or partners are tested even if they have no symptoms. Sexual intercourse must be avoided until the infection is cleared up in both partners.

How is NSU prevented?

Using condoms for vaginal or anal sex provides some protection and should be used with any new partner.

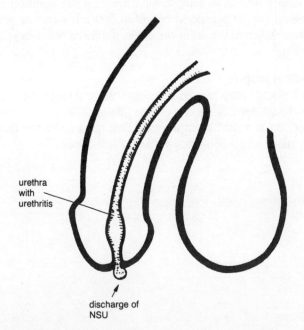

urethra
with
urethritis

discharge of
NSU

Non-specific urethritis in males

Important points

- Chlamydia is a common STD.
- It sometimes causes symptoms in men.
- There may be no symptoms in women.
- It can cause infertility in women (and less commonly in men).
- It is readily treated by antibiotics.
- Treatment takes 10–21 days and may need repeat courses.
- All sexual partners need to be treated.
- Do not have sex until infection is cleared (both partners).
- Condoms provide protection.

Pharyngitis

What is pharyngitis?

Pharyngitis is inflammation and infection of the pharynx, which is that part of the throat at the back of the tongue between the tonsils and the larynx.

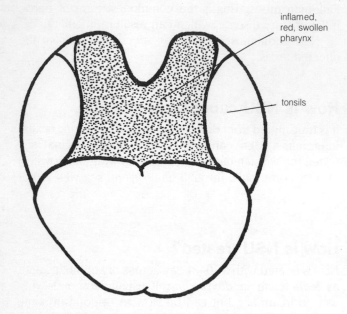

inflamed, red, swollen pharynx

tonsils

What is the cause of pharyngitis?

The commonest cause is a viral infection, which may be part of a common cold or a direct infection. Bacteria and fungi infections are also causes. Irritation and inflammation of the pharynx can also result from irritants such as cigarette smoke, alcohol or excessive use of the voice such as talking above excessive noise. Oral sex may lead to infection with sexually transmitted diseases. Various disorders, such as diabetes, immune deficiencies such as AIDS and poor general health make people prone to pharyngitis.

What are the symptoms?

This depends on whether the infection is acute (sudden onset), which is more severe, or chronic. The following symptoms vary in severity.

- sore throat
- 'tickle' or lump in throat
- difficulty swallowing
- fever (in more severe cases)
- red, swollen throat
- possible muscular aches and pains

How common is the problem?

It is very common and is by far the commonest cause of a sore throat. On average, a person consults a doctor once each year with pharyngitis. It tends to occur in people who are overworked and fatigued.

What is the usual outcome?

With most cases of pharyngitis the throat is extremely sore for 2–3 days and then settles quickly. However, if it is due to a bacterial infection, it usually persists and you tend to feel quite ill with fever. This requires medical attention.

What is the treatment?

Self-help

- You and your throat need a rest.
- Do not smoke.
- Have a fluid or soft diet for a few days.
- Drink extra fluids: at least 8 glasses of fluid daily.
- Take aspirin or paracetamol regularly, e.g. 2 soluble tablets 4 times a day. Children should have paracetamol rather than aspirin.
- Commercial soothing lozenges and mouthwashes may help: avoid those with a topical anaesthetic effect.
- Gargles help give symptomatic relief: a salt solution is useful (mix 1 teaspoon of salt in 500 mL warm or hot water). When the solution cools, gargle as often as you wish.

Medical help

Your doctor may prescribe an antibiotic if inspection of the throat reveals severe pharyngitis due to a bacterial infection. It must be emphasised that most cases are due to viruses and antibiotics make no difference.

John Murtagh, *Patient Education*, Second edition, McGraw-Hill Book Company

Scabies

What is scabies?

Scabies is a highly infectious skin infestation caused by a tiny mite called *Sarcoptes scabiei*. The mite, which is a type of arthropod, burrows just beneath the skin in order for the female to lay her eggs. She then dies. The eggs hatch into tiny mites, which spread out over the skin and live for about 30 days only. The mites cause an allergic rash.

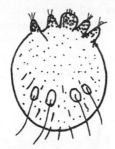

The appearance of an adult scabies mite (actual size is 0.5 mm)

How is scabies spread?

The mites are spread from person to person through close personal contact (skin to skin), including sexual contact. They may also be spread through contact with infested clothes or bedding, although this is uncommon. Sometimes the whole family can get scabies. The spread is more likely with overcrowding and sexual promiscuity.

What are the symptoms?

- intense itching, causing scratching
- a red, lumpy rash

The itching is worse with warmth and at night. The scratching may cause sores and scabs. The allergy may result in eczema.

Where does it occur?

It usually occurs on the hands and wrists. Other common areas are the male genitals, buttocks, elbows, armpits, nipples in females, feet and ankles.

How is it diagnosed?

Scabies is diagnosed by its very itchy, lumpy rash. It is rare to find the tiny mites, but it may be possible to find them in the burrows, which look like small wavy lines. When dug out, they are examined under the microscope.

What is the treatment?

Topical medication

- *All ages* (*except children under 2 years*): permethrin 5% cream
- *Children under 2*: benzyl benzoate 25% solution (can be used for all ages)
  Lindane 1% lotion can be used as an alternative.

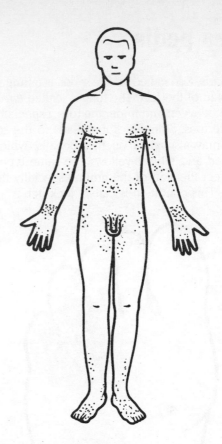

Typical distribution of the scabies rash

Where?

Apply to the entire body from the jawline down to the tip of the toes (even for genital scabies). Make sure you treat under the nails, in all the skin folds and the genitals.

How?

First have a warm shower or bath (not too hot). Use a clean washer and towel, and allow the skin to dry. Paint the lotion on all the skin thoroughly with a brush such as a shaving brush or paint brush. Do not rub your eyes or wash your hands. Put on clean clothes. Leave overnight for permethrin and for 24 hours for benzyl benzoate, then have a shower or bath.

How often?

One treatment is usually enough. It can be repeated in a week if necessary, but check with your doctor.

Clothing and bedding

Remove pillows and sheets, pyjamas and underwear after the second shower and wash normally in hot water as a separate load.

Note

- The whole family must be treated at the same time, even if they do not have the itch (one application is sufficient). Use separate towels and brushes.
- Itching can continue long after successful treatment; resist repeated treatments, but check with your doctor.

Tinea pedis

Tinea pedis, also called *athlete's foot*, is a fungus infection of the skin of the feet. The fungus, called *tinea*, grows in the skin between and under the toes, especially the outer two little toes. Sometimes it spreads to the soles of the feet. It may also grow on the toenails, which become thickened and whitish-yellow. The same type of fungus may infect the skin of the groin, especially the scrotum in men. This condition is called 'jock itch'.

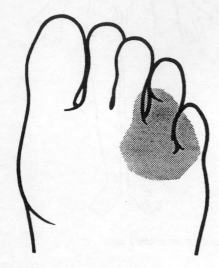

The area most commonly affected

What are the symptoms?

The commonest symptoms are itchiness and foot odour. The skin becomes red, flaky and itchy. Sweat and water make the top layer of skin white and soggy.

How common is it?

Tinea pedis is very common, but many people do not find it troublesome enough to visit their doctor. Men are affected more than women.

Is it serious?

Tinea pedis is a harmless condition.

What is the treatment?

Self-help

- Keep your feet as clean and dry as possible.
- Carefully dry your feet after bathing and showering.
- After drying your feet, use an antifungal powder, especially between the toes.
- Remove flaky skin from beneath the toes each day with dry tissue paper or gauze.
- Wear light socks made of natural absorbent fibres, such as cotton and wool, to allow better circulation of air and to reduce sweating. Avoid synthetic socks.
- Change your shoes and socks daily.
- If possible, wear open sandals or shoes with porous soles and uppers.
- Go barefoot whenever possible.
- Use thongs in public showers such as at swimming pools.

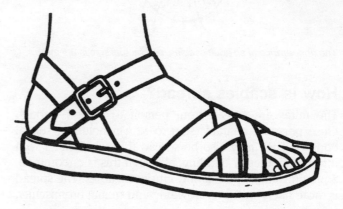

Wear well-ventilated sandals or open shoes to keep the feet dry

Medication

The old-fashioned remedies such as Castellani's paint, Whitfield's ointment and tolnaftate are still useful for mild cases, but the best treatment is one of the new antifungal creams or solutions such as *clotrimazole* or *miconazole*. These should be gently applied after drying 2 or 3 times a day for 2–3 weeks.

If the condition is severe and stubborn, your doctor may prescribe a course of tablets.

John Murtagh, *Patient Education*, Second edition, McGraw-Hill Book Company

Tonsillitis

What is the cause of tonsillitis?

Viruses or bacteria (germs) break through the tonsils' defence and cause red, swollen, painful tonsils, often with pockets of yellow pus. Tonsillitis may be a feature of glandular fever.

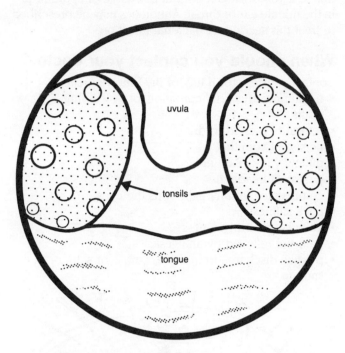

View of the throat with the two tonsils

What are the symptoms?

Symptoms include sore throat, fever, muscle aches, lethargy and swollen glands on either side of the neck. Often children experience abdominal pain and may not complain about a sore throat.

What is the treatment?

Activity

Be as active as your energy permits, but rest if feeling unwell or feverish.

Diet

If your throat is very painful, confine yourself to fluids, including milkshakes and soups. Avoid smoking, and very hot food and drink.

Medication

- *Pain-killers*: Take paracetamol or aspirin for pain relief.
- *Antibiotics*: Penicillin is usually chosen provided the patient is not allergic to it or does not have a viral infection such as glandular fever. Complete any course of antibiotics prescribed. In streptococcal tonsillitis the symptoms usually disappear after 2 days or so of treatment, but it is important to continue penicillin (or other prescribed antibiotic) for 10 days to eradicate the *Streptococcus* organism, which can cause rheumatic fever and glomerulonephritis.

What about tonsillectomy?

Doctors are reluctant to remove the tonsils because they play an important role in the body's fight against infection. Isolated attacks or large tonsils are not grounds for an operation. However, if the tonsils become a focus of chronic infection or if several severe attacks of tonsillitis occur in one year, removal may be required.

Tonsillitis in children

Most children experience attacks of tonsillitis during preschool and early school years, when the tonsils are normally large and defences against infection are not fully developed.

For most children, proper treatment of acute attacks is all that is required. The attacks will become less frequent as the child matures; tonsillectomy is advised only in exceptional circumstances.

Viral infection

What is a viral infection?

Viral infections are caused by *viruses*, which are microscopic germs and are quite different to the larger bacteria germs. They look like tiny crystals under the microscope. They are the commonest cause of infection, but are usually not serious. We eventually get over the infection simply by resting and looking after any troublesome symptoms.

What are examples of viral infections?

They usually cause upper respiratory tract infections (URTIs) such as the common cold and pharyngitis (sore throat). Other examples are influenza, gastroenteritis (especially in children), measles, rubella, mumps, chickenpox, glandular fever and cold sores.

What are the typical features?

- The illnesses are bothersome, but usually not serious.
- Symptoms include feeling unwell, fever, aches and pains (including headache).
- The illness is 'self-limiting'; that is, it gets better naturally.
- The body builds a defence by producing antiviral antibodies.
- Normal routine antibiotics have no effect on the outcome.
- Serious complications are rare, but dehydration can be a special problem in children and we have to watch out for encephalitis (inflammation of the brain) with some viruses (such as mumps and measles).

What is the treatment?

- *Rest* to allow the body to shake off the virus.
- Take *analgesics* (paracetamol or aspirin) for fever and aches or pains. Use paracetamol in children.
- *Take adequate fluids*, especially children. Use clear fluids such as water.
- Use *decongestants* for URTIs.

Why not give antibiotics?

Routine antibiotics do not help viral infections. Bacterial infections are generally more serious and are cleared up by antibiotics.

However, bacteria can attack the affected vulnerable parts of the body during a viral infection and cause problems such as middle ear infection, sinusitis, bronchitis, pneumonia and skin infection. You or your doctor may notice a yellowish-green nasal discharge or sputum, pus in the middle ear or throat. Antibiotics may be prescribed to treat this secondary bacterial infection.

When should you contact your doctor?

Contact your doctor if any of the following occur:
- no improvement in condition or worsening after 48 hours
- refusal of a child to drink
- persistent vomiting
- difficulty in breathing
- persistent headache
- complaints that any light hurts the eyes
- neck stiffness
- paleness and drowsiness
- pain not relieved by analgesics
- pus-like discharge from the ear, nose or skin, or in the sputum

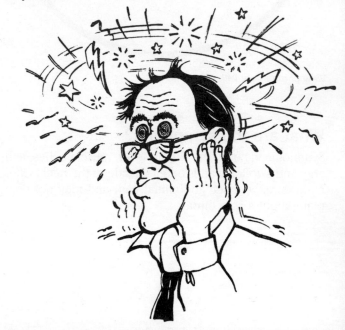

John Murtagh, *Patient Education*, Second edition, McGraw-Hill Book Company

Warts

What are warts?

Warts are lumps on the skin produced by a virus. The virus invades the skin, usually through a small injury, and causes the skin cells to multiply rapidly. Wart viruses are spread by touch or by contact with the shed skin of a wart.

Common types

The *common wart* is a small, hard, flesh-coloured lump with a 'cauliflower' surface. It can grow anywhere on the body, but is most common on the hands. It is usually painless.

The *plantar wart* (papilloma) is a wart that grows on the sole of the foot and tends to become pushed in as you walk. It is usually painful, rather like walking with a stone in your shoe.

Anal warts and *genital warts* are usually spread sexually and tend to multiply very rapidly. They are caused by a different strain of wart virus.

How common is the problem?

Warts are common in children and teenagers but less common in adults. About 1 schoolchild in 20 has 1 or more warts.

Do warts disappear if left alone?

Yes—many warts will disappear, without any treatment, if left alone. However, plantar warts and anal/genital warts take longer, and it is advisable to contact your doctor about these warts.

What is the treatment?

The treatment of warts is slow to provide a cure, but a patient approach is usually rewarding. Do not treat warts on your face and genitals with wart paint, because the skin on these areas is very sensitive. Anal and genital warts require special professional care.

Common warts

1. Soak the wart in warm, soapy water.
2. Rub back the surface of the top of the wart with a pumice stone.
3. Apply the prescribed paint or ointment, but only on the wart. It may be wise to protect the surrounding healthy skin with petroleum jelly (Vaseline).

Note:
- Carry out this treatment every second day.
- Carefully remove the loose dead skin between applications.

Plantar warts

The wart is first shaved back (pared) by your doctor with a sterile blade (this should *not* be done at home). Then use the same steps as for common warts. The use of the pumice stone is very important. Your doctor should check progress in 6 weeks. It is usually a very slow process.

Other methods

Some warts remain stubborn and other methods can be used by your doctor. These include freezing with liquid nitrogen, electrocautery and the application of very strong pastes. Most warts eventually respond to treatment, leaving the skin free of a scar.

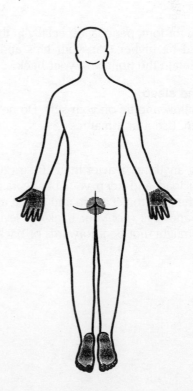

Common sites for warts

John Murtagh, *Patient Education*, Second edition, McGraw-Hill Book Company

10 Musculoskeletal disorders

Backache

What causes backache?

Backache usually is caused by minor strains in the muscles or ligaments, but more serious lower back pain usually is the result of an injury to one of the many joints in the base of your spine. The joints include the *facet joints* and *discs*, which when disturbed push against painful tissue or nerve roots just behind them. The injury usually happens while bending your spine forwards (flexing it), especially while lifting something heavy.

Never bend forward with your legs straight to perform any task. Once you have experienced back trouble, it has a tendency to recur, and so be careful to protect your back.

How can you care for it?

Adjust your activity to your back discomfort. Take care with posture, making beds and so on. Avoid fatigue. Ideally you should perform a set of exercises to strengthen the muscles of your spine and abdomen.

Sport and exercise

Be careful of sudden twisting movements and sudden overloading of muscles, as in cricket, golf, squash, sailing, weightlifting and horse riding. Walking, jogging (avoid hard surfaces) and swimming are good activities if you can manage them.

Sitting

Avoid sitting for long periods, especially in the car. Your knees should be higher than your hips and your back straight. Maintain the hollow in your back.

Bed rest and sleep

Use a low pillow and lie on your side. Do not lie face-up or face-down. Use a firm mattress.

Lifting

Avoid lifting anything heavier than 10 kg (20 lb). Squat close to the load and keep your back straight. Do not stoop over the load to get a grip and pick it up. Lift using your knees and legs (not your back) as leverage. Keep your back straight, not bent forwards or backwards.

Scrubbing floors and gardening

Your hands should be as far forward of you as necessary to keep your back straight. Do not flex your back by having your hands working too close to your knees.

Bending

Take care when bending, for example tying shoelaces or putting on stockings. Put your foot on a stool, chair or box that is near enough to your body and high enough so that you do not have to bend down to your foot.

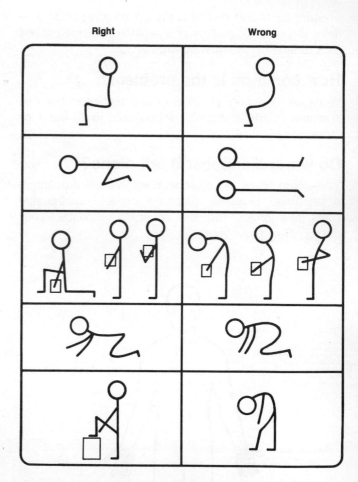

Rules of care for sitting, lying, lifting and bending

John Murtagh, *Patient Education*, Second edition, McGraw-Hill Book Company

Carpal tunnel syndrome

What is carpal tunnel syndrome?

It is a painful disorder of the hand caused by pressure on a very large nerve called the *median nerve* as it passes through a 'tunnel' at the wrist.

The tunnel is formed by a tough membrane that makes a 'roof' to a natural arch produced by a group of wrist bones (known as the *carpal bones*). The purpose of this membrane is to keep the many tendons, arteries and nerves that pass under it in place. When it thickens, it causes too much pressure on these structures, especially the sensitive nerve.

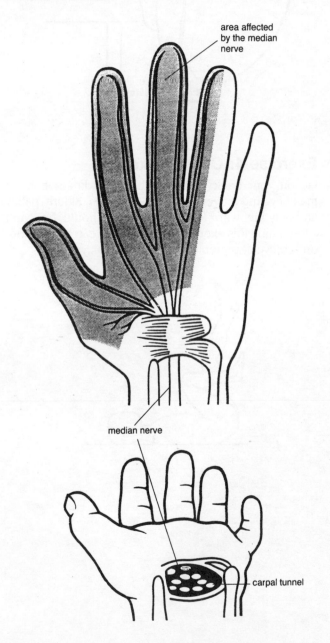

area affected by the median nerve

median nerve

carpal tunnel

Who gets it?

It is quite a common disorder, especially in middle-aged women and in pregnant women. It is thought to be caused by hormone changes causing swelling of the membrane and extra fluid in the tunnel. People doing a lot of hard manual work (such as farmers) seem prone to carpal tunnel syndrome. Sometimes an illness such as rheumatoid arthritis may cause it.

What are the symptoms?

The symptoms are tingling and numbness of most of the hand. The little finger is usually free of symptoms. Pain may shoot up the arm from the wrist. One or both hands may be affected. The pain and tingling is usually worse at night and causes you to wake from a deep sleep. It may be relieved by hanging your hand over the side of the bed and shaking or rubbing it. Warmth seems to aggravate the problem (e.g. under warm bedclothes and washing up in hot water).

What are the risks?

It is not a serious problem, but if not treated it can cause permanent weakness and numbness of the thumb and index and middle fingers.

What is the treatment?

Sometimes the problem clears up without treatment, and in some people fluid tablets may help. In pregnant women a splint worn on the wrist at night is helpful, but once the baby is born the problem usually settles of its own accord.

An injection of cortisone into the tunnel can give dramatic relief for quite a long time.

However, most cases require a small operation to relieve the pressure on the nerve. This is done by cutting through the tough membrane so that more space is created for the nerve in the tunnel. It is a most successful operation, leading to immediate relief of the discomfort.

Exercises for your knee

These exercises are designed to help people who have weakness of their *quadriceps* muscle, which is often caused by any knee disability but especially by problems of the *patella* (kneecap). Following knee disorders, the knee joint muscles and the powerful quadriceps (used for walking, climbing and running) become weak; the joint can become unstable. If done regularly several times a day, the exercises will help the knee regain its normal strength and stability.

Exercise 1: Quadriceps tightener

Sit upright on a couch with your legs stretched out straight in front. Slowly and deliberately tighten the thigh muscles by straightening the knee to position (a) from the relaxed position (b); brace the knee back hard. Count 2, and then relax the muscles completely. This should be done several times a day so that it becomes a habit.

Tightening the quadriceps can be done while you are standing or sitting.

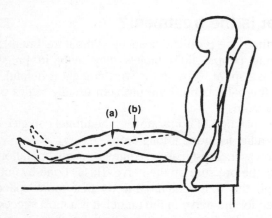

Exercise 2: Leg lifts

Starting from the same position as in exercise 1, brace the knees straight and then lift the whole leg upward (a), outward (b), across (c) and back to the resting position (d).

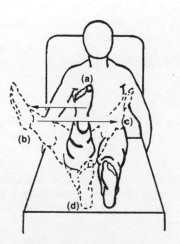

Exercise 3: Alternating leg pushes

Sit on the edge of the couch with a cushion under your knees and your legs hanging down (a). Straighten one knee firmly (b) and at the same time bend the other knee, pushing the calf hard against the couch (c). Slowly and deliberately change position so that the bent knee becomes straight and the other one pushes against the couch.

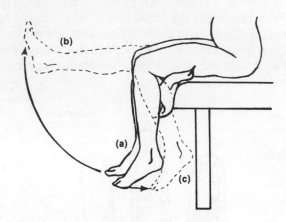

Exercise 4: Cycling exercise

Lie on your back with your hips and knees bent and make cycling movements with your legs. Elderly patients and anyone with lower back pain should be careful when doing this exercise. This exercise can be performed on a bicycle, preferably an exercise 'bicycle'.

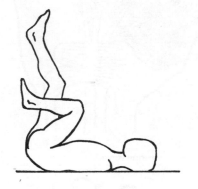

John Murtagh, *Patient Education*, Second edition, McGraw-Hill Book Company

Exercises for your lower back

Back exercises are extremely important because the muscles of the spine and abdomen support the spine better than any brace or corset. If you have chronic, nagging back pain, it is likely that performing these exercises religiously for 3 months will greatly reduce your back pain.

Exercises for the lumbar spine

The purpose of these exercises is to strengthen the various muscles that support the spine, especially the abdominal muscles and the extensor muscles of the spine.

Guidelines

- Do these exercises on a padded or well-carpeted floor.
- Do them at least twice a day for no less than 5 minutes at a time; once a day is better than not at all.

- Rest between each exercise.
- 2 or 3 of the 6 exercises is sufficient.
- Do not strain.
- The exercise may be uncomfortable at first, and initially each one should be repeated *only 2 or 3 times*.
- If there is any problematic pain with a particular exercise, stop doing it.

As the muscles stretch and strengthen, the routine becomes more natural and enjoyable.

Splinting the lumbar spine

It is a good idea to learn how to keep the lumbar spine in a fixed position by using the abdominal muscles and those around the spine.

- Lie face-up with one hand under your neck and your knees bent.
- Draw in your stomach firmly, and press your lumbar region against the floor by slightly raising your buttocks. Hold—count to 6—relax; repeat 10 times.

Note Swimming is the ideal exercise for your back.

Exercise 1: Back arch

Stand up straight, feet pointing directly forwards and apart as wide as your shoulders, hands placed on the small of your back, fingers pointing backwards. Breathe in and breathe out slowly. As you breathe out, bend backwards as far as you can while supporting your back with your hands and keeping your knees straight. Hold your lower back arched for 5 seconds, then return to the neutral position. Repeat 5 times.

Exercise 2: Cat back

Assume a kneeling position, resting on your hands and knees. Arch your back like a cat and drop your head at the same time. Hold for about 5 seconds, then reverse the arch by bringing up your head and forming a 'U' with your spine. Arch and sag your back several times.

Exercise 3: Knee-to-chest raise

Lie flat on your back, bend one leg up, grasping it with your hand just below the knee, and bend your head forward so that your forehead approaches your knee. Hold for 5 seconds. Repeat on the other side.

Exercise 4: Straight-leg raise

Lie on your back. With your leg perfectly straight, raise it as high as you can. Repeat with the other leg. Take this to the limit of pain.

Exercise 5: Straight-leg swing

Lie on your back with your arms spread out on either side. Raise one leg as high as possible, keeping it straight. Swing the leg in an arc from one side to the other. It is important to swing the leg on the side of your back that you feel pain (if you have any). Hold for 5 seconds. Repeat 5 times.

Exercise 6: Pelvic roll

You can get better results if someone pins your shoulders to the floor while you do this exercise. Lie on your back. Lift your legs together in the air and roll them from side to side. Hold for 5 seconds on each side. Repeat 5 times.

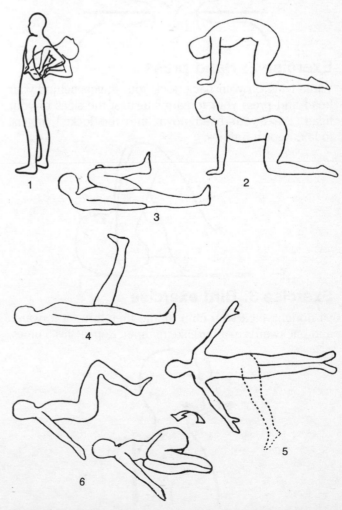

Exercises for your neck

If you have neck pain and stiffness, a course of exercises is important because it loosens the stiff joints (all 35 of them) and strengthens the muscles that control the movements of the neck.

If there is any problematic pain with a particular exercise, you should stop doing it. It is best to keep your head in a neutral position with your chin tucked in before you start.

Do the exercises 2 or 3 times a day. Exercises 1 and 2 can also be done while sitting up, so that all the exercises (except 4) can be done anywhere (such as at the office or in the car when stopped in traffic).

Exercise 1: Neck rotation

Lie on your back on a firm surface such as a floor or bed. Turn your head firmly (but not quickly) to the side by turning your chin towards your shoulders. Hold for 3 seconds and then turn to the opposite side. Repeat 5 times.

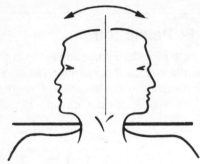

Exercise 2: Hand press

While lying on your back, lock your fingers behind your head and press your forearms against the sides of your head. Press your head down into the locked fingers. Relax. Repeat 5 times.

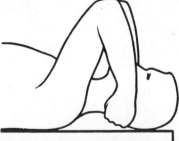

Exercise 3: Bird exercise

Sit upright, tuck your chin in and then thrust it forwards and backwards in a bird-like manner. Repeat this 5 times.

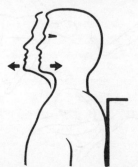

Exercise 4: Resisted side bending

Lie on your side with your head resting on a small, firm pillow. Your head and neck should be in a straight line. Take a deep breath in, hold it and push down hard on the pillow for 7 seconds, then breathe out as you relax. Repeat 3 times. Repeat on the opposite side if this side is tender.

It is important to make sure that you press down on your painful side.

This type of exercise can be used for flexion (lying face downwards), extension (lying on the back) and rotation (lying on the back).

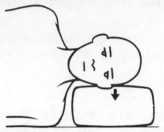

Exercise 5: Resisted side bending

Sit upright in a chair, tuck your chin in and keep your head straight. Place your right hand over the top of your head to grasp the head just above the ear (a right-sided problem is demonstrated). Pull your head down until it first begins to feel uncomfortable. Take a deep breath in, hold it and press firmly against your hand for 7 seconds (you will be pushing to the left). Breathe out, relax and then pull your head firmly towards the right. Repeat this 3–5 times. (Reverse sides for a left-sided problem.)

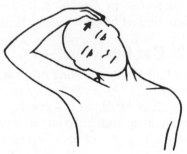

Exercise 6: Resisted rotation

Sit upright in a chair, tuck your chin in and turn it to the left side to the point of discomfort. Then place your right hand on the back of your head and your left on the chin as shown (a left-sided problem is demonstrated). Take a deep breath in—now try to turn your head to the right but hold it in place by resistance from your hands. As you relax and breathe out, rotate your head firmly but gently towards the left. Repeat 3–5 times. (Reverse sides for a right-sided problem.)

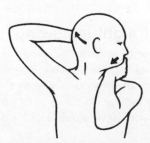

John Murtagh, *Patient Education*, Second edition, McGraw-Hill Book Company

Exercises for your shoulder

A tender, restricted shoulder is caused by inflammation of the tendons and muscles controlling the shoulder or of the main joint. It recovers spontaneously but slowly. The pain subsides, leaving the joint stiff, but it will resolve gradually with use of the limb. These exercises are designed to help recovery.

Exercise 1: Straight-arm rotation

Bend forwards and sideways. Let your arms hang down from your shoulders. Make circular movements clockwise and anticlockwise.

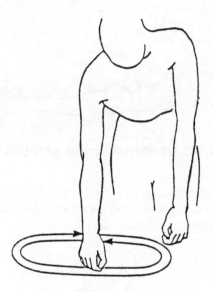

Exercise 2: Shoulder stretch

With the tips of your fingers touching your body, bring the hand of the affected arm across your chest until it reaches the opposite shoulder (a). With the other hand, gently press the elbow of the arm towards the shoulder (b).

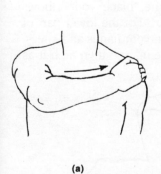

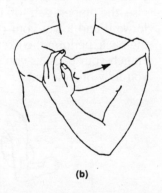

(a)   (b)

Exercise 3: Shoulder winging

Lock your hands behind your head and brace back the elbows. You can do this while standing or lying on your back.

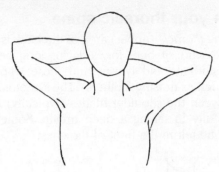

Exercise 4: Coupled armswing

Lie on your back and intertwine your fingers across the front of your body (a). Lift the affected arm with the 'good' arm to bring the hands up and over your head (b). Return the arms to the starting position (a), again carrying the weight of the affected arm with the other hand.

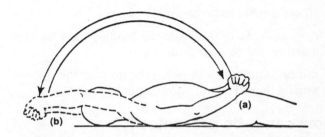

Exercise 5: Towel exercise

When the shoulder is recovering, the following exercise should be done. Put a towel over the normal shoulder and grasp the front end with the normal hand. Place the affected arm up the small of your back and grasp the other end of the towel with it. Make a seesaw movement as if drying your back.

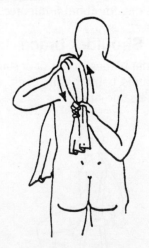

Exercises for your thoracic spine

Pain in your thoracic spine

Pain in the *thoracic* (upper) area of the back is common in people who sit bent forwards for long periods, especially students and typists, and those who lift constantly (such as nursing mothers). The symptoms include pain between the shoulder blades (typically) and possibly difficulty in taking a deep breath. Sometimes the pain can be felt in the front of the chest.

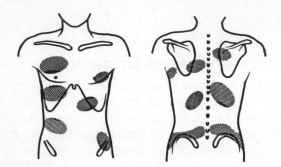

Examples of pain distribution in the thoracic area

There appear to be two main causes:

1. chronic strain of the ligaments binding the vertebrae together due to poor posture
2. stiff or 'jammed' joints where the ribs join the spine—usually due to injury, including lifting and falls

How can it be prevented?

Maintain a good posture by doing the following:
- Keep your head erect.
- Brace your shoulder blades together and then release—practise many times a day.
- Look after your posture at the office; have a good chair with a firm back support.

Exercises

Select at least 2 exercises that suit you and perform them once or twice a day for about 5 minutes.

Exercise 1: Shoulder brace

Brace the shoulder blades as you sit or stand, by swinging your clasped hands behind your back, extending your head back at the same time.

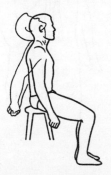

Exercise 2: Back arch

Lie face downwards. Lift your shoulders, hold for 10 seconds, then relax.

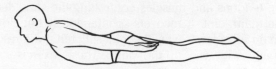

Exercise 3: 'Seal' movement

Lie face downwards. Lift from the waist, and rotate your upper trunk from side to side so that you feel a tight stretch in your back.

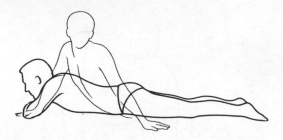

Exercise 4: Broom-handle stretch and swing

Place a long rod, such as a broom handle, behind your neck, grasp it as shown and rotate your body from side to side, reaching maximum stretch.

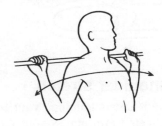

Exercise 5: Knees-to-elbows back arch

Position your back like a cat, as illustrated (a). Support yourself on both knees and elbows. If you need to exercise the upper part of the spine, place your elbows forward and lower your chest (b). For the lower part of the back, perform the exercise on your hands and knees. Hunch your back as you breathe in, and then arch it as you fully breathe out.

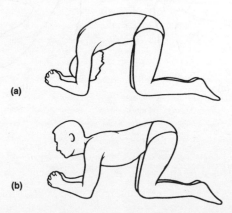

(a)

(b)

John Murtagh, *Patient Education*, Second edition, McGraw-Hill Book Company

Gout

What is gout?

Gout is a type of arthritis that is caused by uric acid crystals getting caught in the spaces between the joints of the feet, the hands and some larger joints. The tissue around the joints becomes inflamed, and this inflammation triggers the sensitive nerve endings at the joint, causing extreme pain.

Uric acid is a waste product from the body, especially from proteins called *purines*. It is passed out in the urine by the kidneys, which sometimes cannot cope with the load of uric acid, and this causes a build-up in the body.

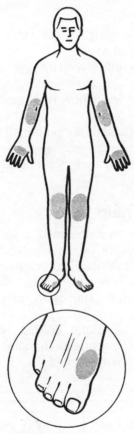

Typical sites of pain in gout

What are the symptoms?

The main symptom is severe pain, usually in the hands or feet, especially at the base of the big toe. Sometimes gout can strike in other joints, such as the elbow or the knee.

The pain usually comes on without warning, often in the early hours of the morning, and soon the joint becomes so tender that one cannot bear even the weight of the bedsheets. The inflamed skin over the joint is often red, shiny and dry. The first attack usually involves only one joint and may last from a few hours to several days, generally about 2 or 3 days depending on how soon treatment is commenced. Sometimes there may be only one attack in a person's lifetime.

Who gets gout?

Almost any person can get gout, because all human beings produce about as much uric acid as the kidneys can handle. However, it does appear to be hereditary and is far more common in men, especially between the ages of 30 and 60.

It is one of the oldest disorders known to humans, and some well-known victims include Alexander the Great, Kublai Khan, Michelangelo, Martin Luther, Isaac Newton, Henry VIII, John Wesley, Francis Bacon and Benjamin Franklin.

What brings on gout?

Contrary to popular belief, it is not necessarily brought on by high living and gluttony. Overindulgence in rich foods and alcohol can certainly bring on an acute attack in those who are prone to gout. It is associated with obesity and high blood pressure. Some drugs, particularly diuretics (fluid tablets), injury, surgery or starvation can bring on gout.

What are the risks?

Gout is a curable disease, but if it is untreated it can cause kidney disease, including kidney stones.

What is the treatment?

The acute attack

The earlier the attack is treated the better. Contact your doctor about the best treatment and the right pain-killer.

Aspirin is not recommended for the pain of gout.

Bed rest is important. Some relief can be obtained by applying a hot compress or ice to the affected joint. Keep the weight of the bedclothes off the foot by placing a bed cradle or similar object under the bedclothes.

Since gout may strike only once, no further treatment is needed apart from following the 'rules of moderation'. If gout keeps returning, it will be necessary to go onto tablets that may have to be taken for a lifetime in order to prevent more acute attacks.

Rules of moderation

Do:
- restrict intake of food high in purines, especially organ meats (liver, brain, kidneys, sweetbread) and tinned fish (sardines, anchovies, herrings)
- reduce your intake of alcohol
- eat a normal, well-balanced diet
- drink plenty of water
- maintain a normal weight, but avoid 'crash' diets
- wear comfortable shoes
- get regular exercise

Don't:
- take your worries to bed
- exercise too strenuously
- overexpose yourself to cold
- drink excessive amounts of alcohol (keep to a modest level only, e.g. 2 standard drinks a day)

Neck: painful neck

What causes neck pain?

Pain in the neck is commonly the result of an injury such as a sharp, sudden jerk of the neck as in a motor vehicle accident. Other causes include blows to the head (such as in boxing and wrestling), striking the head on an overhead object or even simple falls. People often wake up with severe neck pain and blame it on a cold draught, but it is caused by an unusual twist in the neck for a long period during sleep. The pain mainly arises from minor injury to the many small swivel joints in the neck (called *facet joints*) and less often to injury of one of the discs between the vertebrae. In older people, arthritis can develop in these joints.

What are the symptoms?

The main symptom is pain and stiffness in the neck, but the pain can travel to the head, around the eye and ear or to the shoulder and arm. Problems from the *cervical spine* (the first 7 vertebrae in the spine) can also cause 'pins and needles' in the neck or down the arm.

What is the outlook?

Neck pain, which is rarely a severe problem, can clear up very quickly and usually responds very well to physical treatment such as exercises, massage and mobilisation. However, it can be persistent or recurrent, and for that reason regular exercise of your neck is advisable.

What about cervical collars?

Collars are very helpful for a short period for acutely painful necks, but should not be worn for any longer than 7–10 days at a time and not at night. Your neck needs to be mobile and exercised naturally.

Dos and Don'ts

To avoid bouts of further neck pain, the following rules are helpful:

Don't:
- look up in a strained position for long periods (e.g. as when painting a ceiling)
- twist your head often towards the painful side (e.g. as when reversing a car)
- lift or tug with your neck bent forwards
- work, read or study with your neck bent for long periods
- become too dependent on 'collars'
- sleep on too many pillows

Do:
- keep your neck upright in a vertical position for reading, typing and so on
- keep a good posture: remember to keep the chin tucked in
- sleep on a low, firm pillow or a special conforming pillow
- sleep with your painful side on the pillow
- use heat and massage: massage your neck firmly 3 times a day using an analgesic ointment

Professional help

Your doctor may prescribe mild pain-killers such as aspirin or paracetamol or other medicine for a short period, especially if arthritis is developing.

A course of exercises to mobilise stiff joints in the neck and strengthen the supporting muscles is probably the best treatment.

To overcome a painful episode, therapy to the muscles and joints by gentle mobilisation from a trained therapist is highly recommended.

Don't . . .

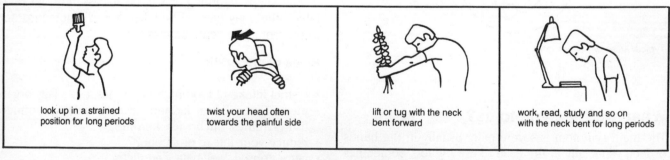

look up in a strained position for long periods

twist your head often towards the painful side

lift or tug with the neck bent forward

work, read, study and so on with the neck bent for long periods

Do . . .

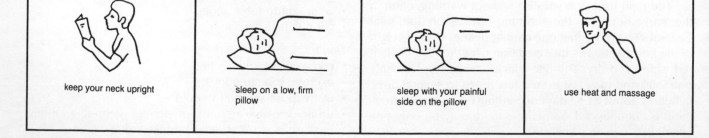

keep your neck upright

sleep on a low, firm pillow

sleep with your painful side on the pillow

use heat and massage

John Murtagh, *Patient Education*, Second edition, McGraw-Hill Book Company

Neck: postaccident neck pain

What is the cause of the problem?

In a rear-end collision, your head is thrown back into overextension and then bends sharply forwards on the rebound. This is commonly called a *whiplash* injury, but it is an overextension injury.

If your car collides with a stationary object, your head bends sharply forwards at first and then rebounds backwards. This results in a similar injury to the neck.

What happens?

1. The ligaments binding the vertebrae together are stretched and torn, rather like a sprained ankle. Some bleeding occurs in the ligaments.

2. The many small joints in the neck are jarred and bruised.

X-rays do not usually show up this injury to ligaments and joints.

What are the symptoms?

At first the neck may feel okay, but later (maybe 2 or 3 days later) becomes painful and stiff (like a sprained ankle). Pain in the arms and headache may follow. Some people have difficulty swallowing. Apart from a sore neck, there is a tendency to feel depressed for about 2 weeks. Talk to your doctor about this feeling if it persists.

What is the outlook?

The outlook is invariably very good with a normal recovery, but it may take some months. It will not be speeded up by repeated X-rays or wearing a cervical collar.

What is the treatment?

Like a sprained ankle, the neck needs time to heal, taking at least 3 weeks.

Self-help

- Apply icepacks for the first 3 days, then warmth and gentle massage.
- *Exercise*: The best treatment is exercising your neck as soon as possible, even though it feels stiff and tender. Mobilisation therapy can certainly help, but manipulation is not recommended in the first 8 weeks. Your therapist will advise on the best exercises, but any slow, deliberate stretching of the neck is good.
- *Pain-killers*: Paracetamol taken every 4 hours for pain is advisable.
- *Cervical collar*: Support for the neck from a 'collar' with the back higher than the front can help for the first 10 days. However, only 2 or 3 days in a collar is preferred. The less time in it the better. Keep the neck in a slightly bent forward non-painful position in the collar. Discard the collar as soon as possible and start moving your neck.

Medication

Your doctor may prescribe a short course of muscle relaxants or anti-inflammatory tablets to make your neck more comfortable.

Osteoarthritis

What is meant by arthritis or rheumatism?

Unfortunately, these common terms produce a considerable amount of fear and concern for many people.

Rheumatism is a vague term used to describe aching in joints and muscles, and the word should be avoided.

Arthritis means inflammation of the joints, but there are over 100 different types of arthritis. The most serious is *rheumatoid arthritis*, which is uncommon. The most common is *osteoarthritis*, which is usually not serious and causes only minor discomfort in some people.

What is osteoarthritis?

This is a condition that occurs during the body's normal ageing process as a result of wear and tear of the joints. It is also called *degenerative joint disease*.

The smooth gristle or cartilage that covers and protects the ends of the bones at the joints is gradually worn away. The joints become rough, and stiffness and inflammation can develop.

X-rays are taken to confirm the diagnosis of osteoarthritis; all other tests done have normal results. X-rays show some degree of osteoarthritis in 1 or more of the joints of 9 out of 10 people over the age of 40.

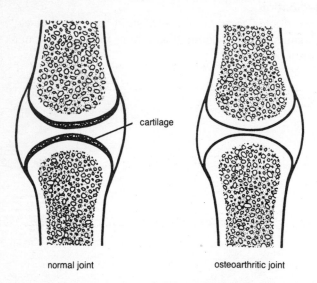

Osteoarthritis: the protective cartilage is worn away

How does osteoarthritis begin?

The most common reason for loss of cartilage is wear and tear due to ageing, but many people never notice it.

It commonly develops in joints that were injured earlier in life (such as with sporting injuries) or joints that have been overworked (such as those in the fingers of a knitter or the feet of a ballet dancer).

Osteoarthritis mostly affects the weight-bearing joints such as the spine, knees and hips (especially in overweight people), but the base of the thumb and the ends of the fingers are common sites also.

What are the symptoms?

The severity of symptoms varies, but usually they are pain, swelling and stiffness of the affected joints. Stiffness is usually worse in the morning. Pain is worse after excessive or prolonged activity such as walking for a long time. Movement may be difficult and interfere with normal activities.

How serious is osteoarthritis?

Osteoarthritis seldom becomes a serious problem and does not threaten one's life. It does not cause the crippling deformities of joints seen in the rarer serious forms of arthritis.

What is the treatment?

There is no cure, but there are many ways to make life more comfortable and keep you mobile and independent. Surgery can relieve a joint that is very stiff and painful.

Diet

Keep your weight down to avoid unnecessary wear on the joints. No particular diet has been proved to cause, or improve, osteoarthritis.

Exercise

Keep a good balance of adequate rest with sensible exercise (such as walking, cycling or swimming), but *stop* any exercise or activity that increases the pain.

Heat

A hot-water bottle, warm bath or electric blanket can soothe the pain and stiffness. Avoid getting too cold.

Walking aids

Shoe inserts, good footwear and a walking stick can help painful knees, hips and feet.

Medication

Aspirin and paracetamol are effective pain-killers for mild osteoarthritis. Your doctor may prescribe antiarthritic medications, but a few may have to be tried to find the one that works best for you. The tablets should be taken with food.

Note: Tell your doctor if you have had a peptic ulcer or get indigestion.

Special equipment

It is possible to increase your independence at home. There is a wide range of inexpensive equipment and tools that can help with cooking, cleaning and other household chores. These can be discussed with people at an Independent Living Centre, with physiotherapists and occupational therapists.

The Arthritis Foundation in each capital city is able to provide information about many aspects of arthritis.

John Murtagh, *Patient Education*, Second edition, McGraw-Hill Book Company

Plantar fasciitis

Plantar fasciitis is a common condition that causes pain under the heel of the foot. It is known also as 'policeman's heel'. The painful area is usually situated about 5 cm (2 inches) from the back of the heel on the sole of the foot.

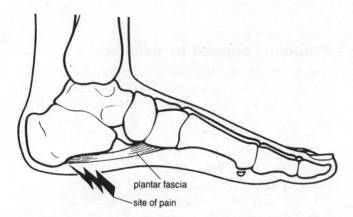

Anatomy of plantar fasciitis

What is the cause?

It is an inflammation of the site where a long ligament called the *plantar fascia* attaches to the main heel bone (the *calcaneus*). It is a condition similar to tennis elbow. One known cause is a tear of this tissue, which can happen, for example, when a runner takes off quickly. Sometimes a spur of bone develops at this spot, but the spur is not a serious problem.

The problem is not thought to be caused by faulty footwear.

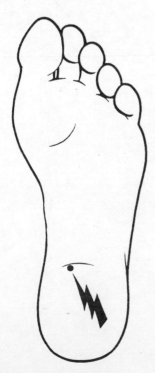

The commonest site of plantar fasciitis

Who gets it?

It occurs typically in people over the age of 40, especially if they start a running activity. It occurs in both sexes. It is common in people who have to stand or walk for long periods in their job, such as policemen on a beat.

It is seen sometimes in young sportspeople.

What are the symptoms?

The pain under the heel is worse when the person first steps out of bed or gets up to walk after sitting for a long time. It is relieved after walking about, but then returns towards the end of the day after a lot of walking. Resting will always ease the pain until you get up and walk. Climbing stairs also hurts.

The painful area on the heel is tender to touch, but not unbearably so.

X-rays may show a small spur on the bone.

What is the outcome?

The pain will usually go away by itself in about 12 months, sometimes as early as 6 months. It is not a serious problem.

What is the treatment?

Rest from long walks and from running is important.

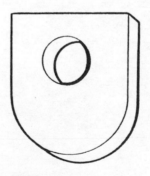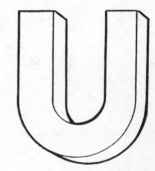

Types of heel pads

Heel pads

The standard treatment is to wear a pad at all times inside the shoe or slipper to cushion the heel. The pad is made from sponge or sorbo rubber and should raise the heel about 1 cm. A hole corresponding to the tender area should be cut out of the pad so that this area does not make direct contact with the shoe. Suitable shapes are illustrated. The best pad is a special inner sole (called an *orthotic aid*) that is moulded for your foot to include the arch as well as the heel.

Injections

If the pain is really bothersome (it is often bad for 2–3 months), an injection given by your doctor can give relief for a few weeks. It is uncomfortable to have but generally well worthwhile.

Plaster instructions

You have had a plaster cast applied to a limb. To allow the plaster to work properly, it is important that you:
- Lie down for the next ... hours.
- Elevate the limb for the next 48 hours.
- Move the fingers or toes around.
- Return tomorrow or whenever advised for a plaster check.

Elevation

Arm
Have the hand raised so that it is higher than the opposite shoulder level (if possible). The arm can be supported on a pillow or in a sling.

Leg
Raise the foot of the bed and place the plaster cast on a pillow or cushion. The patient can lie down or sit up, as long as the leg is elevated.

Other useful tips
- For a fractured leg crutches may be provided, but these are best used after 48 hours of rest.
- The plaster can take up to 2 days to dry.
- You should not stand on a leg plaster before 2 days.
- Contact your doctor if you notice a smell or discharge coming from inside the plaster.

Problems caused by swelling

Sometimes the swelling around the fracture will cause the plaster to become too tight. The patient should be brought back to the doctor or to the emergency department of the hospital *immediately* if any of the following develop:
- marked swelling of the fingers or toes
- blueness of the fingers or toes
- loss of feeling or numbness in the fingers or toes
- a tight pain not eased by elevation of the limb
- inability to move the fingers or toes

John Murtagh, *Patient Education*, Second edition, McGraw-Hill Book Company

Rheumatoid arthritis

What is rheumatoid arthritis?

Rheumatoid arthritis is a disease of the joints, usually the smaller joints of the body. Many people believe wrongly that this is always a disabling, severe condition. In fact, it may be mild and can be well controlled using modern medicine. It is not infectious, but no one is able to say what triggers it. There is no cure for this condition, but all patients can be treated.

What are the symptoms?

The symptoms will vary a great deal from person to person, as well as from day to day. However, some of the common symptoms include:

- stiffness and tenderness of the small joints, especially of the wrist, hands and feet (the base of the fingers, thumbs or toes can be affected; less commonly it can affect the larger joints such as the knee, shoulder, ankle and neck)
- tiredness
- morning stiffness

In summary, the main symptoms are pain, stiffness and swelling of the small joints.

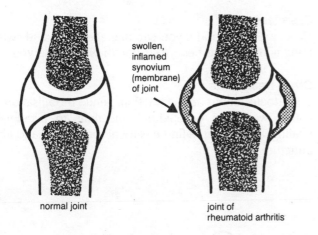

normal joint

swollen, inflamed synovium (membrane) of joint

joint of rheumatoid arthritis

How is it diagnosed?

After being suspected by the doctor upon examination, rheumatoid arthritis can usually be diagnosed by tests, including X-rays of the hands and special blood tests.

How common is the problem?

About 2 persons in 100 suffer to some extent from rheumatoid arthritis. It is more common in females. Most sufferers are between 40 and 60 years of age, but the disease can affect people in any age group. However, the majority of patients have little or no long-term problems and only 1 patient in 10 is severely affected.

What are the risks?

In severe cases the swollen and deformed joints may become partly or completely dislocated, causing considerable discomfort and problems with walking if the knee or foot joints are affected. The tendons may become so weak that they can snap. A special problem is the neck, which can become unstable so that manipulative procedures can be dangerous and cause paralysis.

What is the treatment?

Exercise

It is important to keep fit. Walking and swimming are to be encouraged. Many local councils and physiotherapists offer swimming and other forms of hydrotherapy in heated pools. Home exercise routines to prevent muscle weakening can be provided by your physiotherapist or doctor.

Rest

Rest is important and depends on how you feel. It must be sensibly balanced with exercise. If an exercise causes pain, it should be altered or reduced.

Joint movement

Each joint affected should be put through a daily full range of motion to keep it mobile and to reduce stiffness. Protect any weakened joints or tendons by lifting gently and smoothly rather than in a jerking motion.

Heat and cold

For stiff joints a hot-water bottle, warm water or a heat lamp can help. For morning stiffness an electric blanket or a warm shower can be helpful. Sometimes cold packs or water are appropriate, for example over a hot, tender joint.

Diet

There is no special diet. No specific food has caused arthritis and no specific diet will cure it. However, a nourishing and well-balanced diet including adequate fibre will promote health and a sense of well-being. Maintain a normal weight to lessen the burden on your joints.

Medication

There are many effective pain-killing and anti-inflammatory drugs available to treat rheumatoid arthritis. The basic drug is likely to be aspirin in high doses, but it can cause ringing in the ears and other unpleasant effects. Your doctor may have to experiment for a time before finding the best drugs for you.

Surgery

Occasionally surgery may help if a particular joint is severely inflamed by removing the inflamed lining called the *synovium*. In later stages it may be possible to replace a badly damaged joint with an artificial joint.

Support

Excellent leaflets and practical help are available from the Arthritis Foundation in each capital city. These include information about and access to a wide range of inexpensive equipment and tools that can assist your daily living.

Sciatica

What is sciatica?

Sciatica is a type of *neuralgia* (nerve pain). The *sciatic nerve* is a huge nerve (about the size of an adult's small finger) that controls the function of the leg, especially the foot. It passes from the spine into the buttock, then into the back of the thigh and leg.

What causes sciatica?

It is caused by pressure, usually from a *prolapsed disc*, on the nerve roots from the lower back that form the sciatic nerve. This problem is often called a 'slipped disc', but it is not a good term because the disc is big and only part of it bulges to cause pressure.

Sciatica can be caused also by the nerve roots being trapped in the tunnel at the side of the spine through which they pass. This pinching effect causes the nerve to become irritated and swollen. The tunnel is made smaller by surrounding arthritis or a flattened disc space. This problem is quite common in elderly people.

A rare cause is a haemorrhage around the nerves in people who are taking blood-thinning tablets.

What are the symptoms?

The patient usually feels a burning pain or a deep aching pain in the buttock, the thigh, the calf and the outer border of the leg, ankle and foot. Sciatica is not a pain covering the whole leg like a stocking. It commonly causes a pain around the outer part of the leg into the ankle. The pain may vary from very severe to mild. A 'pins and needles' sensation or numbness may be felt in the lower leg and the foot.

The pain is usually made worse if you sneeze, cough, strain at the toilet or lift something.

What are the risks?

Fortunately most cases of sciatica gradually get better in about 6–12 weeks. Sometimes the pressure on the nerve is so great that the leg, especially the foot, becomes weak and floppy. In such cases, an operation is required to relieve the pressure.

Rarely a disc prolapse will cause severe weakness and numbness in the legs, and lack of control of the bladder or bowels. This is very serious and needs urgent attention.

What is the treatment?

Rest

When the pain is acute, it is most important to rest lying down for 2 or 3 days. You should do nothing but rest on a firm mattress or on the floor, getting up only to go to the toilet.

After the acute phase, you should take things gently to allow the problem to settle. Avoid lifting, bending your back and sitting in soft chairs for long periods.

Medication

Your doctor will prescribe some tablets for your pain and perhaps some tablets to relieve inflammation around the nerve.

Exercises

These are very good if you can manage them, and swimming is one of the best. Your doctor will advise you.

Other treatments

Your doctor could advise traction, gentle mobilisation of your lower back or epidural injections to accelerate healing. Some people find electrical stimulation and acupuncture helpful.

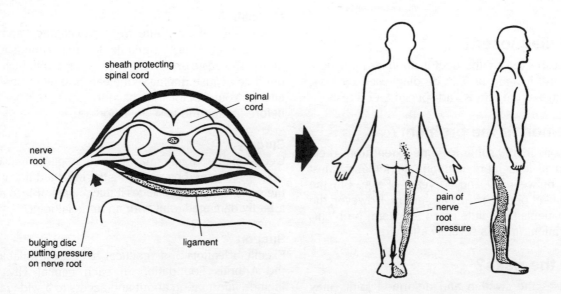

Typical sciatic pain

John Murtagh, *Patient Education*, Second edition, McGraw-Hill Book Company

Spondylosis

What is spondylosis?

Spondylosis is a condition of the spine in which it is hardened and stiffened by osteoarthritis. It is also referred to as *degenerative disease of the spine*. The two areas commonly affected are the neck (*cervical spondylosis*) and the lower back (*lumbar spondylosis*).

What causes it?

Constant wear and tear and injury to the joints of the spine cause arthritis in the joints. The discs, which are like soft rubber shock absorbers between the vertebrae, become hard and stiff as they shrink with age. This causes strains on all the surrounding joints and tissues, leading to stiffness. It is common in people who have worked hard with their backs (such as labourers and farmers) and those who have had injuries (such as in car accidents). The older one gets, the more likely one is to get spondylosis.

What are the symptoms?

Many milder cases cause no symptoms. The common symptoms are stiffness and tenderness in the neck or lower back, especially first thing in the morning or after activity such as gardening or painting.

Cervical spondylosis

This can cause a painful neck with headache and aches and pains in the surrounding areas. The neck feels very stiff, which makes it hard to turn around (while reversing the car, for example). The head can feel like a heavy cannonball.

Lumbar spondylosis

Common symptoms are stiffness and pain in the lower back with poor movements (such as difficulty in bending forwards). Shooting pains in the buttocks and legs resulting in sciatica are common. There may be pain in the back of the legs after a long walk. This uncommon problem is caused by narrowing of the space inside the spine from overgrowth of the bones due to arthritis and may require an operation.

What is the treatment?

It is important to keep active, but do not overdo the activity. A sensible balance between mild to moderate exercise and rest is necessary, but it has to be 'played by ear' as each individual is different. You should be able to live comfortably with spondylosis with exercise, following your physiotherapist's advice and taking medication. It is usual for the discomfort to improve with time, although the stiffness remains.

Exercise

Regular gentle exercise for your neck or lower back will help you. You will be advised by your doctor or physiotherapist about the best exercises for you, but gentle, slow stretching exercises to as far as you can stretch are recommended. Swimming or hydrotherapy will help overcome the stiffness.

Medication

Regular use of mild pain-killers such as aspirin or paracetamol will relieve your aches and pains. Your doctor may prescribe a course of anti-inflammatory drugs.

Sports injuries—first aid

Muscle strains

You can 'pull' (strain or tear) a muscle if you do not warm up properly before exercising or if you have not done enough preseason training.

Management of a pulled muscle is based on 'RICE':

Rest	No exercise, no stretching; rest the injured soft tissue of the muscle.
Ice	Apply an icepack for 20–30 minutes every 2 hours while awake during the first 48 hours.
Compression	Keep the muscle firmly bandaged for at least 48 hours.
Elevation	Rest the leg on a stool or chair (or the arm on cushions or in a sling) until the swelling goes.

- If the injury is severe, see a doctor immediately.
- After resting the muscle for a few days, stretching can begin. Warm the area first with an infra-red lamp or a hot-water bottle. Then stretch your leg or arm about 5 times to contract the muscle gently. Do this twice each day for 14 days.
- Do not return to sport until the pain and swelling have gone, the muscle is strong and you can move the limb freely without discomfort.

Note

Reusable soft-fabric cold compresses that can be stored in a freezer (at least 2 hours) and dual-purpose hot/cold packs are available and are ideal for the athlete to have always available.

Torn leg muscles

For a damaged hamstring or other leg muscle, begin the stretching by lying on your back with the knee straight. Lift the leg to a level where it just starts to hurt and hold the position for about 30 seconds. Do this twice a day for about 14 days.

Then start more vigorous stretching. Strap a 1.5 kg weight to your ankle, lie on your stomach and lift your foot (bending the knee) so that your heel almost touches your buttock. Repeat 5–10 times. Stop if it causes pain; otherwise do this exercise 2 or 3 times a day for 2 or 3 weeks, increasing the weight gradually to 5 kg.

Keep yourself fit with swimming while the muscle is recovering.

Joint sprains

One of the commonest injuries in sport is a joint sprain: stress on the joint stretches its lining or ligaments (or both) beyond normal limits. Most often, damage occurs to the knee, ankle and wrist joints, making them swollen, tender and painful to move. Bruising is not always obvious. Again, first aid is based on 'RICE':

Rest	Rest helps prevent the injured area from moving, reducing pain and speeding healing. Use crutches to take the weight off injured joints in the leg.
Ice	Cold will reduce swelling, pain and stiffness. Use a reusable compress or a packet of frozen peas or beans or wrap ice-cubes in a damp tea-towel (or a thin bath towel); never apply ice directly to the skin. Use the icepack for about 20 minutes every 2 hours for the first 48 hours.
Compression	Compress and support the injury with a firm (not tight) elastic wrap bandage.
Elevation	Elevate the leg on a stool or chair (leg, knee and ankle injuries) or put your arm in a sling (shoulder, arm, wrist injuries) until the swelling goes.

Most minor joint and muscle injuries settle quickly with this treatment. If not, or if the injury was severe, professional assessment and treatment are necessary.

John Murtagh, *Patient Education*, Second edition, McGraw-Hill Book Company

Sprained ankle

What is a sprained ankle?

A *sprain* occurs when there is damage to the ligaments that bind the bones of the ankle joint. The fibres of the ligament that has been overstretched tear and then bleed. The tear is usually minor, involving a small number of fibres, but sometimes the ligament can be completely torn.

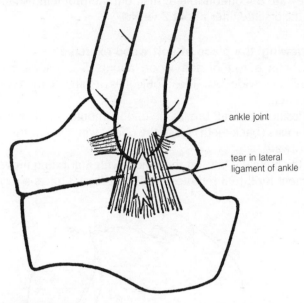

ankle joint

tear in lateral ligament of ankle

Sprained ankle

What is the cause?

The cause is a sudden twist of the foot inwards so that the ligaments on the outside of the ankle are over-stretched, rather like tearing an overstretched piece of material. Sometimes the inside of the ankle is sprained when the foot twists outwards.

What are the symptoms?

The symptoms depend on the extent of the damage. Pain, swelling, bruising and tenderness of the injured area usually occur and vary from mild to severe. With a complete tear the ankle joint will go out of shape and feel unstable.

How common is the problem?

Sprained ankles are very common. In an average year, at least 1 person in 50 consults a doctor about this injury.

What is the treatment?

For a mild sprain, self-help measures are usually sufficient. However, a severe sprain requires an X-ray, since there may be a fracture or a complete tear. Sometimes the discomfort of a sprain settles quickly, but should it persist beyond 3–4 days a visit to your doctor is advisable. Your doctor may apply a special strapping.

Self-help

This includes following the 'RICE' formula:

Rest — Rest as much as possible. If the sprain is severe, use crutches to take the weight off the ankle.

Ice — Apply icepacks and/or soak the ankle in cold water to reduce swelling and pain. Use a special reusable compress (e.g. ACE wrap) or a packet of frozen peas or beans or wrap ice-cubes in a damp tea-towel; never apply ice directly to the skin. Use the icepack for about 20–30 minutes every 3 hours when awake for the first 48 hours. (Icepacks can be placed over a bandage.)

Compression — Compress and support the ankle with a firm (not tight) elastic bandage.

Elevation — Elevate the leg on a stool or chair until the swelling goes.

Exercise program

Exercises started early will help prevent permanent stiffness. Exercise every hour up to the point of discomfort. Do each exercise at least 10 times.

1. Firmly flap your foot up and down at the ankle joint.

2. Rotate your foot inwards and outwards, keeping the foot at right angles to the leg.

3. Combine these exercises so that your foot moves slowly in a circle (clockwise, then anticlockwise).

Pain-killers

Take analgesics for pain, especially at night. Paracetamol with or without codeine is usually sufficient.

Walking

Walking with your ankle supported in comfortable walking shoes is recommended for short distances. Walk as normally as possible, but avoid standing still for long periods. Walking without shoes in sand is an excellent way of strengthening your ankle quickly (after the first 2–3 days).

What is the outcome?

For most sprains you can expect full recovery in 1–6 weeks, but severe sprains with complete tearing take longer, as a plaster cast for 4–6 weeks or surgery may be necessary.

Temporomandibular joint dysfunction

What is temporomandibular joint (TMJ) dysfunction?

It is an abnormal movement of the *mandible* (the jaw bone) in its socket at the base of the skull situated just in front of the ears. It is often caused by dental problems, but in many people there is no obvious cause. Uncommon diseases such as rheumatoid arthritis have to be ruled out.

What are the symptoms?

There is a discomfort or pain in the jaw in front of the ear, especially when eating. A clicking or clunking noise may also occur with movements of the jaw.

Is it a serious problem?

It is an annoying problem rather than a serious problem. Fortunately it responds well to treatment.

What is the treatment?

It is best to try simple methods first before embarking on expensive and sophisticated treatments.

For a very painful problem

The acute problem requires rest and support by following these rules:
- When eating, avoid opening your mouth wider than the thickness of your thumb and cut all food into small pieces.
- Do not bite any food with your front teeth—use small bite-size pieces.
- Avoid eating food requiring prolonged chewing, e.g. hard crusts of bread, tough meat, raw vegetables.
- Avoid chewing gum.
- Always try to open your jaw in a hinge or arc motion. Do not protrude your jaw.

- Avoid clenching your teeth together—keep your lips together and your teeth apart.
- Try to breathe through your nose at all times.
- Do not sleep on your jaw—try to sleep on your back.
- Practice a relaxed lifestyle so that your jaws and face muscles feel relaxed.

For the nagging problem

Once the acute phase has settled it is best to strengthen the muscles and joints by performing a set of exercises. They are uncomfortable at first, but the problem usually starts to settle after about 2 weeks.

'Chewing' the piece of soft wood exercise

- Obtain a rod of soft wood about 15 cm long and 1.5 cm wide. An ideal object is a large carpenters pencil.
- Position this at the back of the mouth so that the molars (back teeth) grasp the object with the jaw thrust forward.
- Rhythmically bite on the object with a grinding movement for 2 to 3 minutes. Do this at least 3 times a day.

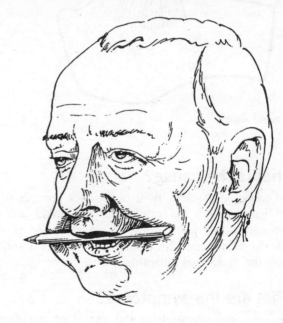

'Chewing the wood' exercise

John Murtagh, *Patient Education*, Second edition, McGraw-Hill Book Company

Tennis elbow

What is tennis elbow?

Lateral epicondylitis ('tennis elbow' or 'backhand tennis elbow') is inflammation of an important forearm muscle tendon at the point of attachment to the outer side of the elbow bone. Tennis players are not the only sufferers. It is common in golfers, carpenters, bricklayers, violinists and housewives, especially those between 35 and 55 years of age.

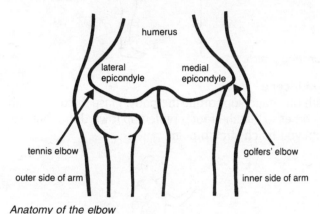

Anatomy of the elbow

What causes it?

Tennis elbow is the result of repeated bending and twisting movements of the arm, such as when playing golf and tennis, using a screwdriver, wringing wet clothes, carrying buckets or picking up bricks. It affects tennis players who use a lot of wrist action in a faulty backhand movement, especially when they are unfit. The force of the ball hitting the racquet is greater than the strength of the muscle; the muscles of the forearm thus become overstrained. The strains, initially painless, cause small tears in the tendon. As they start to heal, more tears occur and painful inflamed scar tissue forms.

What are the symptoms?

The outer bony projection of the elbow (the *lateral epicondyle*) is painful. For some people the pain is constant and can interfere with sleep.

The forearm aches with grasping and lifting movements such as pouring tea, turning stiff handles, ironing clothes and typing. Even simple things like picking up a glass, shaking hands or brushing teeth can cause pain.

What is the treatment?

Tennis elbow is stubborn to treat but almost always curable. The two bases of treatment are:
- rest (avoiding the cause, e.g. stop playing tennis)
- exercise (to strengthen the forearm muscles, which bend the wrist)

Your general practitioner might recommend a cortisone injection to speed recovery. Sometimes it can take 1–2 years to heal.

Exercises

Use a dumbbell or similar type of weight such as a bucket of water. Start with 0.5 kg (1 lb) and build up gradually to 5 kg.

1. Sit in a chair beside a table.
2. Rest your arm on the table so that the wrist is over the edge.
3. With your palm facing downwards, grasp the weight.
4. Slowly raise and lower the weight 12 times. Rest for 1 minute.
5. Repeat twice.

Do the exercise every day until you can play tennis, work or use your forearm without pain.

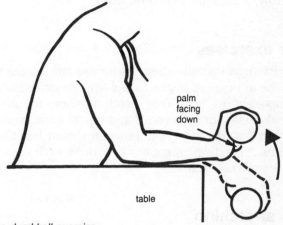

The dumbbell exercise

The towel-wringing exercise

This hurts at first, but usually cures the problem by 6 weeks. Roll up a handtowel and, with your arms straight, grasp the towel, then wring it slowly so that your wrist is fully bent forwards. Hold for 10 seconds, then reverse the wringing action to extend your wrist; hold for 10 seconds. Gradually, increase the time by 5 seconds until you can hold for 60 seconds. Do this twice a day, twice in each direction. Many people prefer to do this exercise using a large face washer while showering.

Tennis

Do not use a tightly strung, heavy racquet or heavy tennis balls. Keep your strokes smooth and try not to bend the elbow. Start the game quietly, taking time to warm up to it.

The 'other' tennis elbow

Medial epicondylitis ('forehand tennis elbow', 'golfers' elbow' or 'pitchers' elbow') is less common and usually less severe. The treatment is the same, but the palm must face upwards for the dumbbell exercise.

Armbands

Some tennis players use a non-stretch band or brace around the arm, about 7.5 cm (3 inches) below the elbow. You might not find it helpful, but it is worth trying. Bands are available from (some) pharmacists, tennis shops and orthopaedic appliance firms.

Warm-up exercises for the legs

The aim of the warm-up period for all athletes is to ensure top performance and reduce the chance of injury, especially early in a sporting event.

- The warm-up should begin with 10 minutes of slower, easier activity such as slow jogging, running on the spot, skipping or cycling.
- The stretching exercises should be gentle at first and should not overstrain or tire or be painful.
- The leg exercises are in addition to general exercises for other parts of the body.
- Ideally, a tracksuit should be worn.

The exercises

The drawings illustrate stretches for the left leg. Stretch until the muscle just begins to feel tight (*stretch point*). It is important to hold the stretch position for 20–30 seconds, relax for 10 seconds and repeat each exercise for each leg. The stretching program should last 10–20 minutes. A practical program is to perform each exercise 2 or 3 times on each leg.

Hip stretching

Adductors

Stand with your feet apart. Bend one knee while keeping the other straight. Bend until a stretch is felt in the groin and inner thigh (stretch point).

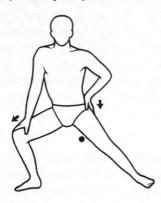

Adductor stretch

Flexors (iliopsoas)

Lie on your side. Grab the ankle of the uppermost leg with your hand. Pull the ankle backwards and slightly to the side.

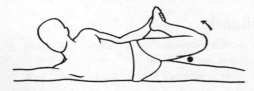

Flexor stretch

Thigh stretching

Hamstrings

Place the heel of the left leg on a low table or chair. Keep the knee straight. Reach forwards with both hands until you reach stretch point.

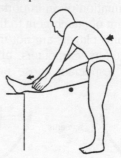

Hamstring stretch

Quadriceps

With one hand supporting the body, grasp the ankle with the other so that the foot is pulled up towards the buttock until you reach stretch point.

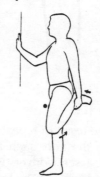

Quadriceps stretch

Calf/Achilles tendon stretching

Calf muscles

1. Stand about 1.5 m from the wall and lean against it. Keep your left knee straight and your left foot flat on the floor. Bend your right knee forwards until you reach stretch point.

2. Stand in a similar position, but bend the left knee so that stretch is felt deeper and lower in the leg.

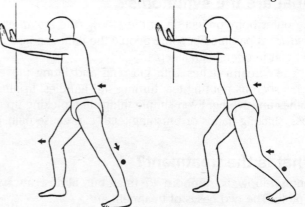

Calf muscle stretch 1   *Calf muscle stretch 2*

> It is very important to *warm down* by repeating the gentle stretching exercises and jogging for several minutes after sporting activity.

John Murtagh, *Patient Education*, Second edition, McGraw-Hill Book Company

11 Common general problems

Alcohol: harmful use of alcohol

What is 'problem drinking'?

People are said to be dependent on alcohol when it is affecting their physical health and social life yet they do not seem to be prepared to stop drinking to solve their problems.

For men, excessive drinking is more than 4 standard drinks of alcohol a day.

For women, drinking becomes a problem at lesser amounts—2 standard drinks a day.

High-risk or harmful drinking occurs at more than 6 drinks a day for men and 4 drinks a day for women.

Measuring your alcohol intake

One standard drink contains 10 g of alcohol, which is in 1 middy (or pot) of standard beer (285 mL), 2 middies of low-alcohol beer or 5 middies of super-light beer. These are equal in alcohol content to 1 small glass of table wine (120 mL), 1 glass of sherry or port (60 mL) or 1 nip of spirits (30 mL).

1 stubby or can of beer = 1.3 standard drinks
1 750 mL bottle of beer = 2.6 standard drinks
1 750 mL bottle of wine = 6 standard drinks

| 1 middy of standard beer (285 mL or 10 oz) | 1 glass of wine (120 mL or 4 oz) | 1 glass of sherry or port (60 mL or 2 oz) | 1 nip of spirits (30 mL or 1 oz) |

Standard drinks

The 0.05 level

To keep below 0.05 blood alcohol level, a 70 kg man or woman should not exceed:
2 standard drinks in 1 hour
3 standard drinks in 2 hours
4 standard drinks in 3 hours

What are the risks?

Heavy drinking damages the body; it may damage all the organs of the body, but will especially damage the liver, stomach, heart and brain. It will cause high blood pressure, gout and pancreatitis (inflamed pancreas). One serious effect is that some drinkers have blackouts of memory; others have blackouts during heavy drinking bouts only. At least 15% of all patients admitted to hospital have an alcohol-related illness and about 50% of fatal traffic accidents involve alcohol. It is a special problem for pregnant women, whose babies can be abnormal: more than 1 drink a day places the baby at risk.

Alcohol also interacts badly with many prescribed medicines, especially sedatives.

How can you get help?

If you experience problems related to drinking in yourself, cut down on the amount and frequency of social drinking. If you find this impossible, seek help without delay—you cannot fight it alone. When you attempt to stop, withdrawal symptoms may be a problem.

Get in touch with your family doctor or your nearest branch of Alcoholics Anonymous or Alanon. Some cities have direct telephone drug and alcohol services. The only way to solve the problem is to realise you have one, admit to it and then do something about it. Experience has shown that the key to success is to quit altogether, and for this reason the help of your family, your doctor and a caring organisation such as Alcoholics Anonymous is essential.

Golden rules to avoid hazardous drinking

- Do not drink daily.
- Aim for less than 12 drinks per week for men and 8 for women.
- Have at least 3 non-drinking days per week.
- Change to low-alcohol beer.
- Avoid drinking on an empty stomach.
- Avoid high-risk situations (e.g. constant parties).
- Mix alcoholic with non-alcoholic drinks.

What are the symptoms?

The possible symptoms or signs are as follows:

Adverse psychological and social effects	Physical effects
loss of self-esteem	brain damage (if severe)
irritability	depression
devious behaviour	insomnia—nightmares
anxiety	hypertension
paranoia	heart disease
stress	liver disease
relationship breakdown	dyspepsia (indigestion)
poor work performance	stomach ulcers
financial problems	sexual dysfunction
accidents	hand tremor
driving offences	peripheral nerve damage
crime—violence	gout
personal neglect	obesity

Anal fissure

What is an anal fissure?

It is a crack or tear at the margin of the anus that extends from the skin into the soft lining of the anus. It can affect all ages and tends to occur in women and infants.

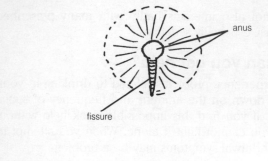

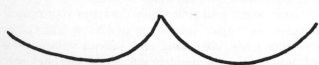

What are the symptoms?

- sharp, often severe pain on opening the bowels
- pain or discomfort when sitting on a hard surface
- spots of blood on the toilet paper or underwear

When the bowels are opened, especially for a hard or large stool, the fissure causes spasm of the circular muscle that controls the anus. The resultant pain can last for several minutes and up to an hour.

What causes an anal fissure?

The tear, which is generally small, usually develops after stretching of the anus from passing a hard, large stool. It is associated with constipation, multiple pregnancies and Crohn's disease. Anal intercourse increases the likelihood of a fissure.

What about infants?

Anal fissures in children usually occur with constipation, and possibly result in refusal to defecate. Recovery usually occurs quickly if the stool is softened. Maltogen 1% can be added to the formula, and fluids should be increased. Treatment includes applying a local anaesthetic ointment to the anus whenever the child shows a desire to defecate, until healing occurs.

What is the usual outcome?

Adults usually recover in about 4 weeks, especially if the fissure is small. More severe cases may not heal without the benefit of a small operation.

How can anal fissures be prevented?

The secret is to avoid constipation and answer nature's call to stool when it comes instead of putting it off. Stools are kept soft by drinking several glasses of water each day, by a high fibre diet and by regular exercise. Some people may find it necessary to use laxatives such as ispaghula (Fybogel, Agiolax).

What is the treatment?

- Prevent constipation; keep the stool soft.
- Gently clean the anus with cottonwool and warm water after each bowel movement.
- Apply a towel soaked in very warm water for painful spasm or take a sitz bath (20 cm of warm water with a small amount of added salt in the bathtub) for about 20 minutes twice a day.
- Take analgesics such as aspirin or paracetamol for pain.
- Apply petroleum jelly (Vaseline) or zinc oxide ointment around the anus to soothe the area.
- A special ointment containing local anaesthetic is usually prescribed by your doctor to relieve discomfort.

Surgical treatment

If the fissure persists despite all the above attention, some minor procedures will certainly allow it to heal quickly in a few days. This may involve stretching the anus under anaesthetic or cutting the anal sphincter (muscle) under local anaesthetic.

John Murtagh, *Patient Education*, Second edition, McGraw-Hill Book Company

Angina

What is angina?

Angina (also known as *angina pectoris*) is the name given to pain in the chest that comes from the heart when it is short of oxygen. The heart is a large muscle that pumps blood about every second, and if it cannot get enough oxygen from its own blood supply (the coronary arteries) it will develop a 'cramping' pain rather like a cramp in the calf of the leg. The main cause of angina is a narrowing of the coronary arteries by a fat-like deposit called *atheroma*. It is a common problem and affects nearly half a million Australians.

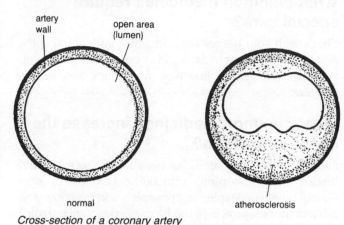

Cross-section of a coronary artery

What are the symptoms?

Angina is typically a dull, heavy discomfort or pain in the centre of the chest. It has been described as 'pressure', 'tightness', 'heaviness' and 'like indigestion'. The pain can spread to the neck (throat), the jaw, the back or the arms (usually the left arm).

Additional symptoms may include shortness of breath, sweating, nausea and tiredness.

What brings on angina?

Angina characteristically appears during physical activity and fades away when the exertion stops. It can also be brought on by highly emotional situations (e.g. anger, fright, excitement), cold weather or after a heavy meal. People who smoke heavily or are overweight are more likely to suffer from angina.

What are the risk factors for angina?

Smoking, high blood pressure, a high blood cholesterol level, obesity and diabetes increase the risk of getting angina. There is also a tendency for it to run in families.

Is angina dangerous?

Angina is a symptom that serves as a warning that the muscle of the heart is not getting enough blood and there is a risk of a heart attack. Angina does not usually cause any damage to the heart.

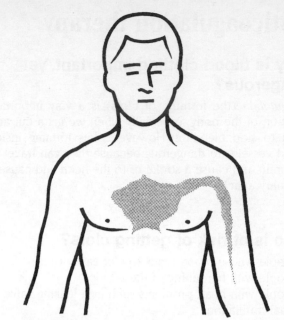

Commonest site of the pain of angina

What tests can be done?

Sometimes it is difficult to be sure that chest pain is true angina, and so an ECG (electrocardiogram) may help the diagnosis. The ECG can be performed while you are lying down (the *resting* ECG) or when stressed, such as cycling on a stationary bike (the *stress* ECG). If surgery is being considered, the state of the coronary arteries can be determined by special X-rays. All patients should be tested for high blood cholesterol.

What is the treatment?

Self-help
- If you smoke, stop.
- If you are overweight, go on a sensible diet.
- If you are inactive, take on an activity such as walking for 20 minutes a day.
- If you are tense and stressed, cultivate a more relaxed attitude to life.

Medical help
There are many tablets that can help. Anginine, which dissolves under the tongue, or a spray of the same substance under the tongue, relieves the pain. It is usual to take half an aspirin tablet each day. Your doctor will advise you about these tablets and other medication.

What are the warning signs of angina?

Patients usually cope well with their angina by using a disciplined approach to life. However, there are some warning signs that mean that the problem is worse than usual and your doctor should be notified:
- angina that lasts longer than 10 minutes
- angina pain that is more severe than normal
- Anginine tablets (up to 3) not easing the pain
- angina becoming more frequent for no apparent reason
- pain coming on at rest for the first time
- new symptoms, such as sweatiness and breathlessness

John Murtagh, *Patient Education*, Second edition, McGraw-Hill Book Company

Anticoagulation therapy

Why is blood clotting important, yet dangerous?

Coagulation (the forming of clots) is a very important function of the body, especially when we get a cut and need to stop bleeding. However, clots forming inside blood vessels are dangerous because they can travel to the brain and cause a stroke or to the heart and cause a coronary attack.

Who is at risk of getting clots?

- people whose blood tends to clot easily (rare)
- people with hardening of the arteries
- people with heart problems such as a leaking valve or atrial fibrillation
- those who have just undergone surgery and are lying idle in bed, who are liable to develop clots (*thrombosis*) in the deep veins of the leg, which can travel to the heart
- those recovering from a heart attack (coronary)

What is anticoagulation?

This is the process of preventing clots in the blood by giving substances that tend to 'thin' the blood by neutralising one of the clotting mechanisms. These substances are called *anticoagulants*. Important types are heparin (given by injection) and warfarin (given orally).

How is anticoagulation regulated?

Thinning of the blood has to be carefully and safely done; otherwise, uncontrolled bleeding (*haemorrhaging*) could develop. The level of thinness is controlled by blood tests. The amount of medication is worked out from these blood tests. Different people require different doses, and so the dose is tailored for each patient.

How should anticoagulants be taken?

The first dose of warfarin is worked out and usually is 10 mg for the first day. The dosage each day is worked out according to a formula that relies on blood testing called the *international normalised ratio* (INR). The tablets should be taken every day at around the same time. Your doctor or laboratory will advise you about the dose.

What about missed tablets?

It is important not to miss taking your tablets, and you should develop a system of taking them at around the same time each day. If you miss a dose, *do not take a double dose*, but take your next dose when it is due.

What should you remember about the INR blood test?

1. Make sure it is done when ordered by your doctor.
2. Call your doctor or laboratory within 24 hours of the test just in case the dose needs adjusting.
3. Record the INR results in the record card provided.

What factors can affect warfarin?

- *Your diet*: It needs to be healthy and balanced.
- *Alcohol*: Use it in moderation and avoid binge drinking.
- *Other medications*: Check with your doctor.

What common medicines require special care?

Check with your doctor regarding the oral contraceptive pill, pain-killers such as aspirin, cough or cold preparations, antacids or laxatives, antibiotics and various vitamins.

What common medicines increase the effect of warfarin?

allopurinol, alcohol, amiodarone, anabolic steroids, antibiotics (most), aspirin, cimetidine, clofibrate, gemfibrozil, metronidazole, miconazole, non-steroidal anti-inflammatories, proton-pump blockers (e.g. omeprazole), phenytoin, quinine or quinidine, ranitidine, salicylates, tamoxifen, thyroxine

What common medicines decrease the effect of warfarin?

antacids, antihistamines, barbiturates, cholestyramine, diuretics, haloperidol, oestrogen, oral contraceptives, vitamin C

What signs of bleeding should you report?

black motions, blood in the urine (red or pink), easy bruising, unusual nose or gum bleeds, unusually heavy periods, unexpected bleeding after minor injury

---

Remember

- Keep to a consistent diet.
- Do not take aspirin or liquid paraffin.
- Always mention that you take warfarin to any doctor or dentist treating you.
- Take tablets strictly as directed without fail and have your blood tests.
- Take the tablets at the same time each day.
- Do not take a double dose.
- Advise your doctor of any illness.
- Avoid pregnancy.

John Murtagh, *Patient Education*, Second edition, McGraw-Hill Book Company

Anxiety

What is anxiety?

Anxiety is an uncomfortable inner feeling of fear or imminent disaster. Most of us experience some temporary degree of anxiety in our lives, sometimes with just cause and at other times without. It can be a common normal human reaction to stress, and being anxious over appropriate things may help to make us more responsible, caring people. Some people, however, are constantly anxious to the extent that it is abnormal and interferes with their lives. Severe cases of anxiety can lead to panic attacks or hyperventilation.

What are the symptoms?

The symptoms can vary enormously from feeling tense and tired to panic attacks. Symptoms include:
- tiredness or fatigue
- dry mouth, difficulty swallowing
- apprehension: 'something awful will happen'
- sleep disturbances and nightmares
- irritability
- muscle tension/headache
- rapid heart rate and breathing
- sweating
- trembling
- diarrhoea
- flare-up of an illness (e.g. dermatitis, asthma)
- sexual problems

What are the risks?

Various physical illnesses—such as high blood pressure, coronary disease, asthma and perhaps cancer—can be related to persistent stress and anxiety. It may aggravate a drug problem such as smoking and drinking excessively. It can cause a breakdown in relationships and work performance. It can lead to the serious disorder of depression. Because an overactive thyroid can mimic an anxiety state, it is important not to overlook it.

What is the treatment?
Self-help
It is best to avoid drugs if possible and to look at factors in your lifestyle that cause you stress and anxiety and modify or remove them (if possible). Be on the lookout for solutions. Examples are changing jobs and keeping away from people or situations that upset you. Sometimes confronting people and talking things over will help.

Special advice
Be less of a perfectionist: do not be a slave to the clock; do not bottle things up; stop feeling guilty; approve of yourself and others; express yourself and your anger. Resolve all personal conflicts. Make friends and be happy. Keep a positive outlook on life, and be moderate and less intense in your activities.

Seek a balance of activities, such as recreation, meditation, reading, rest, exercise and family/social activities.

Relaxation
Learn to relax your mind and body: seek out special relaxation programs such as yoga and meditation.

Make a commitment to yourself to spend some time every day practising relaxation. About 20 minutes twice a day is ideal, but you might want to start with only 10 minutes.
- Sit in a quiet place with your eyes closed, but remain alert and awake if you can. Focus your mind on the different muscle groups in your body, starting at the forehead and slowly going down to the toes. Relax the muscles as much as you can.
- Pay attention to your breathing: listen to the sound of your breath for the next few minutes. Breathe in and out slowly and deeply.
- Next, begin to repeat the word 'relax' silently in your mind at your own pace. When other thoughts distract, calmly return to the word 'relax'.
- Just 'let go': this is a quiet time for yourself, in which the stresses in body and mind are balanced or reduced.

Medication
Doctors tend to recommend tranquillisers only as a last resort or to help you cope with a very stressful temporary period when your anxiety is severe and you cannot cope without extra help. Tranquillisers can be very effective if used sensibly and for short periods.

Recommended reading

Herbert Benson, *The Relaxation Response*, Collins, London, 1984.

Dale Carnegie, *How to Stop Worrying and Start Living*, Rev. edn, ed. Dorothy Carnegie, Angus & Robertson, Sydney, 1985.

Ainslie Meares, *Relief without Drugs*, Fontana, Glasgow, 1983.

Norman Peale, *The Power of Positive Thinking*, Cedar, London, 1982.

Claire Weekes, *Peace from Nervous Suffering*, Angus & Robertson, London, 1972.

Claire Weekes, *Self-Help for your Nerves*, Angus & Robertson, London, 1976.

Aphthous ulcers

What are aphthous ulcers?

These are very painful ulcers that arise in the lining of the mouth, usually in the gums between the lower lip and teeth. The small hole on the surface exposes the sensitive tissue beneath. These mouth ulcers are not herpes infections or cancerous.

What do they look like?

The ulcers are small (about 2–3 mm across), shallow and yellow or grey in colour. Each ulcer is surrounded by a bright red halo.

Who gets aphthous ulcers?

Any person can get the ulcers. However, they occur most often in adolescents and young adults and tend to occur more often in women, especially just before a period. Aphthous ulcers are very common and affect at least 1 person in 10.

What causes aphthous ulcers?

The cause is not precisely known. One theory is that a virus or bacteria is able to ulcerate the gum surface when the immune system is below par. Known associations for this are:
- emotional or physical stress
- being 'run down'
- premenstrual tension
- injury such as from rough dentures, dental work, hot food, toothbrushing or biting the mouth
- irritation from certain foods such as citrus fruits, salted nuts, acid foods and chocolate

What are the symptoms?

The first thing you usually notice is eating something acidic (such as a grapefruit or spicy food) that makes the ulcer smart. Sometimes there is burning or tingling for several hours beforehand. The ulcers may be so painful for the first 3 days that they make eating or speaking most uncomfortable.

What is the usual outcome?

Aphthous ulcers are not a serious problem. Most ulcers heal without scarring within 10–14 days. Recurrent attacks of ulcers are quite common in some people. Any ulcer that lasts beyond 3 weeks is unusual. If the doctor is concerned about an ulcer, a blood test or biopsy may be taken.

What is the management?

In most cases the ulcer will heal without any treatment and only feel uncomfortable for 3–4 days. If the ulcer has a known cause, such as a jagged tooth or rough denture, your dentist should be consulted. Some patients simply 'grin and bear it' and wait for healing to occur without applying any agents to the ulcer; they may just take mild pain-killers. Many choose to have treatment to relieve the discomfort.

Eating and drinking
- Avoid eating spicy or sharp-tasting acidic foods (e.g. grapefruit, vinegar).
- Avoid any foods that aggravate the ulcer.
- Drink plenty of fluids and eat soft foods such as yoghurt, ice-cream and custard.
- Reduce the pain by sipping liquids through straws.

Pain relief
Apply a topical anaesthetic such as lignocaine gel or paint (e.g. SM-33 adult paint formula or SM-33 gel for children every 3 hours). This helps eating if applied before meals.

Healing methods
There are several methods that can help healing. One simple method is to rinse the mouth regularly with a salt solution (1 teaspoon to 500 mL of warm water). One of the following can be tried during the painful period of the ulcer.
- *The teabag method*: Apply a wet, squeezed out, black teabag directly to the ulcer 3–4 times daily. The tannic acid promotes healing.
- *Topical steroid paste*: Apply triamcinolone 0.1% (Kenalog in orabase) paste as soon as the ulcer appears, 3–4 times a day.
- *Topical steroid spray*: The sprays used to treat asthma (such as beclomethasone) can be sprayed onto the ulcer 3 times a day.
- *Tetracycline suspension rinse for several ulcers*: Empty the contents of a 250 mg tetracycline capsule into 20–30 mL of warm water and shake it. Swirl this solution in the mouth for 5 minutes every 3 hours. This has a terrible taste and should be spat out after rinsing.

John Murtagh, *Patient Education*, Second edition, McGraw-Hill Book Company

Asthma

What is asthma?

Asthma is a common chest condition in which there is temporary narrowing of the breathing tubes in the lungs (airways) because they are hyperreactive (oversensitive). In asthma these tubes have inflammation and swelling of their linings, increased mucus inside, tightening of the muscles in their walls and therefore less flow of air in and out.

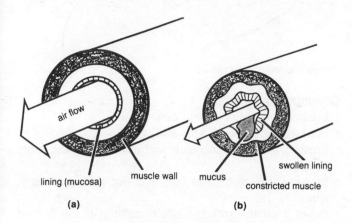

(a) Normal airway; (b) airway in asthma

What causes an attack?

No single cause has been found, but a variety of factors may trigger an attack. A check list of trigger factors is:
- infections, especially colds
- allergies (e.g. to animal fur, feathers, pollens, mould)
- house dust, especially the dust mites
- cigarette smoke; other smoke and fumes
- sudden changes in weather or temperature
- occupational irritants (e.g. wood dust, synthetic sprays, chemicals)
- drugs (e.g. aspirin, drugs to treat arthritis, heart problems and glaucoma)
- certain foods and food additives
- exercise, especially in a cold atmosphere
- emotional upsets or stress

What are the symptoms?

The main symptoms are breathlessness, tightness in the chest, wheezing and coughing (especially at night).

Severe asthma

Symptoms or signs of very severe asthma are anxiety, blue colour of the lips (*cyanosis*), ashen grey colour of the skin, fast pulse, rapid breathing, indrawing of the chest wall, difficulty speaking, no response to asthma medication and feeling very sick. These uncommon severe symptoms mean that you should seek urgent medical attention—they are 'call the ambulance' signs.

How common is asthma?

About 1 child in 4 or 5 has asthma, usually in a mild form. It usually comes on between the ages of 2 and 7. Most children 'grow out of it' by puberty, but a small number get it again as adults. Others continue with it. About 1 in 10 adults has asthma.

What are the risks?

Severe asthma can retard the growth of children, but the biggest worry (although uncommon) is the number of deaths (including sudden deaths), especially in those who do not realise how severe the attack really is. With correct treatment, almost all children should be able to lead normal lives.

What is the treatment?

Prevention of attacks is the best treatment, and all asthmatics and their families should aim to know the disorder very well and become expert in it.

Know your asthma
- Read all about it.
- Try to identify trigger factors and avoid them.
- Become expert at using your medicine and inhalers. A big problem is incorrect inhaler technique (35% of patients).
- Know and recognise the danger signs and act promptly.
- Have regular checks with your doctor.
- Have physiotherapy: learn breathing exercises.
- Work out a clear management plan and an action plan for when trouble strikes.
- Learn the value of a peak expiratory flow meter (for anyone over 6).
- Always carry your bronchodilator inhaler and check that it is not empty. (Learn about the water flotation test.)

Stay at your best

If you need medications, these should be as simple, safe and effective as possible. This is why inhaled medications are most often used for asthma. There are basically two types of inhaled medication that your doctor might advise you to use:
- the 'preventor' (such as Becotide, Aldecin, Pulmicort or Intal)
- the 'reliever' (such as Bricanyl, Respolin, Ventolin or Atrovent), which is called a *bronchodilator*

Key points

- Get to know how severe your asthma is.
- Avoid trigger factors such as tobacco smoke.
- Keep at your best with suitable medicines.
- Get urgent help when danger signs appear.
- Have an action plan for severe asthma.
- Use your inhalers correctly and use a spacer if necessary.
- Get a peak flow meter to help assess severity and work out your best lung function.

Asthma: correct use of your aerosol inhaler

Did you know that 90% of the medication from metered dose inhalers (also known as puffers) sticks to your mouth and does not reach your lungs?

Why all the fuss about inhalers?

It is very important to use your inhaler correctly so that the medication in the spray reaches deep into your lungs to treat your asthma. A faulty inhaler technique is a common cause for medication not working properly. It is important to know that it is your *inhalation* effort—*not* the pressure from the aerosol pushing in—that gets the medication into your lungs. Why not ask your doctor to check your use of your inhaler?

What are the two main techniques?

The *open mouth technique* and the *closed mouth technique* are the main techniques, and both are effective. Choose the technique that suits you best.

Both techniques are suitable for most adults. Most children from age 7 can learn to use puffers quite well.

The open mouth technique

1. Remove the cap. Shake the puffer vigorously for 1–2 seconds. Hold it upright (canister on top) to use it (as shown).
2. Hold the mouthpiece of the puffer 4–5 cm (about 3 fingers' breadth) away from your mouth.
3. Tilt your head back slightly with your chin up. Open your mouth and keep it open.
4. Slowly blow out to a comfortable level.
5. Just as you then start to breathe in (slowly) through your mouth, press the puffer firmly, once. Breathe in as far as you can over 3–5 seconds. (Do not breathe in through your nose.)
6. Close your mouth and hold your breath for about 10 seconds; then breathe out gently.
7. Breathe normally for about 1 minute, and then repeat the inhalation.

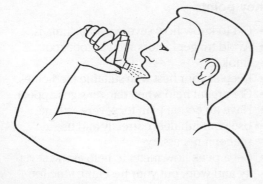

The open mouth method

The closed mouth technique

The method is basically identical to the open mouth technique except that you close your lips around the mouthpiece.

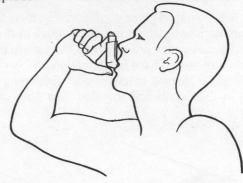

The closed mouth method

Common mistakes

- holding the puffer upside down
- holding the puffer too far away
- pressing the puffer too early and not inhaling the spray deeply
- pressing the puffer too late and not getting enough spray
- doing it all too quickly: not breathing in slowly and holding your breath
- squeezing the puffer more than once
- not breathing in deeply

Large volume spacers

Some people who have trouble using inhalers can have a special 'spacer' fitted onto the mouthpiece of the inhaler. 1 or 2 puffs of the aerosol are put in the spacer. Then you breathe in from its mouthpiece. Take 1 deep inhalation then 1–2 normal breaths, *or* take 4–6 normal sized breaths. This method is useful for adults having trouble with the puffer and for younger children (older than 3). Spacers are very efficient and cause less irritation of the mouth and throat.

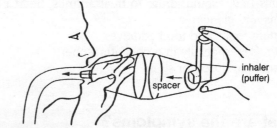

inhaler (puffer)

spacer

Using a spacer

Extra points

1. The usual dose of a standard metered dose aerosol is 1 or 2 puffs every 3–4 hours for an attack.
2. If you do not get adequate relief from your normal dose, you should contact your doctor.
3. It is quite safe to increase the dose, such as to 4–6 puffs.
4. If you are using your inhaler very often, it usually means your other asthma medication is not effective or is not being used properly. Discuss this with your doctor.

John Murtagh, *Patient Education*, Second edition, McGraw-Hill Book Company

Asthma: dangerous asthma

What are the symptoms and signs?

Failure to recognise the development of a severe asthma attack has cost the lives of many people. Most people cope with their asthma nicely, but doctors are concerned about the fact that some die when it could be prevented.

Asthma has to be treated with great care. The more you know about it, the better you can recognise danger.

Who are likely to be at high risk?

People who have experienced one or more of the following are more likely to have a severe attack:

- a previous severe asthma attack
- previous hospital admission, especially if to intensive care
- hospital attendance in the past 12 months
- long-term oral steroid treatment
- carelessness with taking medication
- night-time attacks, especially with severe chest tightness
- recent emotional problems

Remember that severe attacks can start suddenly (even in mild asthmatics) and catch you by surprise.

Why is peak expiratory flow measurement important?

People who have moderate to severe asthma should obtain a *peak expiratory flow* (PEF) meter and measure their PEF. It tells you how well your lungs are working by measuring the amount of air moving through the airways. It is very simple to use. Anyone older than 7 years can test PEF accurately. You should measure your PEF in the morning and at night before inhaling your bronchodilator, and then 10 minutes after. Do this 3 times for each test.

Warning signs using PEF are:

- falling of your PEF and poor control
- readings less than 70% of your normal best
- readings less than 100 L/min
- more morning dipping than normal
- erratic readings
- less response to your bronchodilator than normal

What are the early warning signs of severe asthma or an asthma attack?

- symptoms persisting or getting worse despite adequate medication
- increased coughing and chest tightness
- poor response to 2 inhalations
- benefit from inhalations not lasting 2 hours
- increasing medication requirements
- sleep being disturbed by coughing, wheezing or breathlessness
- chest tightness on waking in the morning
- low peak expiratory flow readings

Contact your doctor if these problems are present.

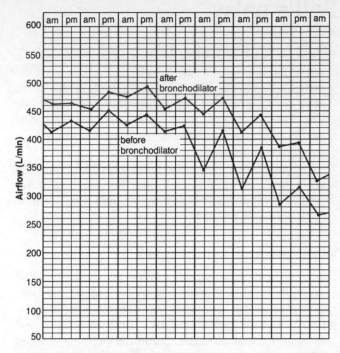

Typical peak expiratory flow record showing signs of worsening asthma

What are the really dangerous signs?

Any of the following problems tell us that asthma is 'out of control':

- marked breathlessness, especially at rest
- sleep being greatly disturbed by asthma
- asthma getting worse quickly rather than slowly, despite medication
- feeling frightened
- difficulty in speaking: unable to say more than a few words
- exhaustion
- drowsiness or 'not with it' feeling
- chest becoming 'silent' with a quiet wheeze, yet breathing still laboured
- blue or blue-grey colour
- chest wall drawing in
- respiratory rate greater than 25 (adults) or 50 (children)

Action plan

If any of these are present, *immediately*:
- Call an ambulance and say 'severe asthma attack' (*best option*).
  or
- Call your doctor.
  or
- If you are having trouble finding medical help, get someone to drive you to the nearest hospital.

Keep using your bronchodilator inhaler continuously if you are distressed.

Bell's palsy

What is Bell's palsy?

It is a condition where the muscles on one side of the face become paralysed because of a fault in the nerve (called the *facial nerve*) that controls those muscles. We are not certain what causes this problem, although a viral infection affecting the nerve or the nearby ear may be a cause in some instances.

The facial nerve leaves the brain through a very small hole in the base of the skull near the ear. The nerve becomes swollen, and because of the tight fit in this hole it does not work properly.

What are the symptoms?

The main symptom, which comes on quite suddenly (maybe overnight), is weakness of one side of the face. The corner of the mouth droops, the eye cannot close properly and actions of the face such as smiling and frowning look out of shape. Some ear pain may be felt just before the problem develops. Drooling of saliva may also occur.

How common is Bell's palsy?

Each year about 1 person in 2000 gets Bell's palsy. It can occur at any age, but is most common in young adults.

What is the outcome?

Although scary, Bell's palsy is usually not a serious or permanent problem. At least 90% make a good recovery. The slow and steady recovery takes about 6 months. Operations to help correct the problem are used occasionally for those rare cases where recovery is not complete.

What is the treatment?

The palsy usually recovers without special treatment. If you see the doctor as soon as it develops, a course of steroid tablets may be prescribed.

Care of the eye

If your eye cannot close fully, it is important to protect it from injury such as dust and grit by wearing goggles and putting a patch over the eye at night. The eye should not be allowed to dry, and artificial tears are usually prescribed. Report any unusual pain in your eye immediately.

Massage and exercises

Massaging and exercising the facial muscles may help recovery. Using oil or cream, massage the muscles of the forehead, cheek, eyes and lips. Exercise these muscles in front of a mirror by screwing up the eyes tightly to close them, smiling widely, baring the teeth and winking.

Heat treatment

If you have pain in the face, apply heat 3 times a day to the painful area. Wring out a face washer after soaking it in hot water and apply for 10 minutes. Make sure your eye is closed or covered.

General care

Continue your normal activities, but choose a good lifestyle by getting plenty of rest and sleep, avoiding smoking and excess alcohol.

Look after your teeth: brush and floss your teeth more often.

Keep a positive outlook on life. Remember that your somewhat embarrassing problem should soon settle.

John Murtagh, *Patient Education*, Second edition, McGraw-Hill Book Company

Bereavement

When a loved one dies, the bereaved person invariably goes through a predictable human process of grieving.

The extent of the reaction will depend on circumstances such as the suddenness and unexpectedness of the death. It will depend also on the age of the deceased and the bereaved, and other factors such as personal, family, national or religious customs and habits. However, no matter what the circumstances, the bereaved will suffer a reaction and the emotions described here are regarded as normal responses.

The first stage
'Shock' or disbelief

The immediate reaction is for you to simply feel numb and empty. For a short time you may feel and behave almost as though nothing has happened—everything is a blur—but eventually extreme grief may take over. During this first stage, delusions of seeing or speaking with the dead person may occur: although this may disturb you, the experiences are normal. There is also a tendency to forget that the person is dead and act as though he or she were alive. You will find it difficult to concentrate and may give vent to spontaneous emotions such as crying, screaming or even laughing.

The second stage
Grief and despair

At this stage the loss of your loved one will really hit you. This sense of loss is reinforced by loneliness, by constant reminders of lost habits and experiences, and by the clothes and other personal effects left behind. You will feel intensely sad and lonely. Friends and acquaintances will not visit you so much now and, in fact, many will feel uncomfortable and embarrassed about approaching you. It is important that you understand this problem. You may actually feel like withdrawing from people.

The sense of presence of the deceased will continue. Two common feelings, anger and guilt, will also surface.

Anger

This may include anger towards those considered responsible for the death and even at the deceased for dying. Your resentfulness may include blaming and accusing the medical attendants of neglect. You will feel like talking a lot about your loved one, and you will probably recall all the vivid memories leading up to the death and constantly churn them over in your mind. Common recurring thoughts include:
- 'Why did it happen to me?'
- 'If only "so and so" had been done, it would be different.'

Guilt and self-blame

You may feel guilty because you did not do more for the person or take more notice of him or her. Such guilt feelings and intense grief are commoner when the death is unexpected. It is important that you do not feel too badly about any apparent neglect on your part—the 'if only I had' feeling.

The feeling of intense grief usually lasts about 6 weeks and the second stage of grief for about 6 months, but it can resurface every now and then over the next few years. During the last 4 months or so of this stage you will feel sad and helpless, then pass into a state of apathy and depression (the third stage).

The third stage
Adaptation or acceptance

After about 6 months you will begin to accept your severe loss. You develop a change in living habits by taking up new roles and activities. You can face up better to disposing of personal effects, establishing new relationships and attending to financial arrangements.

This phase takes a year or so and requires considerable understanding by all concerned. However, the feelings of apathy and depression can be a problem. Physical illness is common and includes problems such as insomnia, wheezing, diarrhoea and stomach pains. It is important to consult your doctor about any worrying physical or mental problems. Despite this, you will adapt and eventually learn to cope.

Self-help

First, you must realise that it is normal to pass through these stages of grieving, and so you cannot fight it. A bereaved person should always try to acknowledge his or her loss and not 'shut it out'. Talking about the deceased to relatives and friends and sorting out the person's possessions will help enormously in coming to terms with your loss, even though it may be painful at first. At the beginning it is good, if possible, to see the dead person, touch them if you want to, attend the funeral and give expression to your emotions.

If you have doubts about the exact cause of death, make sure that you discuss it with your doctor as soon as possible.

If you have prolonged intense grief feelings, make sure that you get professional help. Avoid visiting spiritualists: they seem to aggravate the problem.

You may find considerable support from others who have suffered a similar loss and from various self-help organisations. Most people find that it is helpful to have a break away from the home, especially staying with sympathetic friends or relatives in a different area or in another state.

The first anniversary of a death or the first Christmas spent alone can be a very difficult time, and so it is good to make arrangements to have company at that time.

Bites and stings

Bites and stings from animals, spiders and insects in Australia are commonplace, but fatal bites are uncommon. In fact, only 1 in 20 bites from the funnel-web spider causes a serious problem. The following information is a summary of first aid treatment for some bites and stings.

Snake bites

First aid

1. Keep the patient quite still.
2. Do not wash or cut the wound.
3. Immediately bandage the bite site very firmly, but not too tightly. A crepe bandage is ideal; it should extend above the bite for about 15 cm.
4. Place the limb that has been bitten in a splint: use a firm stick or slab of wood.
5. Get the patient to the nearest doctor or major hospital without delay. If possible, take the dead snake along too.

Tick bites

Ticks may lodge anywhere in the body of humans and their bite can be fatal, especially in children.

First aid

Do not attempt to pull the tick out by grasping the body. Take the patient to someone who is expert at removing them. If this is not possible, loop a strong thread around the tick's head close to the skin and pull it sharply sideways.

Blue-ringed octopus stings

Children playing in small rock pools around sea shores are most likely to be stung.

First aid

Seek medical attention immediately. Mouth-to-mouth resuscitation may be necessary.

Spider bites

The Sydney funnel-web and the red-back spiders are the most dangerous. Unlike bites from snakes, spider bites are painful.

First aid

The first aid for the Sydney funnel-web is exactly the same as for snake bites. For red-back spider bites, apply an icepack but do not bandage. Then seek medical help.

Bee stings

First aid

1. Scrape the sting off sideways with a fingernail or knife blade. Do not squeeze it with the fingertips.
2. Apply ice to the sting site.
3. Rest and elevate the limb that has been stung.

Other bites and stings

These include bites from ants, wasps, bluebottles, scorpions and centipedes.

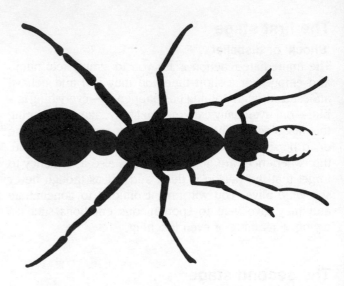

First aid

1. Wash the site with large quantities of cool water.
2. Apply vinegar or Stingose to the wound for about 30 seconds.
3. Apply ice for several minutes.
4. A soothing anti-itch cream then can be used.
5. Medicine is not usually necessary.
6. Seek medical aid if any unusual problems develop.

> **Note**
>
> The box jellyfish (sea wasp) in tropical waters is very dangerous. Liberal amounts of vinegar should be applied as soon as possible.

John Murtagh, *Patient Education*, Second edition, McGraw-Hill Book Company

Body odour

Body odour is an unpleasant smell that is a social embarrassment for many people.

What causes body odour?

It is usually caused by a combination of inadequate or incorrect attention to personal hygiene and excessive perspiration from the armpits and groin. The old saying 'Make sure you do an APC (armpits and crotch) wash' is sound advice. Certain types of bacteria that are present on our skin can cause a strong odour in some people who perspire heavily.

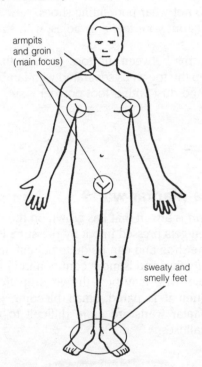

armpits and groin (main focus)

sweaty and smelly feet

Common types of body odour

What medical conditions cause body odour?

Body odour can be caused by an infection in the vagina, by kidney failure or by taking certain social drugs such as marijuana.

What is the treatment?

There are many ways to manage body odour and come up 'smelling like a rose'.

Scrubbing the body

Thoroughly scrub the body, especially the armpits and groin, with water and a deodorant soap. A good deodorant soap is pine soap. It is preferable to scrub morning and night under the shower, since the sweat glands and bacteria are active day and night. If the soap is not working, use an antibacterial surgical scrub (which your pharmacist can supply).

Choose suitable clothes

Choose natural fabrics such as cotton and wool that absorb perspiration better than synthetics. They also allow better evaporation of the sweat from the fabric.

Keep your clothes fresh

Regular washing of clothes is important. Using the same underwear for up to seven days is a certain way to cause bad smells, so change each day, especially in the summer months. A daily change of your shirt or blouse is also advisable and regular laundering or dry-cleaning of stale coats, trousers and skirts is essential.

Underarm antiperspirant deodorants

Ask your pharmacist for the most suitable antiperspirant deodorant. Do not use a deodorant only.

Dietary advice

It is important to watch what you eat, as some foods contribute to body odour. Avoid or reduce the intake of garlic, fish, curry, onions and asparagus. Reduce your intake of caffeine (coffee, tea and cola drinks), which stimulates sweat activity.

Care of smelly feet

If your feet are sweaty and smelly, make sure that you change your socks (should be cotton or woollen) regularly. Use shoe liners such as Odor eaters or charcoal inner soles. Also use a special solution such as Driclor or Hidrosol or the new preparation Neat Feat.

Shaving hair under the arms

Shaving the hair from the armpits is certainly essential in women with a body odour problem.

Surgery

If you perspire heavily from the armpits, the sweat glands can be surgically removed by a simple procedure called *axillary wedge resection*. Ask your doctor to arrange this if necessary.

Desperate measures

If all else fails, you can try the 'old skunked dog trick' by taking a bath in dilute tomato juice. Pour 2 cups of tomato juice in your bath water and sit in it for 15 minutes before scrubbing with a deodorant soap. This is reported to be very effective.

Calluses, corns and warts on feet

Tender skin lumps on the feet are usually caused by *calluses*, *corns* or *warts*. Calluses and corns are areas of skin that have thickened due to constant pressure, while warts are viral infections.

Calluses

What is a callus?

It is simply a thickening of skin caused by some form of repeated pressure and friction. It is usually not painful but can be uncomfortable. It is common on the sole of the foot over the base of the toes. A callus can be found on any part of the body, especially the hands or the knees. When a callus is pared, normal skin is found underneath.

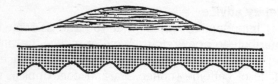

Callus

What is the treatment?

- No treatment is necessary if it is painless.
- Proper footwear is necessary to prevent calluses. Choose shoes that are wide enough and have cushioned pads over the balls of the feet.
- Paring with a scalpel blade by your doctor gives relief. (Avoid using razor blades.)
- Filing with callus files or a pumice stone wears away the callus. Soften it by soaking it in water before peeling the skin.

Corns

What is a corn?

A corn is a small tender raised lump that is round and has a hard centre. Corns usually form over the toes—over the joints, between the toes and on the outside of the little toe. Sometimes they can be very painful. Paring reveals a white circular mass of old skin.

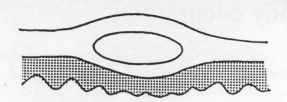

Corn

What is the treatment?

- The treatment is similar to that for a callus.
- A corn pad will reduce pressure.
- The corn can be softened with a chemical (salicylic acid) in commercial corn removers and then pared or peeled.
- Remove the source of friction if possible. Wear wide shoes—do not wear poor-fitting shoes. New shoes can be a cause, but your feet may adjust with stretching of the shoes.
- For soft corns between the toes (usually the last toe-web), keep the toe-webs separated with lamb's wool at all times and dust with a foot powder.

Warts

What is a plantar wart?

A *plantar wart* is a wart that has grown on the sole of the foot and then gets pressed into it by pressure. It feels like a stone in the shoe and can be quite painful. It is caused by a viral infection and is more common in children and young people, who may pick the virus up from public showers. When it is pared, small bleeding points are exposed. Plantar warts are more difficult to treat than corns and calluses.

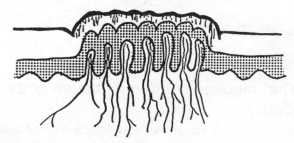

Wart

What is the treatment?

Professional help is usually needed to treat these warts. Many methods can be used, such as freezing with liquid nitrogen, application of chemicals or surgical removal. Special cushions or pads should be worn inside the shoes to relieve pressure.

John Murtagh, *Patient Education*, Second edition, McGraw-Hill Book Company

Cancer

What is cancer?

Cancer is an abnormal disorganised growth of cells in the tissues of a person. The cells multiply out of control and drain vital nutrition from the normal cells. A foetus growing in a mother's womb is a rapid growth of cells, but unlike cancer it is beautifully organised. Cancer is often referred to as a *growth*. There are two types of growth: *benign* and *malignant*. The benign type is more organised and not generally dangerous as opposed to malignant growth (cancer), which can spread from its original site to other areas of the body.

Is cancer a single disease?

No. Cancer is a group or class of diseases that share the main feature of uncontrolled cell growth.

What causes cancer?

Although we are able to identify several triggering factors (such as smoking for lung cancer, sunlight for skin cancer, and nuclear radiation for blood and other cancers), we still do not understand the how and why of what causes some cells to become malignant.

There is no hard evidence that cancer is contagious or is inherited, except for some rare cancers.

How lethal is cancer?

Cancer is still a leading cause of death, accounting for about 1 in 8 deaths of people under 35 and 1 in every 4 deaths of those over 45.

What are the common sites of cancer?

- *In men*: skin, lungs, prostate, bowel, kidneys, testes, bladder, stomach, pancreas.
- *In women*: skin, breast, bowel, lungs, reproductive organs, kidneys, bladder, stomach, pancreas.
- The 6 commonest causes of death from cancer in Australia are cancer of the bowel, lung, breast, prostate, bladder and skin (melanoma).

What are the main warning signs (common symptoms)?

- unusual bleeding or discharge
- a lump or thickening in the breast or elsewhere
- a sore that does not heal
- a change in bowel or bladder habits
- a persistent hoarseness or coughing
- persistent indigestion or difficulty in swallowing
- loss of weight
- a change in a wart or mole

Do these symptoms or signs always mean cancer?

No, not always, but it is dangerous to ignore them because the earlier the treatment (if cancer is the cause) the greater the chance of recovery. Unusual bleeding should always be treated very seriously. If you have any of these listed symptoms or any trouble that persists longer than a month, see your doctor—to be on the safe side. It probably will not be cancer—but whatever it is should be cured!

Is pain an early sign of cancer?

No, not usually. Pain is usually a very late symptom of cancer, when it has grown into the nerves. People often think that persistent pain such as headache and back pain means cancer, but this is rarely the case. However, pain should not be ignored.

Can cancer be cured?

Once cancer has spread, cures are very exceptional, but many cancers if detected and treated early (before the malignant cells have spread) can usually be completely cured. The cure rate for many cancers is steadily improving, particularly cancer of the cervix, testes, skin, large bowel, lymph glands (lymphoma) and blood (leukaemia).

What are the methods used to treat cancer?

There are many methods used to treat cancer, including surgery, chemotherapy (special drugs to destroy fast-growing cells), radiotherapy, laser therapy, cryotherapy and hormone therapy. The specialist will choose the most effective treatment for the particular cancer. It is best not to delay treatment while you try 'quack cures', but there is certainly a place for 'whole person' treatment. Some patients find benefit from meditation, good nutrition and vitamin therapy in addition to specialised treatment.

How may cancer be prevented?

Some areas worth considering (based on studies of communities where cancer is rare) are:
- Do not smoke.
- Have a healthy diet including fruit, vegetables, cereal products and fish.
- Avoid exposure to harmful sun. (Use a hat, long sleeves and 'block out' lotion.)
- Be relaxed—avoid stress and anxiety; practise meditation.
- Avoid exposure to radioactivity and asbestos.

Other than this, screening measures for early detection include:
- 2-yearly Pap smears up to the age of 70
- regular mammography for women over 50
- regular breast or testicular self-examination
- bowel examination for those at risk
- regular inspection of the skin

Cannabis (marijuana)

What is cannabis?

Cannabis is a drug that comes from a plant called *Cannabis sativa* or the Indian hemp plant. It contains a chemical called *tetrahydrocannabinol*, which makes people get 'high'. It is commonly called *marijuana, grass, pot, dope, hash* or *hashish*. Other slang terms are *Acapulco Gold, ganga, herb, J, jay, hay, joint, reefer, weed, locoweed, smoke, tea, stick, Mary Jane* and *Panama Red*. Marijuana comes from the leaves, while hashish is the concentrated form of the resinous substances from the head of the female plant and can be very strong (it comes as a resin or oil).

Is cannabis a new drug?

No. It is a very old drug and was used by the Chinese about 5000 years ago.

What are the effects of taking cannabis?

This depends on how much is taken, how it is taken, how often, whether it is used with other drugs and also on the particular person. The effects vary from person to person.

Effects of a small to moderate amount
- feeling of well-being and relaxation
- decreased inhibitions
- woozy, floating feeling
- lethargy and sleepiness
- talkativeness and tendency to laugh a lot
- red nose, gritty eyes and dry mouth
- unusual perception of sounds and colour
- nausea and dizziness
- loss of concentration
- looking 'spaced out' or drunk
- difficulty remembering things
- delusions and hallucinations
- lack of co-ordination

The effects of smoking marijuana appear in up to 20 minutes and usually last 2–3 hours, then drowsiness follows.

A very serious problem is habitual use with the development of dependence. Another serious problem is the tendency to cause schizophrenia in those who are prone to develop it.

Does cannabis improve one's sex life?

No—quite the opposite. Although one feels less inhibited, it tends to decrease libido. Long-term use suppresses sex hormones, decreases fertility and may result in impotence and loss of normal sex drive.

What happens with dependence and long-term use?

'Pot' has a severe effect on personality and drive. People using it lose their energy, initiative and enterprise. They become bored, inert, apathetic and careless. A serious effect of smoking 'pot' is the loss of memory.

Other serious problems are:
- deterioration of academic or job performance
- crime
- lack of morality—scant respect for others and their property
- respiratory disease (more potent than nicotine for lung disease)
- often a prelude to taking hard drugs
- becoming psychotic (resembling schizophrenia)
- impaired ability to drive a car and operate machinery

What about driving under the influence?

Cannabis affects co-ordination and perception, and so it is dangerous to drive a car or ride a motorbike after using it. In an experiment, several people were given 'pot' to smoke and then asked to drive around a test circuit. Most made a mess of their driving, including crashing into posts and retaining walls. It is particularly dangerous when mixed with alcohol. Activities such as surfing, waterskiing and motorbike riding are also dangerous.

What are the withdrawal effects?

The withdrawal usually starts 12 hours or so after stopping using cannabis. The effects are usually mild and over within a few days in most people. Some of the withdrawal symptoms are:
- irritability
- nervousness (anxiety)
- feelings of depression
- sleep disturbances
- increased sweating
- tremors
- muscle twitching
- restlessness
- nausea and other gastric disturbances

What is the management?

The best treatment is prevention. People should either not use it or limit it to experimentation. If it is used, people should be prepared to 'sleep it off' and not drive.

John Murtagh, *Patient Education*, Second edition, McGraw-Hill Book Company

Chronic fatigue syndrome

What is chronic fatigue syndrome (CFS)?

CFS is a feeling of chronic fatigue that persists or keeps recurring for longer than 6 months and is associated with several other problems, including a reduction in physical activity by at least 50%. Organic disease or psychiatric causes are absent.

What are the symptoms of CFS?

Four or more of these symptoms can be present:
- extreme exhaustion (with little physical effort)
- headache or a vague 'fuzzy' feeling in the head
- aching in the muscles and legs, especially after exercise
- an emotional 'roller-coaster'
- poor concentration
- memory problems
- sleep problems, especially excessive sleeping
- feeling tired on waking
- feelings of depression
- feeling very flat and unwell after exertion
- aching in the joints
- sore throat
- palpitations
- feeling feverish (although temperature normal)
- swollen glands in neck
- various other symptoms, e.g. ringing in the ears

Does CFS have other names?

Yes; CFS is also known by several other names including *myalgic encephalomyelitis (ME)*, *postviral syndrome*, *yuppie flue*, *chronic Epstein–Barr viral syndrome*, *Icelandic disease*, *Royal Free disease*, *Tapanui disease* and *Raggedy Ann syndrome*.

What is the cause?

So far the cause is unknown. We do know that about 2 out of 3 patients have a viral flu-like illness beforehand. No single virus has yet been identified. It is similar to the chronic fatigue that can follow glandular fever. In other patients CFS simply develops out of the blue and the body's immune system responds but in an abnormal way.

Who gets CFS?

The onset usually occurs between the ages of 20 and 40 years, but it can affect people of any age, social status and occupation.

What do the tests show?

All tests will be normal. (There is no single test for CFS available, but a special urine test is being developed.) The main reason that you have tests is to make sure that you do not have an organic cause such as anaemia.

What is the usual outcome and what are the risks?

CFS usually gets better with a slow, steady improvement, but relapses can occur on and off for some time. There are usually no complications and the main concerns are feelings of anger, frustration and depression.

What is the management?

There is no magic drug treatment, so the management is mainly support and care. It is important to be reassured that CFS is usually a self-limiting problem. In some cases it can clear up in 2 years but in others it can last for 10 or more years. The patient is the major carer of his or her body and must 'listen' to it and work out a day-to-day plan of what to do, in conjunction with the doctor. It is important not to get onto a merry-go-round of visiting many practitioners.

Self-help guidelines
- Rest seems to be the best way to cope, although it does not cure it.
- Take pain-killers such as aspirin for aches and pains.
- Pace yourself—don't overdo it, and rest when you can.
- Avoid things such as stress that aggravate the fatigue.
- Avoid long distance travel if possible.
- Good supportive relationships are important.
- Attend a local support group.
- Undertake a realistic, regular, graduated exercise program.
- Join a meditation class and practise it at home.

Drug treatment
Drugs are generally not helpful, and using them is based on a 'wait and see' trial. Some patients respond to certain drugs such as antidepressants, evening primrose oil or vitamin B12 injections, while others do not seem to get any benefit. Your doctor will guide you.

Circulation to legs: poor circulation

Poor circulation to the legs (known as *peripheral vascular disease*) is caused usually by *atherosclerosis* (hardening of the arteries). It is quite common in older people, and the likelihood of it occurring increases with age. It is known to be caused by smoking, high blood cholesterol, high blood pressure and diabetes.

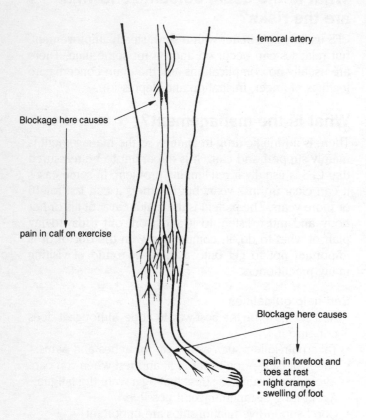

femoral artery

Blockage here causes

pain in calf on exercise

Blockage here causes

- pain in forefoot and toes at rest
- night cramps
- swelling of foot

What are the symptoms?

Pain in the calves and other muscles
The reduced blood flow to the legs can cause pain, usually in the calves but also in the buttocks and thighs. The pain is a cramping or ache felt only when the legs are active, such as when walking a long distance or running, and it disappears soon after rest. The cramping pain is caused by a lack of oxygen, which is carried to the muscles in the blood.

Pain in the foot
Some patients feel pain in the foot, especially the toes, forefoot and heels. Unlike pain in the muscles, it affects the skin and comes on at rest. It is generally worse in bed at night, is constant and hard to relieve.

Other symptoms
Other symptoms or signs include loss of normal hair on the legs, shiny skin, nail changes, coldness of the feet and discolouration of the foot (such as red, white or blue).

What aggravates the problem?
Certain drugs, such as beta-blockers (used to treat high blood pressure), smoking and anaemia aggravate this condition.

What are the risks?
The legs are subject to thrombosis, infections, wounds that do not heal (may develop into ulcers) and gangrene.

What tests are done?
There are special investigations to measure the blood flow to your legs. If surgery is being considered, an X-ray of the arteries will be arranged.

What can be done?
The most important thing to do is change your lifestyle so that the problem does not get worse. If you smoke, you must stop. If you are overweight, reduce your weight to ideal weight and have a healthy diet. Regular moderate exercise is recommended. Try to keep your legs warm and dry. If you have rest pain in the feet, sleep with your legs dangling over the edge of the bed.

What are the special precautions?
Care of your feet is important, especially care of the toenails. When cutting toenails, avoid cutting the flesh; any wound is likely to get infected. It is advisable to have a podiatrist (chiropodist) care for your feet. Avoid injury to the legs and feet. Any simple wound is likely to break down and form an ulcer, which can take months to heal. Consult your doctor if you have any problems, especially an unusual change in the colour of your feet or a sudden onset of pain.

John Murtagh, *Patient Education*, Second edition, McGraw-Hill Book Company

Constipation

What is constipation?

Constipation is:
- hard, often very small stools
- infrequent bowel movements

  or
- a feeling of unsatisfied emptying of the bowel

What are the causes?

It is mainly caused by simple things such as:
- neglecting the habit of attending the toilet
- not responding to 'nature's call'
- overuse of laxatives
- overuse of pain-killers
- a poor diet with a lack of fibre
- lack of exercise
- insufficient fluid intake

Apart from slack habits, there are other important causes such as bowel cancer, drugs, thyroid disease, depression, anorexia nervosa and lead poisoning. Any medicine that you are taking should be suspected of causing constipation.

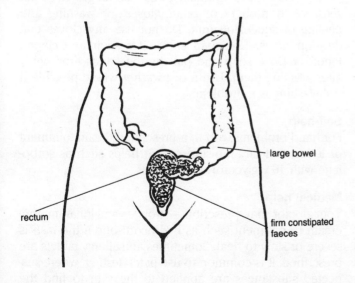

large bowel

rectum

firm constipated faeces

What are the risks?

Constipation can cause a lot of discomfort in the stomach and rectum and may cause blockage of the bowel. It can lead to problems of the anus such as piles and itchiness, and to hernias.

Very important points

- If an obvious change occurs in your bowel habit, consult your doctor for advice.
- Bowel regularity can vary from person to person. Some people believe that just as the earth rotates on its axis once a day, so too should their bowels open daily to ensure good health. This may be ideal, but it can be normal to 'go' every second day or even twice a week.

Useful hints to avoid constipation

Activity
Adequate exercise, especially walking, is important.

Diet
Take plenty of fluids, especially water and fruit juices. Eat foods that provide bulk and roughage, for example vegetables and salads, cereals (especially bran), fresh and dried fruits, and wholemeal bread. Some examples of food with good bulk (from least to most) are potatoes, bananas, cauliflower, peas, cabbage, lettuce, apples, carrots and bran. Fruit has good fibre, especially in the skin, and some have natural laxatives (e.g. prunes, figs, rhubarb, apricots).

Habit
Answer nature's call to empty your bowels as soon as possible. Develop the after-breakfast habit. Allow time for a good relaxed breakfast and then sit on the toilet (up to 10 minutes if necessary) while reading! Eat meals slowly in a relaxed manner at regular times.

Laxatives
Avoid laxatives, codeine compounds (tablets or mixture) and neglecting the call of nature.

Many laxatives can actually aggravate the problem in the long run and should be avoided. If absolutely necessary, your doctor may recommend one of the hydrophilic bulk-forming agents such as isphagula and psyllium.

Contact dermatitis

What is contact dermatitis?

It is a skin inflammation caused by an allergic or irritating reaction to certain substances coming into contact with the skin. The reaction can be *acute* (sudden), within minutes to hours, or *chronic*, which comes on slowly (such as the reaction to the nickel in a watchband).

What are the symptoms?

- redness of the skin
- itchiness
- bright red weeping areas or blisters (if severe)

The dermatitis can actually range from a faint redness to 'watermelon' swelling of the face.

What areas are usually affected?

- the face, especially around the eyes
- the genital area
- the hands and feet

What substances commonly cause dermatitis?

Irritants

- acids and alkalis
- detergents or soaps
- sprays
- solvents or oils

Allergens

- plants (e.g. rhus, grevillea, primula, poison ivy, mango skin, parsnips)
- chemicals in some perfumes and cosmetics
- some metals in jewellery, especially nickel (e.g. nickel buttons or studs); chromate (in cement and leather)
- rubber and latex
- some topical medications (e.g. antibiotics, anaesthetics, antihistamines)
- resins and glue
- dyes
- coral

What is occupational dermatitis?

Occupational dermatitis is a very common form of contact dermatitis. It is caused by a whole range of irritants and allergens used in industry that come into contact with the skin of workers. Most problems occur on the hands.

What is housewife's dermatitis?

This is a common form of dermatitis on the hands of women (and men) who regularly use detergents, washing-up liquids and various household cleaners, especially with hot water. The skin becomes red, sore, dry and rough, especially over the knuckles. It may itch and crack, leading to extreme soreness.

What is the treatment?

The obvious thing to do is work out the cause and remove it or avoid it if possible.

Prevention

Always try to avoid the cause: an example is to get someone to remove any offending plants from the garden. Cut down the use of irritating substances such as solvents, soap, detergents, paint and thinners, scouring powder and pads, turpentine, various polishes. A barrier cream can be rubbed into the hands before work.

For dermatitis of the hands, wear protective work gloves such as cotton-lined PVC gloves.

For housewife's, dermatitis wear rubber gloves (if not sensitive to rubber) or other gloves for washing and peeling or squeezing fruit. Do not use any gloves that develop holes. Use soap substitutes such as Cetaphil lotion or Dove soap and pat dry the hands thoroughly after washing them. Use a dishwasher where possible if dishwashing is a problem.

Self-help

For hand problems, rub in a prescribed cream, ointment or lotion and any moisturiser that helps such as sorbolene with 10% glycerol or Nutraplus.

Medical help

Your doctor may prescribe a stronger anti-inflammatory cream or ointment such as hydrocortisone if the rash is severe or slow to heal. Sometimes anti-allergy tablets are prescribed. It is common to use patch testing, where suspected substances are applied to the skin to find the exact cause. If the patch test is positive, you should avoid the particular substance.

John Murtagh, *Patient Education*, Second edition, McGraw-Hill Book Company

Coping with a crisis

The harsh reality

No matter how sound and healthy your normal state of mind and body, there is every chance that at some stage during your life you will face some sort of crisis. It may be brought on by a build-up of stress or it may be sudden and unexpected, such as becoming the victim of a crime or by suffering the sudden loss of something or someone precious to you.

Normal reactions

You will naturally feel terrible and react with disbelief and a whole range of emotions and physical feelings that are quite unfamiliar to you. These reactions include fear, helplessness, sadness, anger, shame, guilt, frustration and a terrible let down. The 'why me?' feeling is very real. The feelings usually last for only a few minutes at any one time. All this is a normal response to a crisis, and then you go through a recovery cycle.

Recovery

You may not think so at the moment, but you will soon learn to cope; nature heals in time. The human body has a remarkable ability to cope both physically and mentally with extreme stress. It is therefore important for your own sake and that of your loved ones who rely on you that you cope and keep on an even keel until time heals your misfortune. There is light at the end of the tunnel.

Rules to help you cope

1. Give expression to your emotions
You simply must accept your reactions as normal and not be afraid to cry or call out. Do not bottle up feelings.

2. Talk things over with your friends
Do not overburden them, but seek their advice and listen to them. Do not avoid talking about what has happened.

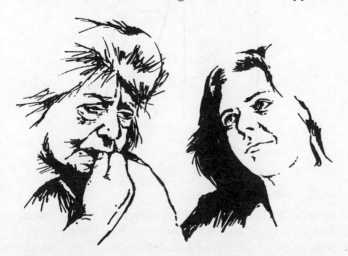

Talking with a friend can help you cope

3. Focus on things as they are now—at this moment
Do not brood on the past and your misfortune. Concentrate on the present and future in a positive way.

4. Consider your problems one at a time
Do not allow your mind to race wildly over a wide range of problems. You can cope with one problem at a time.

5. Act firmly and promptly to solve a problem
Once you have worked out a way to tackle a problem, go for it. Taking positive action is a step in allowing yourself to get on with life.

6. Occupy yourself and your mind as much as possible
Any social activity—sports, theatre, cards, discussion groups, club activity—is better than sitting around alone. Many people find benefit from a holiday visit to an understanding friend or relative. Religious people usually find their faith and prayer life a great source of strength at this time.

7. Do not nurse grudges or blame other people
This is not easy, but you must avoid getting hostile. In particular, do not get angry with yourself and your family, especially your spouse.

8. Set aside some time every day for physical relaxation
Make a point of doing something physical such as going for a walk, swimming or enjoying an easy exercise routine.

9. Stick to your daily routine as much as possible
At times of crisis a familiar pattern of regular meals and chores can bring a sense of order and security. Avoid taking your problems to bed and getting sleepless nights. Try to 'switch off' after 8 pm. Taking sleeping tablets for those few bad nights will help.

10. Consult your family doctor when you need help
Your doctor will clearly understand your problem, because stress and crisis problems are probably the commonest he or she handles. Consult your doctor sooner rather than later.
- Remember that there are many community resources to help you cope (e.g. ministers, social workers, community nurses, crisis centres, church organisations).
- Take care: drive carefully to avoid accidents, which are commoner during this time.

John Murtagh, *Patient Education*, Second edition, McGraw-Hill Book Company

Cramp

What is cramp?

Cramp is a painful spasm in the muscle, usually the calf muscles of the leg. It can also occur in the foot. The affected muscle feels hard and tense, and it is almost impossible to control it.

Who gets cramp?

Cramp happens from time to time in almost everyone, but some are more prone than others to regular cramps. Pregnant women are prone to cramps. They are common in athletes and footballers, especially after long periods of intense running. They are also common after unaccustomed exercise. Many people, especially the elderly, are often roused during sleep by sudden and severe cramps in the calves.

What is the cause?

There is usually no underlying cause other than unaccustomed exercise. It is thought that a type of natural acid substance builds up in the muscles and initiates the cramp. It can also be caused by a prolonged period of sitting, standing or lying in an uncomfortable position. Uncommon causes are more serious medical conditions such as hardening of the leg arteries, thyroid troubles, lack of salt (sodium chloride) in the cells and various drugs.

What is the treatment?

The usual cramp lasts no longer than a minute or so and will usually clear up of its own accord. It can be eased by firmly massaging the affected muscle and flexing the foot back towards you. It is easier if you can get someone to do this for you. Some people claim that they can quickly terminate their cramps by applying firm finger pressure in the webbing between the first and second toes.

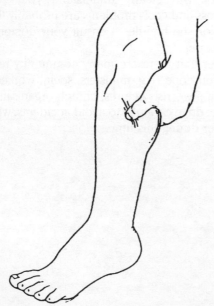

Massage the affected muscle

How can night-time cramps be prevented?

Medication

Doctors often prescribe quinine sulphate tablets to take before retiring, but it may be worth trying a glass of tonic water instead.

Pillows at the foot of the bed

It is worth trying to keep the bedclothes off the feet and placing a doubled up pillow under the sheet at the foot of the bed so that the feet are kept bent back towards you during sleep. Some people find that raising the foot of the bed about 10 centimetres helps prevent cramps.

Exercises

Certain muscle stretching and relaxation exercises help prevent cramps.

Exercise 1: Stand barefoot about 1 metre from a wall, lean forward with the back straight and your outstretched hands against the wall (as in the diagram). Lift your heels off the floor and then force them into the floor to produce tension in the calf muscles. Hold this position for 20 seconds and repeat about 5 times. Do this exercise 2–3 times a day for a week and then each night before retiring.

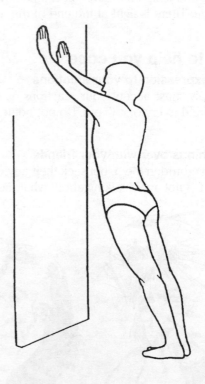

Exercise 2: This usually follows exercise 1 before retiring. Rest in a chair with your feet and legs horizontal and with support under your Achilles tendon. Keep this position for 10 minutes.

John Murtagh, *Patient Education*, Second edition, McGraw-Hill Book Company

Dandruff

What is dandruff?

Dandruff is the excessive production of small flakes of dead skin on the scalp. It is a normal process, because the cells of the outer layer of scalp skin (the *epidermis*) die and are replaced constantly, like all other cells in the body. The dead cells then move to the outer edge of the skin and flake off after about 1 month.

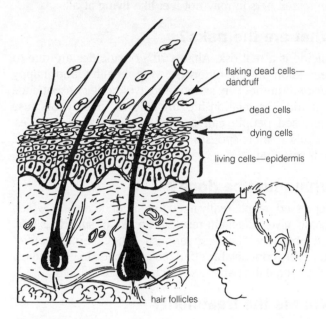

flaking dead cells—dandruff

dead cells

dying cells

living cells—epidermis

hair follicles

Skin of the scalp

What does it mean?

Dandruff is a common, normal condition and carries no risk to health whatsoever. Everyone has it to some degree, and some people only notice it when they wear a dark suit, dress or collar. There is an old saying that 'nothing stops dandruff like a blue serge suit'. It is not contagious and does not cause baldness.

What aggravates dandruff?

Dandruff seems to be made worse by a variety of factors such as emotional stress, poor diet, poor hygiene (including rarely washing or shampooing the hair), allergies, and various chemicals and cosmetics applied to the scalp. The skin inflammation called *seborrhoeic dermatitis* is considered to be a most important cause of dandruff.

Does hormone imbalance cause dandruff?

This is thought to be a factor, because it runs a similar course to acne. It is rare under the age of 12, is most common in adolescence and worse around the age of 20.

What about very severe dandruff?

In some people the dandruff is severe and persistent and itchy. Two causes of this are dermatitis of hair-bearing skin (*seborrhoeic dermatitis*) and *psoriasis*. There is usually evidence of these skin disorders on other parts of the body.

What is the treatment?

There are many shampoos that are suitable for the treatment of dandruff, but no one particular shampoo suits everyone. The shampoo selected depends on the severity of the dandruff. The sulphide preparations upset some people because of staining of necklaces and after odour, but they are effective. If you find a shampoo that suits you, stick with it.

Mild cases

Suitable shampoos are zinc pyrithione (e.g. Dan-Gard), selenium sulphide (e.g. Selsun) and mixed preparations (e.g. Ionil).

The shampoo is massaged into the scalp, left for 5 minutes, then rinsed thoroughly. Use it 2–3 times a week.

Stubborn scaling and itching

This often is due to seborrhoeic dermatitis and psoriasis. Coal tar shampoos are effective for psoriasis. Examples are:
- Ionil T or Ionil T Plus shampoo, followed by Ionil rinse conditioner
- Sebitar shampoo, followed by SebiRinse conditioner

Nizoral shampoo is ideal for seborrhoeic dermatitis. The best way to use it is to start with a milder shampoo, rinse off, then use Nizoral, leave it for 4–5 minutes and then rinse off. Use it twice a week.

If itching is a problem, a cortisone scalp lotion such as Diprosone or Betnovate scalp application can be used.

Depression

What is depression?

Most people feel unhappy or depressed every now and again, but there is a difference between this feeling and the mental illness of depression.

Depression is a very real illness that affects the entire mind and body. It seriously dampens the five basic activities of humans: their energy for activity, sex drive, sleep, appetite and ability to cope with life. They cannot seem to lift themselves out of their misery or 'fight it themselves'. Superficial advice like 'snap out of it' is unhelpful, because the person has no control over it.

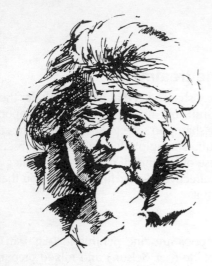

What is the cause?

The cause is somewhat mysterious, but it has been found that an important chemical is present in smaller amounts than usual in the nervous system. It is rather like a person low in iron becoming anaemic.

Depression can follow a severe loss, such as the death of a loved one, a marital separation or a financial loss. On the other hand it can develop for no apparent reason, although it may follow an illness such as glandular fever or influenza, an operation or childbirth. Depression is seen more commonly in late adolescence, middle age (both men and women), retirement age and in the elderly.

How common is depression?

It is one of the commonest illnesses in medicine and is often confused with other illnesses.

What are the symptoms?

The patient can experience many symptoms, both physical and mental. On the other hand, the classical symptoms of being depressed (crying and not sleeping) may be absent—we call this 'masked depression'. Usually some of the following are present:

- a feeling of not being able to cope with life (e.g. hopelessness, helplessness)
- continual tiredness
- sleeping problems (e.g. early waking)
- eating problems (e.g. poor appetite)
- loss of interest in things such as sex
- inability to enjoy normally enjoyable things
- tension and anxiety
- irritableness, anger or fearfulness
- feelings of guilt or worthlessness or being unwanted
- difficulty in concentrating and making decisions
- headache, constipation or indigestion

The symptoms may vary during the day, but are usually worse on waking in the morning. If they are severe, the depressed person may not feel like living at all.

What are the risks?

Suicide is a real risk. Almost 70% of suicides are due to depression in an otherwise very healthy and happy person. Another very serious and avoidable consequence is marital or relationship breakdown, mainly because depressed people can be unpleasant to live with, especially if their spouses or friends do not understand their suffering.

What must be done?

Depressed people really need urgent medical help, which usually gives excellent results. The risk of suicide is real, and threats must be taken seriously—they are often carried out. Every conceivable effort must be made to get medical help, even if the patient is reluctant to see a doctor.

What is the treatment?

The basis of treatment is to replace the missing chemicals with antidepressant medication. Antidepressants are not drugs of addiction and are very effective but take about 2 weeks before an improvement is noticed. If the person is very seriously depressed and there is a risk of suicide, admission to hospital will most likely be advised. Other more effective treatments can be used if needed. The depressed person needs a lot of understanding, support and therapy. Once treatment is started, the outlook is very good.

Special counselling is also very important. Simply talking about your feelings is most helpful.

Important points

- Depression is an illness.
- It is commoner than is realised.
- It just happens; no one is to blame.
- It affects the basic functions of energy, sex, appetite and sleep.
- It can be lethal if untreated.
- It can destroy relationships.
- The missing chemical needs to be replaced.
- It responds well to treatment.

Recommended reading

Paul Hauck, *Overcoming Depression*, The Westminster Press, London, 1987.

John Murtagh, *Patient Education*, Second edition, McGraw-Hill Book Company

Depression: medication for depression

What is the purpose of your medication?

The medicine is prescribed to correct the chemical changes in your nervous system that have caused your depressive illness. It is known that an important chemical is present in smaller amounts than usual. It is rather like a person low in iron becoming anaemic and being given iron until the system is restored to normal. Most people have an excellent response to the medication.

What is the nature of the medication?

The pills are called *antidepressants*. They are not tranquillisers, pep pills, nerve pills or drugs of addiction. They are designed to lift you out of your depression—to lift your mood and energy and your ability to cope with life.

How soon will the medication work?

It usually takes 2–3 weeks before you notice an improvement. Sometimes it is sooner, sometimes longer, depending on the medicine and the individual person. Because it is difficult to predict your chemistry, the pills may have to be juggled for the first few weeks or even changed if they do not suit.

What is the dosage?

The dose will be clearly explained in the directions on the bottle. The lowest effective dose will be prescribed and the tablets will be gradually increased as required. It is common to start with a smaller dose and then build up the medication.

What time of day should it be taken?

The timing is not important to get the desired results, but it is usual to take most (if not all) of the tablets at nighttime. This ensures that you will have a good sleep, because drowsiness is one of the side effects. If you feel too drowsy in the morning, you will have to spread them out during the day. It does not matter when they are taken with respect to meals (during, before or after).

How long will the treatment last?

It is usual to take the tablets for about 6–9 months, and then they will be reduced slowly. Even if you feel much better after 3 weeks or so, it is important to keep taking the tablets to allow your chemical balance to steadily consolidate. Knocking off the tablets too early may cause a relapse.

What side effects can I expect?

You may experience no bothersome side effects, but you could get some of the following:

- sleepiness or drowsiness: avoid driving or operating machinery if you feel drowsy
- dry mouth: this is common; you can chew sugarless gum, have sips of water, suck ice or have gargles
- increased appetite: weight gain is common; choose your food carefully (low fat, low sugar, high fibre)
- constipation or difficulty passing urine (in older men)
- difficulty reading fine print
- dizziness on standing or getting up quickly
- sexual problems, mainly with ejaculation in men

If you do experience some of these milder effects, it is usually a sign that the medication is working. You soon adapt to most of these side effects, which can settle after 2–3 weeks. Contact your doctor about any problems.

What about alcohol?

Alcohol can interact with the tablets, making you more sleepy or more drunk! A small amount will not hurt you, but do not drink and drive.

What about pregnancy?

It is not advisable to take these tablets if you are planning to become pregnant.

Important points

- Take the tablets as instructed.
- Side effects tend to improve.
- Improvement takes about 2–3 weeks.
- Plan to take them for about 6 months.
- Do not drink and drive.
- Keep the tablets away from children.
- Contact your doctor about any concerns.

Diabetes

What is diabetes?

Diabetes mellitus is a disorder in which there is too much sugar in the blood. It is caused by a lack of an important hormone called *insulin*, which is made by a gland behind the stomach called the *pancreas*. *Diabetes* comes from a Greek word meaning 'to pass or flow through' and *mellitus* means 'sweet'. Insulin controls the balance of sugar (glucose) in the body.

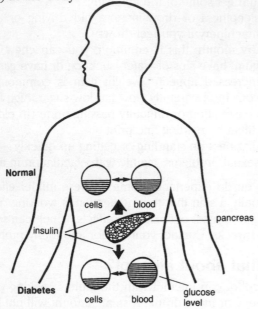

Glucose balance in the body

What are the two main types of diabetes?

Type I diabetes is known as *juvenile-onset diabetes* or *insulin-dependent diabetes mellitus*. It occurs mainly in young people, and because their pancreases produce very little insulin they require injections of insulin. The cause is not known exactly.

Type II diabetes is known as *maturity-onset diabetes* or *non-insulin-dependent diabetes mellitus*. It mainly affects people over 40, many of whom are overweight and have a diet with excess calories. It is usually controlled by a proper diet only, but sometimes tablets may have to be used.

What are the symptoms?

The classical symptoms of untreated diabetes are:
• excessive and frequent urination (every hour or so)
• excessive thirst
• loss of weight (mainly in type I)
• tiredness and lack of energy
• a tendency to get infections, especially of the skin

How common is the problem?

About 1 person in 30 gets diabetes. It tends to increase as we get older because the pancreas, like other organs, tends to wear out.

What are the risks?

Modern treatment is very effective for diabetes, but the results depend on the patient following the treatment, especially the diet. If diabetes is untreated, the complications are very severe and include coma (from the blood sugar being either too high or too low), kidney disease, blindness and heart disease. The feet and eyes are at special risk and need special care and regular checks.

Can diabetes be cured?

No, not yet, but it can virtually always be controlled by a proper diet and regular exercise, and if necessary insulin or special tablets. Although the diagnosis comes as a shock to patients, it is not the major problem that it is generally believed to be—most patients lead normal lives.

Is diet the main treatment?

Yes; all diabetics require a special diet in which carbohydrate and fat intake is controlled. The objectives of the diet are:
• to keep to ideal weight (neither fat nor thin)
• to keep the blood sugar level normal and the urine free of sugar

This is achieved by:
• eating good food regularly (not skimping)
• spacing the meals throughout the day (three main meals and three snacks)
• cutting down fat to a minimum
• avoiding sugar and refined carbohydrates (e.g. sugar, jam, honey, chocolates, sweets, pastries, cakes, soft drinks)
• eating a balance of more natural carbohydrates (starchy foods) such as wholemeal bread, potatoes and cereals
• eating a good variety of fruit and vegetables
• cutting out alcohol or drinking only a little

Is exercise important?

Yes—it really benefits your health. Exercise is any physical activity that keeps you fit. Good examples are brisk walking (e.g. 2 km per day), jogging, tennis, skiing and aerobics. Aim for at least 30 minutes 3 times a week, but daily is ideal. Go slowly when you start.

Good advice

• Exercise is important.
• Do not get overweight.
• A proper diet is the key to success.
• A low-fat, no-sugar diet is needed.
• Do not smoke.
• Minimise alcohol.
• Take special care of your feet.
• Self-discipline will help make your life normal.

John Murtagh, *Patient Education*, Second edition, McGraw-Hill Book Company

Diabetes: blood glucose monitoring at home

How do you check blood glucose levels?

Put blood from a finger prick on a strip. Blot off excess blood with a tissue. Read the strip either by comparing the colour with the colour chart on a bottle or by using an electronic meter. It is important to follow the instructions on the bottle or meter carefully.

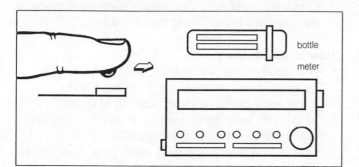

When should you check the levels?

Routinely

For type II diabetes (usually controlled by diet and tablets, or by diet alone), 2–3 times each week at different times of the day is enough.

For type I diabetes (which requires insulin), more regular checking is required; that is, at least once a day, usually first thing before breakfast and then about 2 hours after a meal.

Your blood glucose levels are likely to be *low* before meals, and *high* 2 hours after meals.

Special circumstances

Stress, illness or too much food will push your blood glucose *up*. Exercise and your medications will pull the blood glucose *down*.

When you are ill or under a lot of stress or exercising more than usual, you may need to check your blood glucose level more often than usual.

What are the ideal levels?

Ideal blood glucose levels are 3–6 mmol/L before meals and 3–8 mmol/L 2 hours after meals.

Fair control is 6–8 mmol/L before meals and 8–11 mmol/L after meals.

Poor control is over 8 mmol/L before meals and over 11 mmol/L after meals.

Key points

1. Check your blood glucose regularly, and record the result and the date and time of the test.

2. Be careful to follow the instructions accurately.

3. Ideal blood glucose levels are between 3 and 8 mmol/L.

4. If you are ill or under stress, your blood glucose level is likely to go up. You should check it more often than usual, and see your doctor if it does go up.

Don't forget to record the date, time and result of your blood tests.

Diabetes: foot care for diabetics

Why are doctors so concerned about your feet?

Problems with the feet are common complications that diabetics suffer from and need special attention. A foot problem can be very difficult to heal once it has set in. Diabetes can decrease the circulation to your feet so that healing is relatively poor. Diabetes can also affect the nerves to the feet so that they are less sensitive to pain, touch and temperature. Diabetics are also prone to infection because the feet are almost 'out of sight and out of mind' and problems can develop without your being aware of them. Very special care of your feet is essential, and they should be checked every day.

What type of problems occur?

Pressure sores can develop on the soles of your feet from things such as corns, calluses and stones or nails in your shoes. Minor injuries such as cuts and splinters can become a major problem through poor healing. Problems with toenails such as *paronychia* (infection around the nail) and ingrowing nails can get out of control. Prevention of these problems is the best way.

What should you do?

1. Keep your diabetes under good control and do not smoke.

2. Check your feet *daily*. Report any sores, infection or unusual signs. Make sure you check between the toes.

3. Wash your feet daily:
   - Use lukewarm water (beware of scalds).
   - Dry thoroughly, especially between the toes.
   - Soften dry skin, especially around the heels, with lanoline.
   - Applying methylated spirits between the toes helps stop dampness.

4. Attend to your toenails regularly:
   - Clip them straight across.
   - Do not cut them deep into corners or too short across.

5. Wear clean cotton or wool socks daily; avoid socks with elastic tops.

6. Exercise your feet each day to help the circulation in them.

7. Check the insides of your shoes each week to make sure no nails are pointing into the soles.

How to avoid injury
- Wear good-fitting, comfortable leather shoes.
- The shoes must not be too tight or too loose.
- Do not walk barefoot, especially out of doors.
- Do not cut your own toenails if you have difficulty reaching them or have poor eyesight.
- Avoid home treatments and corn pads that contain acid.
- Be careful when you walk around the garden and in the home. Sharp objects such as stakes in the garden, protruding nails and sharp corners of beds at floor level should never be in the home of a diabetic.
- Do not use hot-water bottles or heating pads on your feet.
- Do not test the temperature of water with your feet.
- Take extra care when sitting in front of an open fire or heater.

Visit the expert
If you have problems with your foot care and especially if your physical condition makes attending to toenails, corns and calluses difficult, you should visit a podiatrist. Your doctor will advise you.

John Murtagh, *Patient Education*, Second edition, McGraw-Hill Book Company

Diabetes: healthy diet for diabetics

Four golden rules

1. Don't get fat
Stay trim, taut and terrific. A healthy diet and regular exercise will keep you, your body and your blood glucose in balance. If you don't know what your weight should be, or need some help to trim down, talk to your doctor.

2. Don't eat fat
Fatty foods like meat, cheese, butter and cream will make you fat and increase your blood fat levels. Nutritionists recommend low-fat foods like grains, cereals, fruit and vegetables.

3. Eat complex carbohydrates
Complex carbohydrates are starches, for example from the bread and cereals group of foods. They are slowly broken down by the body to gradually release glucose. They provide a steady, gradual source of glucose for the body.

Simple carbohydrates, such as sugar, are more quickly taken into the body and cause quicker and higher increases in the blood glucose level. They should be avoided, and complex carbohydrates should be eaten instead.

4. Spread your complex carbohydrates
If you eat three large meals during the day, there may not be enough insulin to allow your body to use the large load of glucose each meal provides. Therefore the blood glucose level rises quickly after the meal and then falls steeply before the next meal.

It is preferable to prevent your blood glucose level from swinging too high or too low. It is better to keep it steady. To do this, you need to eat three small meals during the day, with snacks in between. This allows the body's insulin to use the smaller loads of glucose, so that your blood glucose level will not rise or fall as much.

If you need advice and help in changing to a diet low in fat and high in complex carbohydrates or in losing weight, speak to your doctor. Advice from a dietitian or nutritionist is also helpful, particularly if you have specific problems with your diet.

Diet check list

This chart will help you determine which foods are high in sugar or fat. It suggests alternatives. You may want to look over the chart with your doctor, so that he or she can see what changes you will be making to your diet.

Foods to avoid or limit	Suitable alternatives
High in sugar	
sugar, honey	tablet or liquid artificial sweetener
spreads: jam, marmalade, syrups, Nutella	low joule jam/marmalade, Promite, Vegemite, meat/fish paste
sweet drinks: cordial, soft drink, flavoured mineral water, tonic water, fruit juice drinks, ordinary flavoured milk, milkshakes	low joule cordial/soft drink, plain mineral/soda water, pure fruit juice (limit to 1 small glass a day), coffee, tea, herbal teas
sweet wine/sherry, port, liqueurs, ordinary beer	dry wine or spirit or low alcohol beer (1 to 2 drinks a day)
confectionery: lollies, cough lollies, chocolate (ordinary/diabetic/carob), muesli/health bars	low joule pastilles
sweet biscuits (e.g. cream, chocolate, shortbread), cakes, doughnuts, iced buns, sweet pastries	crispbreads, Cruskits, wholemeal crackers, wheatmeal or coffee biscuits, scones, 'no added sugar' fruit loaf
sweet desserts: ordinary jelly, fruit in sugar syrup, fruit pies, cheesecakes, puddings, ordinary flavoured yoghurt or ice-cream, ice-cream toppings	low joule jelly, fresh or tinned/stewed fruit without added sugar, custard or junket made with liquid sweetener, plain or diet-lite 'no added sugar' yoghurt, plain ice-cream (1 scoop occasionally), low joule ice-cream topping
sweet cereals: some mueslis, Nutrigrain, Cocopops, Honeysmacks, Sugar Frosties	most other cereals, e.g. porridge, Weetbix, All-Bran, Ready Wheats
High in fat	
mayonnaise, oily dressings, cream sauces, fatty gravies, sour cream	low joule dressings, vinegar, lemon juice, low joule Gravox, plain yoghurt
fat on meat, chicken skin, fatty meats (sausages, bacon, salami)	lean cuts of meat with skin and fat removed
deep-fried foods, pies/pasties	foods cooked without fat, or with a minimal amount of vegetable oil
snack foods: nuts, crisps, corn chips	crisp, raw vegetables, fruit, plain popcorn
large amounts of margarine, butter, oil, cream, peanut butter, dripping, lard, ghee	limit to 3–6 teaspoons a day, preferably polyunsaturated margarine or oil

Diabetes: insulin injections

The proper injection of insulin is very important to allow your body, which lacks natural insulin, to function as normally as possible. You should be very strict about the way you manage your insulin injections and have your technique down to a fine art.

Common mistakes

- poor mixing technique when mixing insulin
- wrong doses (because of poor eyesight)
- poor injection technique—into the skin or muscle rather than the soft, fatty layer
- not taking insulin when you feel ill

When to inject insulin

Develop a set routine including eating your meals on time and giving the injections about 30 minutes before your meal.

Where to inject insulin

The injection should go into the fatty (*subcutaneous*) tissue between the skin and muscle. The best place is the abdomen below the navel. Other suitable areas are the buttocks and thighs. These areas have a good layer of fat under the skin and are free of large blood vessels and nerves. It is advisable to stick to one area, and the abdomen is recommended. Avoid giving injections into your arms, near joints, the navel and the groin.

Do not inject too often into the same small area (it can damage the tissue). Give the injection at a different place each time. Keep a distance of 3 cm (1½ inches) or more from the last injection.

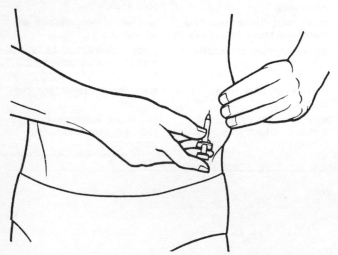

How to inject insulin

- Lift up or pinch a large area of skin on your abdomen between your thumb and fingers.
- Hold the syringe in your other (dominant) hand between your thumb and middle finger: this leaves the index finger free to push the plunger.
- Insert the needle straight in (like a dart) at right angles to the skin (push the needle well in but not into the muscle).
- Push the plunger all the way down.
- Quickly withdraw the needle.
- Press down firmly (do not rub or massage) over the injection site for up to 60 seconds.

Drawing up the insulin

Make sure your technique is checked by an expert.

You may be using either a *single insulin* or a *mixed insulin*. A mixed insulin is a combination of shorter and longer acting insulin and is cloudy.

Rules for mixing

- Always draw up clear insulin first.
- Do *not* permit any of the *cloudy* insulin to get into the *clear* insulin bottle.
- Do *not* push any of the *clear* insulin into the *cloudy* insulin bottle.

Drawing up rules

- Wash and dry your hands beforehand.
- Gently roll the insulin bottle between your hands to mix—do not shake it.
- Always draw up air equal to the dose of insulin into the syringe.
- Always expel air bubbles and ensure you do not inject air.

Storing insulin

- Keep insulin stores (unopened bottles) in the refrigerator, *not* the freezer.
- Opened bottles can be stored in a cool, dark place; refrigeration is not necessary.
- Keep insulin out of heat and sunlight.
- Keep an eye on expiry dates on the bottles.

Golden rules

- Take your insulin every day, even if you feel ill.
- Do not change your dose unless instructed.

John Murtagh, *Patient Education*, Second edition, McGraw-Hill Book Company

Diarrhoea: acute diarrhoea in adults

What is diarrhoea?

Diarrhoea is the passage of many loose, watery, offensive bowel movements. It is a symptom, not a disease. It is usually associated with colic-type abdominal pain and vomiting.

What causes it?

Diarrhoea usually is caused by a viral or a bacterial infection. Most episodes last for such a short time that a search for the cause is not necessary. However, if it lasts for 12 hours or longer, medical attention is needed.

Uncommon infections to be excluded are typhoid and food poisoning as well as parasite infestations with *Giardia lamblia* and amoebae. If you have diarrhoea on returning from overseas, it must be checked out.

Other possible causes are acute appendicitis, rich food, alcohol, emotional upset and excess vitamin C.

What is the treatment?

Rest

Your bowel needs a rest and so do you. It is best to reduce your normal activities until the diarrhoea has stopped.

Diet

It is vital that you starve but drink small amounts of clear fluids such as water, tea, lemonade and yeast extract (e.g. Marmite) until the diarrhoea settles. Then eat low-fat foods such as stewed apples, rice (boiled in water), soups, poultry, boiled potatoes, mashed vegetables, dry toast or bread, biscuits, most canned fruits, jam, honey, jelly, dried skim milk or condensed milk (reconstituted with water).

Avoid alcohol, coffee, strong tea, fatty foods, fried foods, spicy foods, raw vegetables, raw fruit (especially with hard skins), Chinese food, whole-grain cereals and cigarette smoking.

On the third day introduce dairy produce such as a small amount of milk in tea or coffee and a little butter or margarine on toast. Add also grilled lean meat and fish (either grilled or steamed).

Medication

Diarrhoea usually settles without the need for medicine. If it is socially embarrassing, kaolin-based preparations can help.

Antibiotics should be avoided unless directed by your doctor.

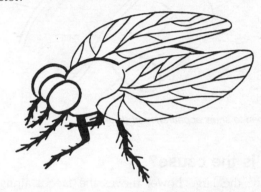

Diverticular disease

What is diverticular disease?

Diverticular disease is a problem of your large bowel (colon) and is related to a lack of fibre in your diet. About 1 person in 3 over the age of 60 years throughout the Western world has this problem.

It is not really a disease, but a condition in which small pouch-like swellings hang from the bowel wall. Infection in such a pouch is called *diverticulitis*.

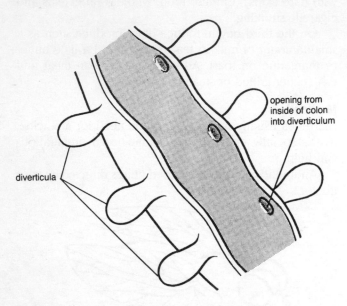

diverticula

opening from
inside of colon
into diverticulum

Colon open to show appearance of diverticula

What is the cause?

Normally, the large bowel moves the faeces along its length with gentle rhythmic contractions of muscles in the bowel wall—this is called *peristalsis*. Without adequate fibre in the diet the motion is dry, small and difficult to move along. The intestinal muscles must therefore perform strong contractions and generate high pressure. This high pressure may push the inner lining through the weaker spots in the wall, rather like blowing up a balloon. The pockets or pouches formed are called *diverticula*. You may have many of these diverticula along the length of the large bowel.

What are the symptoms?

Diverticular disease rarely causes symptoms. A lack of fibre in the diet can cause you to experience bloating, flatulence (desire to pass wind) and abdominal pains.

Are there any tests?

There are two tests done to confirm diverticular disease. The first is *sigmoidoscopy*. A hollow tube is passed into the back passage, through which your doctor can see the bowel lining. The second is a *barium enema*. Barium dye is forced into the back passage; a series of X-ray films clearly show diverticula outlined by use of this dye.

Are there any complications?

Complications are infection and bleeding, which are uncommon. If infection (diverticulitis) develops, you will experience abdominal pain, nausea and fever. These symptoms or any bleeding require prompt attention by your doctor.

What is the treatment?

The gradual introduction of fibre with plenty of fluids (especially water) will improve any symptoms you may have and reduce the risk of complications. Your diet should include:

1. cereals, such as bran, shredded wheat, muesli or porridge

2. wholemeal and multigrain breads

3. fresh or stewed fruits and vegetables

Bran can be added to your cereal or stewed fruit starting with 1 tablespoon and gradually increasing to 3 tablespoons a day. Fibre can make you feel uncomfortable for the first few weeks, but the bowel soon settles to your improved diet.

> **Note**
>
> Any unusual symptom, such as bleeding, constipation, diarrhoea and other changes in your normal habit, may be a sign of bowel cancer. If they occur, report to your doctor.

John Murtagh, *Patient Education*, Second edition, McGraw-Hill Book Company

Dry skin

Dry skin is a common problem, especially in people with atopic dermatitis (eczema). It is rough, scaly skin that is dry to touch and less elastic than normal skin. Some people describe it as feeling like sandpaper. It is especially common in cold, dry climates.

What causes dry skin?

The main feature is a lack of water or moisture in the skin surface. It also appears to be caused by a relative lack of natural oils. However, the main problem is insufficient water to moisturise the skin.

What are the effects of dry skin?

It is not a serious medical problem. One of the worst irritating effects is itching. Cracking of the skin (particularly of the legs) can occur in older people, especially in winter. People often complain of a 'crawling' sensation in the skin. Dry skin does *not* cause wrinkles.

What makes dry skin worse?

- too much washing and bathing (too long and too often)
- use of very hot water
- use of traditional alkali soaps
- cold weather
- low humidity and artificial heating
- dry air
- overexposure to wind and cold
- poor diet

What is the treatment?

Washing and bathing

It is important not to have frequent long baths or showers. Reduce the number and length of baths and showers. It is probably better to avoid baths, swimming in pools and bathing in spa baths. Concentrate on having short showers and perhaps at times have the so-called APC (armpit and crutch) scrub with soap and water instead of a shower or bath.

Use tepid water instead of hot water.

Bath oils

The addition of oils to baths helps to seal in moisture in the skin. However, you must be careful not to slip getting in and out of the tub, as bath oils make the tub surface slippery.

Soaps

Avoid using the traditional alkali soaps and harsh soaps. Use soap substitutes such as Dove, Neutrogena or Cetaphil lotion. Less expensive soaps such as oatmeal soap, which are readily obtained from health shops, can also be used.

After showering

After you shower, do not rub hard with a towel but pat dry and then rub a bath oil or mild baby oil into the skin.

Clothing

Avoid wearing wool next to the skin. Do not wear heavy woollen clothing. Wear cotton clothing.

Skin softeners and lubricants

Apart from various mineral oils and Vaseline intensive care, preparations that soften, lubricate and soothe the skin include QV skin lotion, Alpha keri lotion and Nutra-D cream.

Moisturisers

Although skin softeners act as moisturisers, the urea-based moisturisers can help make the skin more soft and supple. Examples are Nutraplus, Calmurid and Aquacare HP. Another suitable moisturising agent is QV cream.

Diet

Eat a well balanced diet. Drink ample water during the day.

Key points

- Dry skin lacks surface moisture.
- Avoid excessive bathing and showering.
- Take shorter and cooler showers.
- Apply skin softener or moisturiser after showering.
- Use soap substitutes.
- Avoid wool and heavy clothing next to skin.
- Avoid overheating and dryness in rooms.
- Follow a good diet.
- Drink plenty of water.

Ear: otitis externa

What is normal?

The outer ear canal is a tunnel that runs from the ear hole to the eardrum. It is about 3 cm long and is lined with normal skin containing hairs and glands that produce wax (see diagram). The outer ear canal is a blind (closed) tunnel and normally drains only through the ear hole.

What is otitis externa?

Otitis externa is a condition in which the skin lining the outer ear canal becomes red and swollen due to infection. This infection occurs commonly because of water entering the ear canal and is sometimes referred to as 'swimmer's ear'. In the tropics, the heat and high humidity cause people to perspire excessively in summer, and this moisture may also play a part in causing otitis externa or 'tropical ear'.

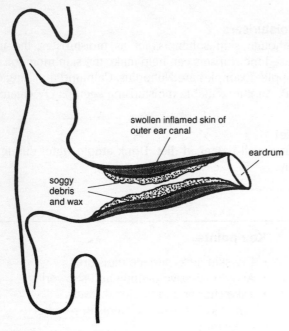

swollen inflamed skin of outer ear canal

eardrum

soggy debris and wax

The ear canal is subject to infection

What are the symptoms?

Pain and tenderness of the ear canal are typical, and in severe cases the pain and tenderness may spread to the outer ear and surrounding skin. Other symptoms include discharge from the outer ear canal, itching and reduced hearing.

Why does it occur?

Water entering the outer ear canal can drain only through the ear hole. The outer ear canal is horizontal and curved; it may contain wax. Water may not drain freely and can cause skin to become soggy, so allowing bacteria or fungi, normally present on the skin, to cause infection.

Who is more prone to otitis externa?

You are more likely to suffer from otitis externa if your outer ear canal is narrow or long, or if the skin lining the canal is in poor condition (i.e. if it is not waterproofed by the wax and is wet by regular swimming). Incidentally, chlorinated fresh water is more damaging than salt water.

The skin lining will deteriorate too if it is prone to dermatitis or eczema and if exposed to chemicals (e.g. hair shampoo, hair dyes and ear ointments). The ear canal can be damaged by attempting to clean it with a hairpin.

What is the treatment?

The basis of successful treatment is to clean the canal and keep it empty and dry. In mild cases your doctor will treat the infection by cleaning the outer ear canal using suction or a probe and then prescribing cream to insert several times a day. The ear cream is used for about 5 days and contains chemicals that kill the bacteria or fungus causing the infection.

If the infection is severe and the outer ear canal is swollen, the doctor may insert a cotton wick coated with the healing cream into the ear canal.

How can otitis externa be prevented?

You can take a number of steps to prevent otitis externa. Among them are:

- Avoid getting water in your ear.
- If water enters, shake it out or use Aquaear drops.
- Use moulded earplugs or a bathing cap when swimming.
- Use earplugs or a cap when showering.
- Use earplugs when washing your hair.
- Coat cottonwool with petroleum jelly (Vaseline) before insertion in ears.
- Avoid poking objects such as hairpins and cotton buds in the ear to clean the canal.

The ear usually cleans itself naturally. Do not attempt to clean it and risk infection of the canal or damage to the eardrum. If you have a problem, contact your doctor for advice and treatment.

John Murtagh, *Patient Education*, Second edition, McGraw-Hill Book Company

Ear: wax in your ear

What is normal?

The outer ear canal is a tunnel that runs from the ear hole to the eardrum. It is about 3 cm long and lined with normal skin containing hairs and small glands that produce wax. The purpose of the wax is to protect the skin of the ear canal and give it a waterproof coating.

Wax is therefore quite normal and people should not feel embarrassed about it building up in their ears. Excessive wax is one of the commonest problems seen by doctors, who are aware of the discomfort it can cause.

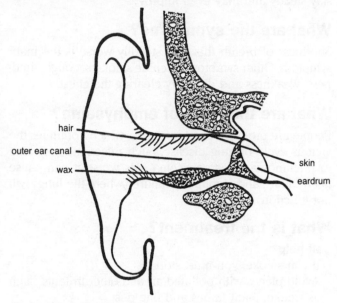

Excessive wax in the ear

How does excessive wax develop?

The glands can produce too much wax or there can be a problem preventing normal drainage of the wax out of the ear.

What are the symptoms?

Most people are not aware that their ear is full of wax until they have a hearing problem or a waxy discharge, but if an infection develops in the skin under the wax the ear might itch and ache.

Hearing can be affected by the wax pressing against the eardrum, making it rigid; even a small amount of wax can cause this.

The wax can be pressed onto the drum by:
• water (when swimming or showering)
• earplugs
• objects inserted in the ear, such as cotton-tipped applicators

What is the treatment?

The doctor can remove excess wax by syringing the ear with water, using a suction instrument or cleaning it out with a fine probe.

Before treatment you might be asked to use wax-softening drops for a couple of days. Some patients find that the drops cause a burning sensation. If this happens, stop using them immediately and notify the doctor.

How can wax problems be prevented?

If you have a tendency to build up wax in the ear, you might be advised to use the ear drops regularly to soften the wax so that it can drain out.

Cleaning the ear

The ear canal has a self-cleaning action that allows natural and unnoticeable removal of the wax. So, the ear should be left alone: 'Never put anything smaller than your elbow in the ear'.

If you have a wax problem, see the doctor for advice and treatment. Do *not* try to fix it yourself: you might cause an infection in the ear canal, or damage the eardrum and affect your hearing permanently.

Emphysema

What is emphysema?

Emphysema is a lung disorder in which the healthy elastic sponge-like tissue is damaged and does not squeeze the air in and out properly. It is as though the lung tissue has become perished, similar to an old flabby football bladder or car tyre tube. This means that the air cannot move in and out of the air sacs easily. The elastic function of the lungs is lost. Air is life to the body, and if we cannot get our normal supply of oxygen into the blood from the lungs they have to work harder to circulate the air.

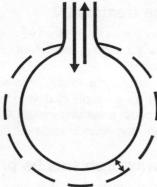

The air sac in a normal lung

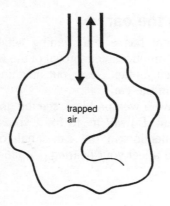

trapped air

A damaged air sac with emphysema

What causes emphysema?

Emphysema is almost always caused by cigarette smoking. Emphysema is 13 times commoner in smokers than non-smokers.

There are other irritating things that can cause emphysema, although these are not as severe as smoking. These irritants include industrial fumes and dusts. Therefore damp mining and industrial towns are not good for people with chest troubles.

How do cigarettes affect the lungs?

When cigarette smoke is inhaled, 80–90% remains in the lungs and causes irritation, increased mucus production and damage to the deep parts of the lungs. Eventually mucus and tar clog up the air tubes, causing chronic bronchitis and emphysema. If you continue to smoke, the problem will get worse. If you stop, the disease may stay steady and may even improve.

What are the symptoms?

Shortness of breath that gets steadily worse is the main symptom. Other symptoms include smokers' cough, tiredness, weakness and difficulty clearing the chest.

What are the risks of emphysema?

People are prone to chest infection, which continues the vicious cycle of lung disease. Such infections may lead to pneumonia. As emphysema gets worse it can cause heart failure and respiratory failure (where the lungs will not function).

What is the treatment?

Self-help

• If you smoke, you must stop.
• Avoid places with polluted air and other irritants, such as smoke, paint fumes and fine dust.
• Go for walks in clean, fresh air. (Keeping physically active is good for the lungs and heart.)
• Get adequate rest.
• Avoid contact with people who have colds and flu.

Medical help

• Visit your doctor regularly for checkups and if you get a chest infection.
• If your chest is tight or wheezy, a bronchodilator spray may help.
• If you have a chest infection, antibiotics will help clear it up.
• Visit your doctor without delay if you get a cold or bronchitis, or start coughing up sputum.
• Annual influenza vaccination is recommended.

John Murtagh, *Patient Education*, Second edition, McGraw-Hill Book Company

Epilepsy

What is epilepsy?

Epilepsy is a disorder that comes in various forms and shows up as a fault somewhere in the complex electrical circuits of the brain and nervous system. This minor fault results in the brain being unable to work properly for a brief period—the various symptoms depend on what part of the brain is affected.

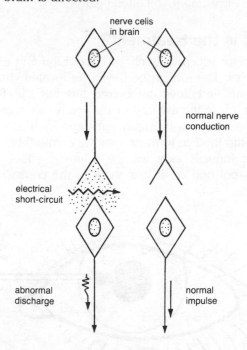

nerve cells in brain

normal nerve conduction

electrical short-circuit

abnormal discharge

normal impulse

In epilepsy there is a fault in the 'electrical' discharge of the cells

What are the symptoms?

Some people will experience convulsions (fits or seizures) while others have unusual sensations. Some children just stare for a brief period (absence seizures) or have sudden feelings of anxiety.

The convulsion

In this type of seizure, patients suddenly become unconscious and fall to the ground. Their bodies go stiff, and then may twitch or jerk briefly. The tongue may be bitten and the bladder usually empties. They then may be drowsy or sleep for half an hour or so. Such a convulsion usually causes no problems.

Dos and don'ts for the onlooker
- *Don't* move the person (unless necessary for safety).
- *Don't* force anything into the person's mouth.
- *Don't* try to stop the fit.
- *Do* roll the person on to his or her side with the head turned to one side and chin up.
- *Do* call for medical help if the convulsion lasts longer than 10 minutes or starts again.

Note: The convulsion in itself will not cause death or brain damage.

What are the causes?

In most cases the cause is unknown and studies show that the brain appears normal in structure. However, it can be caused by damage from previous infections, scars from previous head injuries and, at times, tumours or problems relating to birth.

How common is it?

Epilepsy is common and affects about 1 person in 100. Both sexes are equally involved, and it seems to run in some families. Famous people who have had epilepsy include Julius Caesar, Agatha Christie, Thomas Edison and Handel.

What is the outlook?

Epilepsy can now be controlled to varying degrees by the careful use of medicine. Most patients can achieve complete control. Most people with epilepsy lead a normal life—they can expect to marry, have a normal sexual life and have normal children.

What about driving?

One has to be very careful about driving. However, most people with epilepsy can drive. The usual rule is that they can drive if they have not had a convulsion for a period of from 1 to 2 years.

What about employment?

People with epilepsy can hold down most jobs, but if liable to blackouts they should not work close to heavy machinery, in dangerous surroundings, at heights (such as climbing ladders) or near deep water. Careers are not available in some services, such as the police, military, aviation (pilot, traffic controller) or public transport (e.g. bus driver).

What about sport and leisure activities?

Most activities are fine, but epileptics should avoid dangerous sports such as scuba diving, hang-gliding, parachuting, rock climbing, car racing and swimming alone, especially surfing.

What is the treatment?

It is important to have medical treatment to help lead a full and normal life. Tablets or capsules should be taken regularly. Regular checkups are needed to watch for any side effects of the medicine (usually minor) and to have blood tests to check the level of the drug in the blood. Quite often, once complete control has been established for several years, the medication can be gradually withdrawn and stopped.

Avoid trigger factors such as fatigue, physical exhaustion, stress, lack of sleep and excess alcohol. You must not drive if these factors apply to you. Take special care with open fires.

John Murtagh, *Patient Education*, Second edition, McGraw-Hill Book Company

Eye: foreign body in the eye

What is a foreign body in the eye?

It is any particle such as dirt, metal or sawdust that lodges on the surface of the eye or inside the eye. The main causes are dust carried by wind, metal fragments from grinding, and wood particles from drilling or cutting.

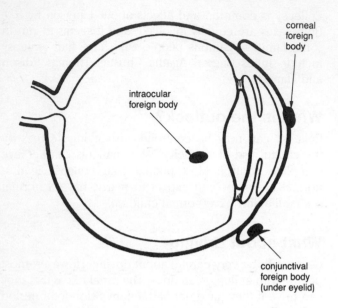

intraocular foreign body

corneal foreign body

conjunctival foreign body (under eyelid)

What are the different types of foreign body?

- A *corneal foreign body* is on the clear surface of the eye.
- A *conjunctival foreign body* is on the skin of the eye, especially under the eyelids.
- An *intraocular foreign body* is inside the eye (a very serious problem).

What are the symptoms?

The main symptoms are eye pain or discomfort, watery eye, blurred vision, redness in the white of the eye and sensitivity to bright light. These may occur straightaway or, more commonly, after about 8 hours. The symptoms are usually worse for an intraocular foreign body, but can be surprisingly mild at first. If you are in doubt, it is better to err on the side of safety and go to your doctor.

Who gets foreign bodies in the eye?

Anyone can, although it tends to be commonest in young adults. Those at most risk are tradespeople such as boiler-makers, woodcutters, fitters and turners, and labourers.

What are the dangers?

The biggest danger is an intraocular foreign body, which can be missed if not suspected. It is diagnosed by X-ray of the eye.

The main problem with metal on the cornea is rusting, which causes a dark spot on the clear part of the eye and can cause a scar, which affects vision.

Infection is a problem, especially if you use unsterile drops in the eye.

What should you do?

If you get a foreign body in your eye, go to your doctor as soon as possible. It is easier to remove and has less chance of rusting if you attend early.

What is the treatment?

The doctor will usually check your vision and examine your eyes. The foreign body will be located (however, sometimes it comes out before this but still feels as though it is in the eye). Since the eye is very sensitive to pain, the doctor will usually put some local anaesthetic drops into the eye to make removal comfortable.

The foreign body will be removed either with a cottonwool bud or, if it is stuck in the cornea, with a needle.

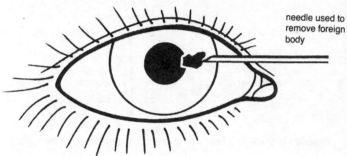

needle used to remove foreign body

What is the follow-up treatment?

If a metal foreign body has been removed from the cornea, some eye drops will be placed in the eye. The drops should be put in regularly as directed by your doctor.

Then an eye pad or patch will be placed over the eye. It is important to keep this pad on, because it allows the small defect in the cornea to heal. Once the local anaesthetic wears off (about 5 minutes), you will have some discomfort in the eye. This can be relieved by taking aspirin or paracetamol. You should not drive with an eye patch on.

You should come back for review as specified by your doctor.

The eye will not heal in less than 48 hours after removal of the foreign body.

How can foreign bodies be prevented from entering the eye?

Wear good eye protection, preferably close-fitting plastic eye glasses with protective sides. Do not walk or stand close to someone who is grinding or drilling. Have eye protection in a dusty, windy area.

John Murtagh, *Patient Education*, Second edition. McGraw-Hill Book Company

Fever

What is fever?

Fever is present when the temperature of the body (measured inside the mouth) rises above 37.2°C. The normal body temperature is up to 37°C. Most fevers are due to an infection in the body and are an important part of the body's defence against infection. Fever is usually caused by a virus but sometimes by bacteria. The temperature returns to normal when the infection settles.

Fever in children

Fever is common in children, in whom the temperature may rise quickly to 38.5°C or higher. It does not mean the child has a serious illness. It is normal for children, especially infants and toddlers, to have at least 5 or 6 episodes of fever a year.

Management of fever

Adults

- Do not overheat with too many clothes or blankets.
- Drink a lot of light fluids, especially water.
- Take aspirin or paracetamol tablets for relief.
- Fan or sponge the patient if the fever is severe.
- Seek medical attention for the following:
  - severe headache or neck stiffness
  - twitching, shaking or convulsions
  - excessive drowsiness
  - signs or symptoms that worry you

Children

- Dress the child in light clothing.
- Do not overheat with too many clothes, rugs or blankets.
- Keep the child cool, but avoid draughts.
- Give the child small drinks of light fluids, especially water, often. Do not worry if the child will not eat.
- Give paracetamol syrup every 4 hours until the temperature settles.
- Give the child plenty of tender loving care, with reassurance that they will soon feel well.

Note: Cooling measures such as completely undressing the child, sponging with lukewarm water and using fans are not necessary.

Seek immediate medical help for the following:

- severe headache or neck pain (with stiffness)
- light hurting the eyes
- repeated vomiting
- a convulsion or the child acting 'odd'
- undue drowsiness or difficulty waking up
- refusal to drink
- the child looking sicker
- no improvement in 48 hours
- earache or other pain

Key points

- Fevers fight infection.
- Fevers are common in children.
- Give them paracetamol mixture every 4 hours.
- Keep them cool.

Gallstones

What are gallstones?

Gallstones are small, hard stones that develop in the gall bladder in a similar way to which pearls grow inside oyster shells. They usually vary in size from that of a grape seed to the size of a marble.

How are they formed?

The gall bladder is a small bag about the size of a fig that collects *bile*—a green liquid produced by the liver. A small bit of sediment in the bile can act as a collecting spot for more sediment and cause it to gradually grow into a stone.

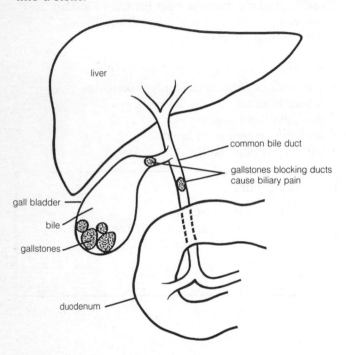

What are the symptoms?

About one-half of people with gallstones do not get any pain because the gallstones simply lie out of the way in the bottom of the gall bladder.

The rest suffer very severe pain, which builds up to a peak over a few hours and then fades. This *biliary pain* is usually felt in the upper abdomen on the right side just under the ribs. It can be felt in the back or middle of the abdomen. Nausea and vomiting often accompany the pain.

What causes the pain?

The pain is caused by the gallstones getting jammed in the *cystic duct* or the *common bile duct*. This leads to raised pressure in the hollow tube from the build-up of bile.

The pain is relieved if the gallstone is pushed forwards into the duodenum or if it falls back into the gall bladder.

Who gets gallstones?

Almost anyone, including children, can grow gallstones. About 1 or 2 in every 10 adults in Western society has 1 or more gallstones. The problem increases with age, so that 1 in 3 elderly people have gallstones. It is related to a diet high in fats. There is an old medical saying that the typical patient suffering from gallstones is 'female, fair, fat and forty'. This is a reasonably accurate picture.

What are the risks?

Gallstones are capable of causing unpleasant complications such as inflammation of the gall bladder and bile ducts, jaundice and acute pancreatitis. Jaundice is caused by the stones remaining stuck in the common bile duct and stopping the flow of bile to the duodenum.

How are gallstones detected?

Gallstones can be detected by having an ultrasound examination, which is simple, safe and painless, or by a special X-ray called a *cholecystogram*.

What is the treatment?

Self-help

Diet is very important. Avoid overeating and eating fatty foods, or any foods that may bring on attacks of biliary pain. A sensible low-fat diet usually keeps the problem under control.

Medical help

Strong pain-killers are needed to relieve the attacks. Sometimes the stones can be dissolved by a special chemical or shattered with special shock waves, but most troublesome gallstones need to be removed by surgery. This usually involves removing the gall bladder and its stones and, if necessary, removing stones from the bile duct.

John Murtagh, *Patient Education*, Second edition, McGraw-Hill Book Company

Glaucoma

What is glaucoma?

Glaucoma is a common eye disorder caused by increased fluid pressure within the eyeball. This high pressure can damage the delicate blood vessels and nerve fibres in the eye. The pressure in this watery fluid builds up because the drainage system gets blocked. Glaucoma, which runs in families, is the second commonest cause of blindness in Australia.

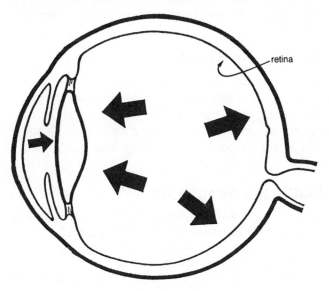

Increased fluid pressure in the eye

What are the two types of glaucoma?

1. *Acute glaucoma*: This develops suddenly and painfully.
2. *Chronic glaucoma*: This is the common type, which develops slowly and may not be noticed by the patient.

What are the symptoms?

Acute glaucoma

Blurred or foggy vision, rainbow halos around lights, pain (may be severe) in the eye, nausea and vomiting, a red eye.

Chronic glaucoma

Loss of side vision at first, gradually increasing to partial or total blindness.

How common is it and who gets it?

Anyone at any age can get glaucoma, but the older you are the more likely you are to get it. Most people are over 40 years when it comes on. Those over 65 are at greater risk, with 1 person in 20 being affected and 1 in 10 at 75 years.

What are the risks?

Blindness is the end result without treatment. If detected early, it can be cured.

How is it diagnosed?

It is detected by routine examination of the eye and by a special instrument being placed on the surface of the eye to measure the pressure of the fluid in the eyeball. It is a simple and painless test that is usually done as a routine screening test by doctors, especially eye specialists.

How can it be picked up early?

Visit your doctor when you suspect eye trouble such as:
- frequent changes of glasses that are unhelpful
- blurred or fogged vision
- loss of side vision
- recurrent pain
- inability to adjust eyes to a darkened room
- coloured halos around lights

Have regular eye examinations (e.g. everyone over 35 should have routine tests and in particular those over 60 should have glaucoma tests every 2–3 years). If you have a close relative with glaucoma, you should have yearly inspections.

What is the treatment?

Special eye drops are usually used to treat glaucoma. Oral medications, laser treatments and sometimes surgery are used also. The eye drops are instilled 2–4 times a day and will have to be taken for life.

Remember
- Glaucoma is common.
- It causes blindness.
- It can be treated successfully.
- It may be symptomless at first.
- Always have unusual eye problems checked.

Haemorrhoids

What are haemorrhoids (piles)?

They are knobbly varicose veins of the rectal or anal area, which can prolapse outside the anus and hang as small grape-like lumps.

What are the different kinds of haemorrhoids?

Internal haemorrhoids are those that form inside the rectum near the beginning of the anus. They are generally not painful and often are only noticed when they bleed.

Prolapsed haemorrhoids are internal haemorrhoids that protrude through the anus when the stool is passed or when a person stands or walks. They are usually painful.

External haemorrhoids are small, painful haemorrhages under the skin around the anus. They form a hard clot after 24 hours. Their proper medical name is *perianal haematoma*. When they settle, they sometimes leave a small skin tag.

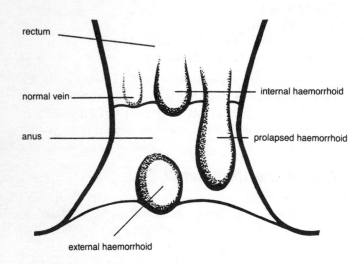

Haemorrhoids

What causes haemorrhoids?

The commonest cause is constipation, mainly due to the excessive straining at toilet because of hard faeces. Some experts say that sitting on the toilet for long periods causes haemorrhoids, but this problem is related to constipation.

It is important to get into the habit of answering the 'call of nature'. The problem tends to run in families. Other associations are heavy manual work, sitting for long periods (such as bus driving) and pregnancy.

How common is the problem?

Haemorrhoids are common and tend to develop between the ages of 20 and 50. About 1 out of 4 Westerners suffer from them at some stage of life.

What are the symptoms?

Bleeding is the main and in many people the only symptom. The word *haemorrhoid* means 'flow of blood'. The blood is bright red and appears when you defecate. You may notice it as streaks on toilet paper or in the faeces.

Piles often cause a mucous discharge and itching around the anus. Any consequent scratching makes the irritation worse.

What are the risks?

Haemorrhoids are not dangerous, but continuous bleeding may result in anaemia. Any bleeding from the anus, especially in someone over the age of 40, should be reported to your doctor. Occasionally the bleeding attributed to haemorrhoids can come from cancer of the bowel.

What is the treatment?

The best treatment is prevention, and softish bulky faeces that pass easily prevent haemorrhoids. Train yourself to have a diet with adequate fibre by eating plenty of fresh fruit, vegetables, and whole-grain cereals or bran.

Try to complete your bowel action within a few minutes and avoid using laxatives.

If you have haemorrhoids, clean yourself thoroughly but gently after each bowel action (using soft toilet paper and soapy water) and dry yourself carefully.

Special astringent ointments or suppositories (advised by your doctor) may relieve the congestion and shrink the haemorrhoids. Mild cases may clear up completely.

If the problem persists, your doctor may advise injections or minor surgery. Occasionally surgery to remove the piles—called *haemorrhoidectomy*—may be the only answer.

John Murtagh, *Patient Education*, Second edition, McGraw-Hill Book Company

Halitosis

What is halitosis?

Halitosis is unpleasant smelling or 'bad' breath. It is common in healthy people, especially in the morning when they first awaken from sleep.

What are the causes?

Dental problems

Halitosis is mainly caused by dental problems, usually tooth decay or plaque and food trapped in the gaps between the teeth. The bits of food undergo decay by bacteria, just like food left to rot, and this process causes an unpleasant smell. This problem can also occur in dentures when food particles stick to them.

Another common dental problem is inflammation of the gums (*gingivitis*), which is usually caused by dental plaque at the base of the teeth as we get older. The gums tend to be sore and bleed on brushing.

Plaque and gingivitis often appear together, and both contribute to halitosis.

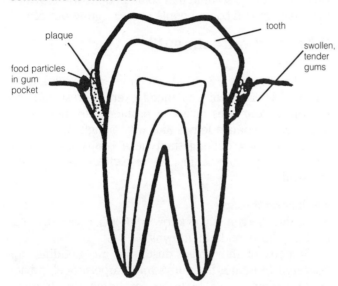

plaque

food particles in gum pocket

tooth

swollen, tender gums

Gases from the stomach

Another cause is gases and smells coming from the stomach due to the breakdown of some foods. Certain people seem to be prone to this problem. It is worse when fasting. Foods that tend to cause problems are onions, garlic, peppers, alcohol, spicy salami and similar meats.

Medical causes

Medical disorders that cause halitosis include:
- tonsillitis
- chronic nose and sinus infections
- lung disorders (e.g. TB and bronchiectasis)
- cancer
- general infections with fever (e.g. glandular fever)
- diabetes
- liver disease
- kidney disease
- drugs, including smoking

Other possible causes
- anxiety and stress
- habitual mouth breathing, which dries saliva in the mouth
- sulphur compounds from the back of the tongue

What are the effects?

It is not a serious problem, but it can seriously affect the personal and social life of sufferers, including their self-esteem.

How is it managed?

Dental and mouth care

The most important thing is to clean the teeth and mouth regularly, especially with a toothbrush and dental floss. To get rid of plaque and tiny food particles it is important to:
- Brush the teeth regularly during the day, immediately after each meal if possible.
- Rinse the mouth out with water after meals.
- Use dental floss each day to clean the teeth.
- Gargle with an antiseptic mouthwash (e.g. Listerine, Cepacol).
- Gently brush the back of the tongue with a soft toothbrush.

Nutrition
- Ensure you have at least 3 healthy meals a day. Regular eating helps.
- Avoid foods such as onions, garlic, peppers and spicy salami.
- Avoid strong cheeses.
- Avoid excessive alcohol (maximum 4 standard drinks a day for men, 2 for women).
- Chewing fresh parsley, especially after eating onions and garlic, is helpful.

Lifestyle
- Avoid fasting for long periods during the day.
- Avoid smoking.
- Avoid excessive coffee (maximum 3 cups a day).

Special tip

A proven method is to gargle an oil and water mixture. Make up a mixture with equal volumes of aqueous Cepacol and olive oil. Gargle a well shaken mixture and expel, 4 times a day.

Hay fever

What is hay fever?

Hay fever (also known as *allergic rhinitis*) is an allergic reaction of the nose, throat and eyes to irritating particles in the air. It is similar to asthma, except that the over-sensitive (allergic) reaction occurs in the upper respiratory tract instead of the lungs.

There are two types of allergic rhinitis:
* *seasonal rhinitis*, which occurs only during certain seasons, usually spring
* *perennial rhinitis*, which is present throughout the year

What are the symptoms?

Symptoms are sneezing, running and itching nose, itching dry throat and itching eyes. Sufferers usually feel generally listless and irritable and may find it difficult to concentrate.

What is the cause?

The airborne irritants, also known as *allergens*, enter the nose, throat and eyes and cause sensitive cells (*mast cells*) to become active (rather like a dormant volcano erupting). These cells release a substance called *histamine*, which causes the symptoms.

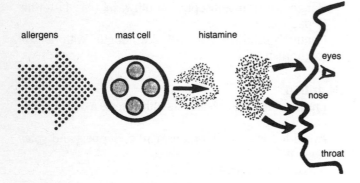

allergens   mast cell   histamine

eyes

nose

throat

What are the allergens?

The allergens are either foreign proteins (tiny invisible particles from plants and animals) or chemicals. They include:
* pollens from trees (in spring) and grass (in summer)
* house dust mites (cause perennial rhinitis)
* mould
* hair, fur or feathers (from cats, dogs, horses or birds)
* some foods (such as milk, eggs, peanuts and peanut butter)

Many people do not know what they are allergic to.

Do any other things aggravate hay fever?

Chemicals such as smoke, paints and sprays, cosmetics and aspirin can make hay fever worse. Emotional upset, fatigue, alcohol, chilly damp weather and air-conditioning can aggravate it also.

Is it inherited?

It does tend to be hereditary. Children whose parents are allergic have an increased chance of getting hay fever.

It is a common disorder, and people can grow into it and out of it at any age.

What are the risks?

Hay fever is not a serious disease but, if not treated, it can lead to asthma, nasal polyps and hearing problems.

Can hay fever be cured?

No, but modern treatment can control the problems and relieve the symptoms. People do not have to suffer with it and should contact their doctor if it is troublesome. Hay fever can be so mild that some people do not realise they have it; and some people seem to grow out of it.

What is the treatment?

Self-help

Keep healthy, eat a well-balanced diet, avoid 'junk food' and live sensibly with balanced exercise, rest and recreation. If your eyes give you problems, try not to rub them, avoid contact lenses and wear sunglasses.

Avoid using decongestant nose drops and sprays: although they soothe at first, a worse effect occurs on the rebound.

Avoidance therapy

Avoid the allergen, if you know what it is. (Consider pets, feather pillows and eiderdowns.)

Sources of the house dust mite are bedding, upholstered furniture, fluffy toys and carpets. Seek advice about keeping your bedroom or home dust-free, especially if you have perennial rhinitis.

Pets, especially cats, should be kept outside.

Avoid chemical irritants such as aspirin, smoke, cosmetics, paints and sprays.

Medical help

Your doctor has many treatments available, ranging from antihistamine pills to desensitisation (after skin testing reveals your allergens). The newer antihistamine pills do not cause as much drowsiness as did the older ones. Sprays for the nose and drops for the eyes, available by prescription, are very effective.

John Murtagh, *Patient Education*, Second edition, McGraw-Hill Book Company

Head injury

What happens?

The patient has sustained a head injury that appears to be mild. He or she has been observed and is showing no serious signs of damage, so can go home and expect that rapid recovery will follow. However, very rarely, complications may follow at any time over the next few days.

What causes complications?

The brain is housed, very compactly, in a rigid case—the skull—and cannot tolerate any increase in pressure. If this occurs due to bleeding or swelling, pressure is exerted on the base of the brain, which contains the vital centres controlling such functions as breathing and heart action.

The problem may occur gradually, and certain warning signs will develop that indicate the pressure will have to be relieved.

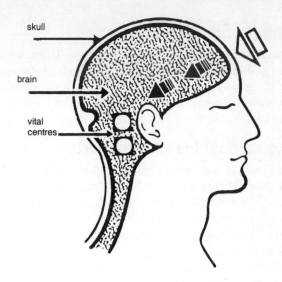

What should you do?

Someone in the household should keep the patient under close observation over the next 24 hours (at least) and bring him or her back to the surgery or to the casualty department of the nearest hospital *immediately* if they notice any of the following features:

1. unconsciousness or undue drowsiness, such as difficulty waking up
2. confused, irrational or delirious behaviour
3. headache that continues
4. bleeding or discharge from the ear or nose
5. repeated vomiting
6. fits or spasms of the limbs or face
7. blurred or double vision

In children

Children should be allowed to go to sleep, but should be woken every 4 hours to see if they are rousable and conscious.

Other points

Diet
Any food and drink can be taken in moderation, but avoid alcohol.

Pain-killers
Paracetamol or aspirin can be taken in the usual doses for headache.

Drugs
Avoid sedatives; take no medication unless instructed.

Icepacks
Icepacks can be used over swollen or painful areas of the head.

Rest
- Stay resting *in bed* for 2 days.
- When you start getting up, return to bed if you feel giddy or get a headache.
- Rest quietly at home and do not return to work or your normal activities until after 7 days.

Heart failure

What is heart failure?

Heart or *cardiac failure* occurs when the heart, which is a muscular pump, fails to pump enough blood around the body. The heart becomes inefficient either because the muscle is weakened or because there is a mechanical fault in the valves controlling the flow of blood.

The mechanics of the heart

The heart is basically a series of two pumps, with the smaller right side pumping blood (returning to the heart) to the lungs to get oxygen. The left side of the heart has the big job of pumping blood rich in oxygen around the body. Heart failure may affect only one side of the heart but more usually affects both sides, in which case it is called *congestive cardiac failure*.

In left-sided failure, the lungs become congested with fluid, causing breathlessness; in right-sided failure, the blood pools in the veins, causing swelling in the tissues, especially of the legs and abdomen.

What are the symptoms?

The main symptom is breathlessness, usually after exertion. Other symptoms are tiredness, lethargy, nausea, and swelling of the ankles and abdomen.

What causes it?

Coronary artery blockage, high blood pressure, faulty heart valves and alcohol abuse are the main causes.

What are the risks?

Despite its name, heart failure is not usually an immediately life-threatening disease; it generally responds to treatment and can be held in check for a long time. If untreated, it puts a great strain on all the body, which tends to become waterlogged. If treated successfully, the only danger comes from the underlying cause such as coronary artery disease or alcohol abuse.

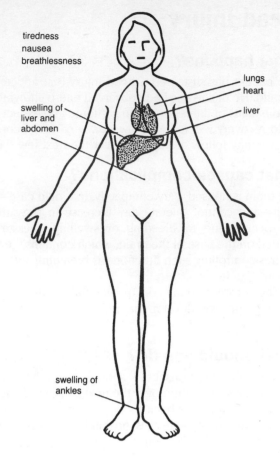

Symptoms of right-sided failure

Self-help

• Reduce your physical activity: rest if your symptoms are severe but take exercise such as walking if your symptoms are mild or absent. • Cut down your salt intake: have a salt-free diet. • Limit your fluid intake to less than 1½ litres a day. • Reduce your weight if you are overweight. • Avoid smoking. • Take no alcohol or small quantities only.

Medication

The most commonly used medicines are fluid tablets (*diuretics*) and *vasodilators* to open up the blood vessels. This helps take the load off the heart. A drug called *digoxin* may be used to improve the strength of the heart. Your doctor will advise you about other drugs.

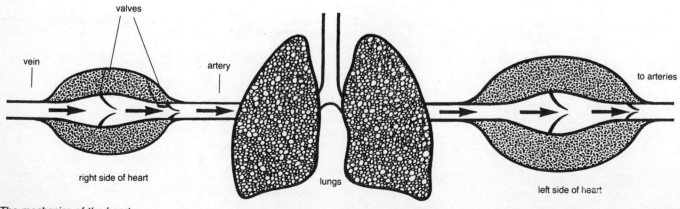

The mechanics of the heart

John Murtagh, *Patient Education*, Second edition, McGraw-Hill Book Company

Heartburn

What is heartburn?

Heartburn is not a disease but a symptom of burning discomfort in your chest, usually associated with an acid taste in the mouth. It is also referred to as *indigestion* or *dyspepsia* and is associated with drinking and eating.

What causes heartburn?

It is caused by the reflux of the acid contents of the stomach back up the oesophagus (gullet) and sometimes into the throat. It may be caused by a peptic ulcer. Reflux occurs because the valve made by a ring of muscle at the junction of the oesophagus and stomach does not close fully, and may be associated with a hiatus hernia.

Factors that bring it on are:
- particular foods (e.g. cabbage, onions, cucumber, curries, pastries—especially pies and pasties, fruit cake)
- certain drinks (e.g. wine—especially red wine, beer, carbonated drinks, coffee)
- eating too fast
- rich or big meals
- chewing gum long and hard
- stress and anxiety
- pregnancy
- old age
- certain drugs (e.g. antirheumatism drugs, aspirin)
- obesity (a common factor)

What tests are done?

Tests may not be necessary, but if it persists or your doctor is concerned about an ulcer, X-rays may be taken or a tube called a *gastroscope* may be passed down into the stomach to inspect it.

How can it be prevented?

Don'ts
- Bolt your food down.
- Eat standing up.
- Smoke.
- Eat fatty foods (e.g. pastries)
- Eat spicy foods.
- Eat large or rich meals.
- Bend over for work.
- Strain at toilet.
- Drink wine with meals.
- Eat foods that 'burn'.
- Drink coffee or alcohol late at night.

Dos
- Eat in a slow and relaxed manner.
- Eat sitting down.
- Avoid foods that 'burn'.
- Eat small or moderate meals.
- Squat rather than bend.
- Keep your bowels regular.
- Avoid stress: relax!
- Relax for half an hour after a meal.
- Reduce your alcohol intake.

What is the treatment?
- Attend to the above preventive advice.
- Learn what brings on your heartburn and deal with it.
- Take antacids when you feel heartburn coming on and before bed at night.
- Make sure that you get to your ideal weight, should you be overweight.
- Your doctor may prescribe other medicine to help.

Hiatus hernia

What is a hiatus hernia?

A *hiatus hernia* occurs when the upper part of the stomach, which is joined to the oesophagus (gullet), moves up into the chest through the hole (called a *hiatus*) in the diaphragm. It is common and occurs in about 10% of people.

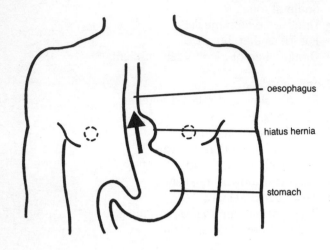

What are the symptoms?

Most people are not troubled by a hiatus hernia, but if reflux of the acid contents of the stomach occurs (called *gastro-oesophageal reflux*), heartburn results. This is a painful burning sensation in the chest, which can sometimes be felt in the throat. Sudden regurgitation of acid fluid into the mouth can occur, especially when you lie down or bend forward. These symptoms are a problem when you go to bed and can wake you up. Other symptoms include belching, pain on swallowing hot fluids and a feeling of food sticking in the oesophagus.

Who gets a hiatus hernia?

It is most common in overweight middle-aged women and elderly people. It can occur during pregnancy. The diagnosis is confirmed by barium meal X-rays or by passing a tube with a camera on the end into the stomach (*gastroscopy*).

What are the risks?

Hiatus hernia is usually not serious; however, it can cause inflammation of the lower end of the oesophagus. This is called *reflux oesophagitis*, and it may cause bleeding (perhaps anaemia) or a stricture. Cancer in a hiatus hernia is very rare, but there is a slight increased risk of it developing in the inflamed area.

What is the treatment?

Self-help

- Keep to your ideal weight.
- Avoid stooping.
- Avoid smoking.
- Reduce alcohol and coffee.
- Avoid tight corsets.
- Adjust your bed.
- Take antacids.
- Have small meals.
- Avoid spicy food.
- Avoid hot drinks.
- Avoid having supper.
- Avoid gassy drinks.

Losing weight nearly always cures it. Eating several small meals each day instead of 2 or 3 large ones helps. You must have a light evening meal without alcohol and avoid supper so that your stomach is empty on retiring. It takes about 1–2 hours for the stomach to empty.

Smoking certainly aggravates it, as do coffee and alcohol, especially spirits. If symptoms occur at night, you are advised to use extra pillows to prop up your head and shoulders. If this fails, you should raise the head of your bed about 10 cm (4 inches) to prevent acid reflux at night.

Medical help

If over-the-counter antacids and other measures do not help, your doctor may prescribe a special mixture or tablets to reduce reflux. If your problem persists, an operation (which has good results) may be necessary.

> The key to coping with a hiatus hernia
> is to keep at ideal weight.

John Murtagh, *Patient Education*, Second edition, McGraw-Hill Book Company

Hypertension

What is hypertension?

Hypertension means high blood pressure and is present when your blood pressure is greater than normal levels for the population. There are two types of blood pressure (BP) that we measure: *systolic* and *diastolic*. The systolic BP is the pressure at the moment the heart pumps the blood and the diastolic BP is that when the heart relaxes and takes in blood.

BP is measured in millimetres of mercury (mm Hg). We have hypertension if our pressure is greater than either the normal systolic pressure (140) or the normal diastolic pressure (90). The diastolic level is the more important, and so we aim to keep this pressure below 90.

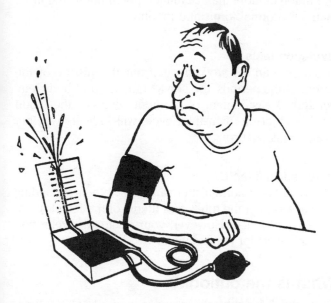

What causes it?

In most cases (95%) there is no identifiable cause—it just happens that way. The pressure in our arteries is high because the heart pumps too hard and the arteries are too narrow. This is like the pressure in a hose—the further we turn up the tap and the narrower the hose, the greater the pressure. Sometimes hypertension is caused by a kidney problem or some other rare disorder. Drinking excessive amounts of alcohol is an important cause.

Who gets hypertension?

Anyone can get it. It is very common and affects about 15–20% of the adult population in Western countries. BP tends to rise as we get older. However, most people are not aware they have it.

What are the symptoms?

Usually there are none. People with very high BP can feel quite well. It is rare to feel headache, palpitations or sick until complications set in.

What are the risks of having it?

You are more likely to have strokes and heart attacks than people with normal BP. The risk increases as the BP rises. With time the pressure can cause the heart and kidneys to wear out, that is heart failure and kidney failure. By keeping the BP within normal limits, we reduce the risks of strokes and heart trouble, including coronary attacks.

What is the treatment?

Medication (called *antihypertensive* medication) can reduce your high BP, but it might be possible to lower your BP to normal by leading a sensible, healthy lifestyle. This self-help may avoid a lifelong commitment to drugs.

Self-help
- *Diet*: Follow a nutritious, low-fat diet.
- *Salt*: Put away the salt shaker; use only a little salt with your food.
- *Obesity*: Aim to keep to your ideal weight.
- *Alcohol*: Aim for either none or only small amounts.
- *Stress*: Avoid stress and overwork. Consider relaxation or meditation classes.
- *Exercise*: Exercise regularly.
- *Smoking*: This does not seem to cause high BP, but is a risk factor for heart disease—so please stop.

Medication
If natural measures do not bring down your BP, tablets will be necessary. The tablets act by softening the strong pumping action of the heart or relaxing the tight arteries or reducing the body chemicals that control your BP. The tablets must be taken regularly as directed and never stopped unless advised by your doctor.

How often should your BP be checked?

It should be measured every 1–2 years by your doctor. If you are over 40 years, it is wise to have it checked every year because it tends to creep up with age. Women on the pill need to be checked regularly.

Infertile couple

What is infertility?

Infertility is the inability to conceive after a period of 12 months of normal unprotected sexual intercourse; that is, not getting pregnant after a year of trying.

A more preferable term is *subfertility*, which is the situation where a couple has problems achieving conception. *Sterility* is the extreme case when conception can never occur.

What is necessary for pregnancy to occur?

Three basic features are essential:

1. The right number of healthy sperm has to be placed in the right place at the right time.

2. The woman must be *ovulating*; that is, producing healthy ova (eggs).

3. The tubes must be patent and the woman's pelvis sufficiently healthy to allow fertilisation of the egg and then implantation in the uterus.

What are the statistics?

About 1 in 10 couples are infertile. The incidence increases with age, so that it gradually increases after the age of 32. About 100 000 couples in Australia have this problem. 100 infertile couples will include:
- 40 with a female factor
- 30 with a male factor
- 15 with an unknown factor
- 15 with a combined female and male factor

What are the main specific causes?

- faulty egg or sperm production that can be related to previous infections (such as mumps) or drugs (such as cancer treatment drugs and anabolic steroids)
- blockages or other structural problems of the reproductive tract that could be congenital (present from birth) or acquired from infections
- psychological factors, such as stress, anxiety or adverse lifestyle
- problems with intercourse and the timing of intercourse

What can be done?

If a couple has not conceived in 12 months, they should both visit their doctor. At first the doctor will work out whether intercourse is frequent enough and suitably timed, and determine whether there is a sexual difficulty such as partial or occasional impotence or premature ejaculation. If a correctable condition comes to light, the couple will be given advice and told to try again for several months. If there is still a problem, the main tests that will be done are the sperm test in the male and the ovulation tests in the female.

The sperm test

The male is required to provide a complete ejaculate of semen, preferably by masturbation, after at least 3 days abstinence from sex. This fluid is placed in a clean bottle, kept warm and examined under the microscope within 1 hour.

Normal values are more than 3 mL with a sperm concentration of more than 20 million per millilitre and more than 60% normal forms and motility.

Ovulation tests

Ovulation can be worked out from the history of the nature of the periods, the cervical mucus and body temperature. Measurement of hormone levels in the blood on day 21 of the menstrual cycle will indicate whether ovulation is occurring.

Other special tests

If these tests are normal, there are many others (including special X-rays of the tubes and uterus of the female) that can be performed. However, your doctor will refer you to a specialist for management.

What is the outlook?

The outlook for subfertile couples improves all the time. Current specialised treatment helps 60% of couples to achieve pregnancy.

The emotional trauma of infertility

Infertility is certainly associated with deep emotional problems that can flare up as crises from time to time. Unfortunately the emotional stress includes taking blame or placing blame on the other partner, and results in guilt feelings. Common feelings of infertile couples are surprise, denial and fear at first, and then frustration, anger, guilt, resentment, depression and loss of self-esteem. It cannot be emphasised enough that you should talk openly and honestly about your feelings and seek the help of a counsellor such as your family doctor.

John Murtagh, *Patient Education*, Second edition, McGraw-Hill Book Company

Ingrowing toenails

An *ingrowing toenail* occurs when the nail of the big toe curves under at the sides of the nail so that it grows into the skin.

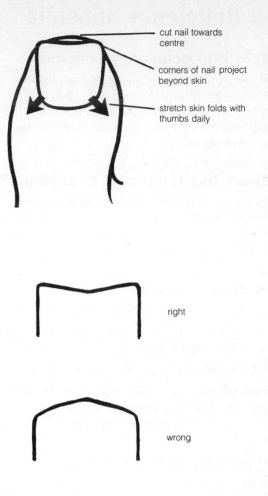

cut nail towards centre

corners of nail project beyond skin

stretch skin folds with thumbs daily

What is the cause?

The two main contributing causes are the wearing of tight shoes and the incorrect cutting of the nails. If the nails are cut on a curve and down at the sides, the nail edges grow into the skin. A spike of nail gets embedded in the skin and causes problems. However, some people, despite cutting their nails properly and using good foot-wear, have very wide nails that tend to be ingrown.

What are the symptoms?

Most ingrowing nails do not cause discomfort, but some-times when they are not attended to they cause pain, especially if tight shoes are worn. The problem is most troublesome when the skin around the ingrowing toenail becomes infected.

right

wrong

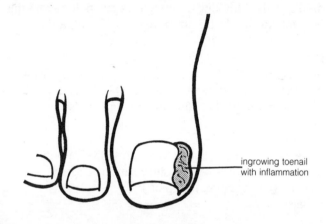

ingrowing toenail with inflammation

How can ingrowing nails be prevented?

It is important to fashion the toenail so that the corners project beyond the skin. The nail should be cut across so that the cuts slope towards the centre of the nail and not down towards the edges.

Each day, after a shower or bath, use the pads of both thumbs to stretch the nail folds at the base as shown.

What is the treatment?

If you have an ingrowing toenail, wear good fitting shoes, cut the nail as described and be careful not to leave spikes at the edges. It is especially important not to dig the scissors into the ingrowing corners and injure the tissues. This injury, which tends to cause minor bleeding, often leads to a nasty infection that can take weeks to heal.

Make sure you wear good fitting shoes and keep the area clean and dry at all times.

Your doctor may choose to use one of several methods to remove the ingrowing nails, including remov-ing the wedge of nail or skin fold so that the leading edge of the nail lies free.

John Murtagh, *Patient Education*, Second edition, McGraw-Hill Book Company

Iron deficiency anaemia

What is iron deficiency anaemia?

Iron is one of the vital chemicals of *haemoglobin*, which is the red pigment in red blood cells. If iron is deficient in the body, the production of haemoglobin is reduced, the red cells are therefore reduced or weak, and this is known as *anaemia*.

What are the symptoms of anaemia?

There may be no symptoms at first, then tiredness, weakness, breathlessness, faintness and loss of interest in things are the main symptoms. Pallor, especially of the lining of the lower eyelid, is a sign.

What are the causes?

Lack of iron is due to 1 or more of 3 main reasons:

1. not enough iron in the diet, especially in growing infants and vegetarians

2. poor absorption of iron from the bowel

3. excessive loss of blood, such as menstrual loss, bleeding from cancer or ulcers in the bowel or stomach or from haemorrhoids (piles)

Who is likely to get anaemia?

- premature infants
- children, especially those 6–36 months old with a diet high in cows milk and low in iron-containing foods
- women, especially those with heavy periods and lack of dietary iron (3 in 10 have low iron reserves)
- the elderly (e.g. through poor diet and chronic illness)
- vegetarians
- athletes, who lose iron in sweat and urine

Anaemia can also develop in those with rapid growth spurts (e.g. adolescents). Those taking certain drugs, such as aspirin or anti-inflammatories, are prone to slow gastric bleeding, which can lead to anaemia. The commonest cause of iron deficiency in the world is from hookworm infestation of the bowel in tropical areas.

How is anaemia diagnosed?

Anaemia is diagnosed by taking a blood sample and sending it to a laboratory for testing. Iron deficiency can be diagnosed by the appearance of the blood and size of the cells. If this is so, further blood is taken to measure the level of iron stores in the body.

What are the main problems?

Iron deficiency anaemia is unlikely to be fatal, but the cause is the concern. In older adults the possibility of bleeding from cancer of the bowel or stomach must be considered. The ideal tests for this are looking directly into the empty organs with a viewing scope. The outlook for those with iron deficiency anaemia is usually very good.

What is the treatment?

The most important thing to do is correct the underlying cause. If investigations give the all clear for a serious bleeding problem, it is likely that the cause is lack of iron in the diet and this is easily corrected. Sometimes a blood transfusion is necessary to correct severe anaemia, especially if you are facing surgery.

Medication

Iron supplements: Iron tablets are preferred to injections of iron but have a reputation for causing gastric upsets such as indigestion and nausea.

- Take 1 tablet a day or 2 tablets every second day.
- Take iron on an empty stomach (e.g. 30 minutes before meals).
- Take vitamin C to help absorption.
- Wait 2 hours before taking other medications such as antacids.
- Take iron tablets with a small amount of food (not milk) if they upset the stomach.
- Continue the tablets for at least 3 months.

In children iron is best given daily before meals with orange juice (not milk). Liquid iron can discolour children's teeth—drinking it through a straw helps avoid this. Milk intake should be no more than 500 mL a day.

Diet

Adults should limit milk intake to 500 mL a day while on iron tablets. Avoid excess caffeine, fad diets and excess processed bread. Eat ample iron-rich foods (especially protein).

Protein foods
- meats: beef (especially), veal, pork, liver, poultry
- fish and shellfish (e.g. oysters, sardines, tuna)
- seeds (e.g. sesame, pumpkin)
- eggs

Fruits
- dried fruits (e.g. prunes, figs, raisins, currants, peaches)
- juices (e.g. prune, blackberry)
- most fresh fruit

Vegetables
- greens (e.g. spinach, silver beet, lettuce)
- dried peas and beans (e.g. kidney beans)
- pumpkin, sweet potatoes

Grains
- iron-fortified breads and dry cereals
- oatmeal cereal

For better iron absorption, add foods rich in vitamin C (e.g. citrus fruits, cantaloupe, brussel sprouts, broccoli, cauliflower).

Prevention of iron deficiency

- Aim for a well-balanced diet with adequate iron.
- Give bottle-fed infants an iron-fortified formula and iron-containing foods as soon as solids are started.

John Murtagh, *Patient Education*, Second edition, McGraw-Hill Book Company

Irritable bowel

What is it?

An *irritable bowel* (also known as *irritable colon* or *irritable digestive system*) is one that does not work smoothly and causes abdominal problems such as colicky pain and disturbed bowel actions. The bowel is a muscular tube that propels the food along in waves (called *peristalsis*). This muscular action may become overactive and cause spasms or tight contractions rather like a cramp in the leg muscles.

What are the causes?

There is no clear-cut proven cause but the main factor is considered to be emotional stress, especially in those people who tend to 'bottle things up inside'. Other possible causes are:

- infection of the bowel
- food irritation (e.g. spicy food)
- food allergy (e.g. milk)
- lack of bulk in the diet
- overuse of laxatives
- pain-killing drugs and antibiotics

What are the symptoms?

The main symptom is a cramp-like pain in the abdomen (in the centre or lower left side). This pain is usually relieved by passing wind or by a bowel movement.

Diarrhoea or constipation may occur, and sometimes the motions will be like small, hard pellets.

You may also feel mildly nauseated, off your food, bloated or flatulent (windy).

How common is it?

At least 1 person in every 100 has it, and many simply learn to live with it.

What are the risks?

The irritable bowel is harmless, but it is common for those with it to worry that they have cancer. It is usual to carry out investigations to ensure that there is no disease in the bowel.

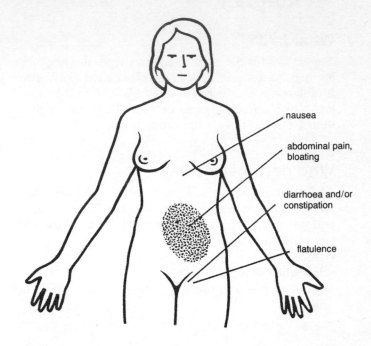

Symptoms of irritable bowel

What is the treatment?

Self-help

Anyone with an irritable bowel should try to work out the things that make the symptoms worse. If you recognise stresses and strains in your life, try to develop a more relaxed lifestyle. You may have to be less of a perfectionist in your approach to life.

Try to avoid any foods that you can identify as causing the problem. You may have to cut out smoking and alcohol. A high-fibre diet may be the answer to your problem. This can be helped by adding 2 teaspoonfuls of unprocessed bran to your diet each day if increased fibre and fluids have not quite settled the problem.

Medical help

If self-help measures are not controlling the problem, your doctor will be able to give you medicine to settle the painful spasm of an irritable bowel. You should avoid taking any medicines not recommended by your doctor.

Melanoma

What is it?

A *melanoma* is the most dangerous type of skin cancer. It grows from special cells in the skin called *melanocytes*. A melanoma is usually brown or blackish in colour and looks like a freckle, mole or spot. They can begin in moles, but most begin in normal skin.

Who gets melanoma?

About 1 in 60 people will get melanoma. It is seen most often in people aged 30–50 years, but it can occur in younger people. People at increased risk are those with:
• several dark moles
• freckles
• fair white skin
• skin that reacts to sunlight (burns easily and does not tan)

Why do they occur?

We do not know why all of them begin, but they are much more likely to occur in people who have a lot of exposure to the sun. Queenslanders have one of the highest rates of melanoma in the world. In spite of this, they do not only occur in areas exposed to the sun—they can occur all over the body.

How do I know if I have a melanoma?

Only a few moles go on to become melanomas. Any changes that occur in a mole should raise suspicion. Changes may include:

• any change in the colour of the mole
• an increase in size, or spread to surrounding skin
• thickening of the mole
• bleeding
• itching

In fact, any change in a mole may be a warning, and should be discussed with your doctor.

What can be done?

Once suspicion is raised about a mole, it should be removed by your doctor. It will then be sent away to be looked at under a microscope, to check if it is a melanoma. Further treatment depends on the result of this test.

Can it be cured?

If melanomas are removed early, they can be completely cured. Over 95% of patients are cured with early removal.

Prevention is the best cure!

To decrease your chances of getting a melanoma, you should protect yourself from the sun. These rules should be followed:
• Try to avoid direct sunlight when the sun is strongest (from 10 am to 3 pm standard time, i.e. from 11 am to 4 pm daylight-saving time).
• Always wear a broad-brimmed hat and T-shirt in the sun.
• Use a factor 15+ sunscreen on exposed skin and renew it regularly.
• Sunbaking might give you a good tan, but it is also going to increase your chances of getting a melanoma, and so you should avoid it.

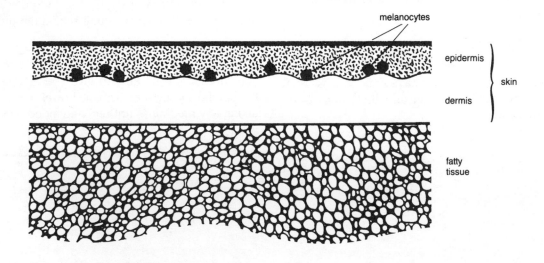

melanocytes

epidermis

skin

dermis

fatty tissue

John Murtagh, *Patient Education*, Second edition, McGraw-Hill Book Company

Ménière's syndrome

What is Ménière's syndrome?

It is a disorder of the balance system in the ear causing attacks of severe dizziness and other unpleasant symptoms. It was described by a French physician, Prosper Ménière, in the nineteenth century.

What are the symptoms of the attacks?

- vertigo (dizziness), lasting for minutes or hours
- tinnitus (ringing or buzzing in the ear)
- a fullness or pressure in the ear
- nausea and vomiting
- loss of balance
- sweating and pallor

In most cases only one ear is affected.

Attacks come on suddenly and may even cause the person to fall over. The attacks usually last from 30 minutes to several hours. They may come on as often as twice a week (unusual) or twice a month to as few as one every year or so.

What is the cause?

The cause is an increase in the amount (and therefore pressure) of fluid in the labyrinth of the ear. The cause of this is unknown but certain risk factors are:

- tension or stress
- high salt diet
- noise
- head injury
- aspirin in high doses
- allergies (e.g. to alcohol, chocolate, dairy products)

Who is usually affected?

It is equally common in both sexes and usually affects adults between the ages of 30 and 60. It is uncommon, affecting only 1 person per 1000.

What are the risks?

It is not a life-threatening problem. Many cases are mild, but in the few cases that have many attacks complete deafness and persistent tinnitus can develop over time. In these people it can be frustrating to treat and cause them embarrassment, loss of confidence, tension and anxiety, especially as the attacks come without warning.

How is Ménière's managed?

You will need to have special diagnostic tests, mainly to check your hearing and the condition of the labyrinth.
During the attack:
- Rest quietly.
- Avoid sudden changes in position.
- Do not read. Avoid glaring lights.
- Do not walk without assistance if unbalanced.
- Do not climb ladders, drive or work around dangerous situations.
- Take medicines as ordered; however, you may require an injection.

Preventive measures include:
- Avoid caffeine, smoking and alcohol.
- Have a low fat, low salt diet.
- Seek out stress management/meditation classes.

You may be prescribed diuretics (fluid tablets) or special tranquillisers. Rarely surgery can be used for severe cases.

Seek out a support group, such as Ménière's Australia Inc., Moonah, Tasmania.

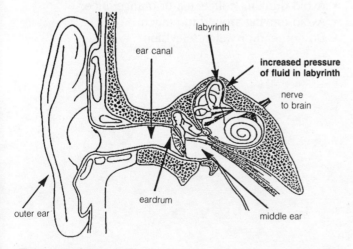

The cause of an attack

John Murtagh, *Patient Education*, Second edition, McGraw-Hill Book Company

Migraine

What is migraine?

Migraine or the 'sick headache' is derived from the Greek word meaning 'pain involving half of the head'. It is a common problem that affects about 1 person in 10. It is commoner in females and is worse between the ages of 20 and 50 years.

What are the symptoms?

Migraine can take several different forms, but the headache is usually preceded by altered vision followed by nausea and vomiting. This is called *classic migraine*. Another type is *common migraine*, which does not have the so-called 'aura' of altered vision but has headache with nausea and vomiting. Children may have recurrent abdominal pain rather than a headache, and can suffer an attack even as early as 6 months of age. The length of each attack is variable, but an attack usually lasts for several hours.

What is the cause?

Migraine is caused by dilation or swelling of blood vessels inside and outside the scalp in people who have very sensitive blood vessels. This results in more blood pumping through the vessels, causing a throbbing sensation like blood to an infected sore on a finger. Hence it is also called *vascular headache*.

Trigger factors
- tension and stress
- unpleasant smells
- certain foods, such as cheese, oranges, tomatoes, chocolates and wines, especially red wine
- fatigue
- hunger
- constant physical stress
- hormonal changes: just before menses or when taking the pill
- bright lights, glare and flickering lights (e.g. television)
- changes in the weather
- excessive noise
- strong perfume

What is the treatment?

There is no cure, but your problem can be considerably improved. Try to think deeply after each attack about what may have caused it—what you were doing, feeling, eating or drinking beforehand.

Some people find their attacks are related to neck problems. If you have such a problem, have your doctor attend to it. Cervical mobilisation or manipulation may help.

Prevention
- *Adopt* a healthy lifestyle.
- *Avoid* tension, fatigue, constant physical and mental stress.
- *Avoid* red wine; otherwise, restrict only those items in your diet that you suspect trigger the problem.
- *Relaxation techniques*, including meditation, may help prevent the attack. It is worth entering a meditation program.
- *Medication* may be necessary to prevent attacks and will be prescribed by your doctor.

Actual attack

You may be able to fend off the attack or modify it by taking 2 soluble aspirin or paracetamol tablets and an antiemetic (has to be prescribed), lying in a quiet, darkened, cool room and trying to relax, maybe meditating or listening to your favourite, soft, relaxing music.

Take any other antimigraine medication (as prescribed) as soon as you suspect an attack is going to occur. The earlier you start treatment the better.

Some people find quick relief from simply 'sleeping off' an attack. Doctors usually prescribe mild sleeping tablets for these people.

Other helpful points
- Place cold packs on your forehead or neck.
- Avoid drinking coffee, tea or orange juice.
- Avoid moving around too much.
- Do not read or watch television.

John Murtagh, *Patient Education*, Second edition, McGraw-Hill Book Company

Nose: stuffy, running nose

What is the cause?

Your nose is lined by a delicate tissue called *mucosa*, which produces mucus to protect your nose. If this tissue is irritated, it becomes inflamed and swells up, causing blockage and a lot of mucus.

This is most commonly caused by a viral infection. Other causes are allergies and dust. Bacterial infection may then develop, and this tends to cause yellow-greenish mucus and sometimes pain.

What are the symptoms?

The commonest symptoms are profuse mucus (running nose) and stuffiness that may cause you to breathe through the mouth.

What are the complications?

Complications are nose bleeding, ear pain and sinusitis.

What is the treatment?

Blowing the nose

Clear excess mucus by blowing into a clean handkerchief or disposable paper tissue. First clear one nostril, keeping the other closed by gently pressing on its side. Then repeat for the other nostril. A common mistake is to press both nostrils almost closed as you blow. This forces air and mucus inwards, causing ear troubles.

Nasal decongestants

These over-the-counter preparations may help but should be used with care. These sprays or drops are designed to shrink and dry out the swollen mucosa, but can cause a 'rebound' reaction and eventually make the problem worse. If necessary, use these for a short period of 2–3 days only, and never exceed the maximum dose advised on the packet. Simple cold-soothing 'lollies' containing menthol can be just as effective.

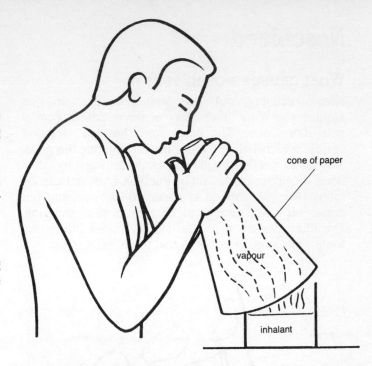

A good method of steam inhalation

Steam inhalation

Steam inhalation is a simple and excellent way of clearing the nose cavities and sinuses. There are several preparations (such as friar's balsam, Vicks VapoRub or other menthol substances) that can be dissolved in hot water. Add 1 teaspoon of the inhalant to 500 mL (1 pint) of boiled water (just off the boil) in an old container such as a wide-mouthed bottle or plastic container. Rather than using the old-fashioned method of a towel over the head, use a paper cone to direct the vapour to the nose and mouth.

Inhale the vapour slowly and deeply through the nose, and then exhale slowly through the mouth. Do this for 5–10 minutes 3 times a day, including before going to bed (the most important time). When you finish the inhalation, blow your nose as described.

Nosebleed

What causes nosebleeds?

Nose bleeding (*epistaxis*) occurs from the tiny veins that are just under the thin surface of the middle or central part of the nose. The nasal lining has lots of blood vessels, which help to warm the air entering the nose. This tissue is rather fragile and easily damaged by infections, including colds, and by injury. A crust that usually forms over the surface is meant to help healing but comes off easily through picking the nose or sneezing. The blood vessels then bleed easily, but a blood clot forms after a few minutes to seal the bleeding vein.

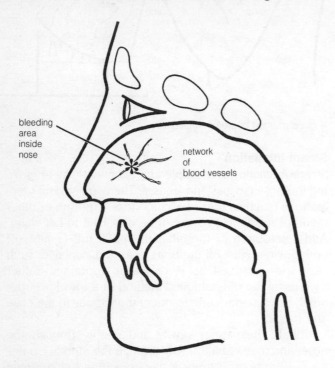

bleeding area inside nose

network of blood vessels

What are the features of nosebleeds?

The bleeding usually occurs quite suddenly and from only one nostril. It may occur only once or twice but can occur many times over weeks. As a rule it just happens 'out of the blue' without any injury. Only a small amount of blood is usually lost before bleeding stops. Nose bleeding can affect all ages but is twice as common in children.

What are the risks?

There is rarely cause for concern as it is usually a passing problem confined to the nose only. Sometimes in the elderly bleeding can occur from the back of the nose, and this can be a major problem. Sometimes nose bleeding can be caused by a generalised bleeding disorder, but there is usually unusual bleeding elsewhere in the body.

What is the treatment?

Self-help

You can stop virtually all nosebleeds yourself with a simple method.

- Sit down and bend your head forward. Hold a bowl under your nose.
- Firmly pinch the lower soft part of your nose between your thumb and finger for 5 minutes non-stop. Breathe through your mouth and do not let go for 5 minutes.

It helps to have someone apply an icepack to the bridge of your nose, but the pressure you apply with your fingers is more important (it allows a blood clot to form).

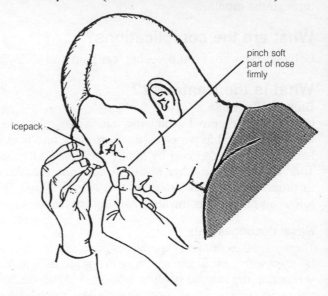

pinch soft part of nose firmly

icepack

Rules

- Do not blow your nose for about 12 hours afterwards, as it may dislodge the clot.
- Avoid picking your nose.
- If bleeding stops then recurs, pinch your nose for 10 minutes.
- Try to avoid swallowing the blood.
- If bleeding continues after 20 minutes or more, report to your doctor or nearest casualty department.

Medical help

If the bleeding keeps coming back, your doctor can do many things to stop the bleeding such as:

- special gauze packing
- cauterising with a special chemical or diathermy
- applying an ointment with an antiseptic or a chemical that constricts blood vessels

John Murtagh, *Patient Education*, Second edition, McGraw-Hill Book Company

Peptic ulcer

What is a peptic ulcer?

A *peptic ulcer* is a raw area or small hole in the lining of the stomach or the *duodenum* (the first part of the small intestine). Most ulcers occur in the duodenum (*duodenal ulcers*); a smaller number develop in the stomach (*gastric ulcers*).

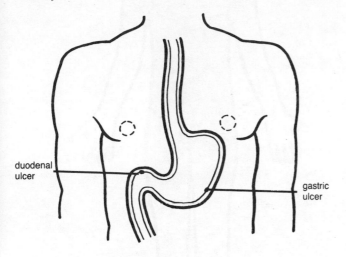

duodenal
ulcer

gastric
ulcer

What causes a peptic ulcer?

Gastric juice produced by the lining of the stomach contains acid and an enzyme (called *pepsin*) that digests protein in our food. This acidic juice can cause an erosion of the lining of the stomach or duodenum if it is excessive. This lining is normally protected by a layer of thick mucus, like a coating of slime. Once it is broken, the raw area of an ulcer can form. It is now known that bacteria in the stomach called *Helicobacter pylori* is associated with this breakdown.

A common modern cause is the use of drugs to treat pain and arthritis, known as *non-steroidal anti-inflammatory drugs* (NSAIDS).

What are the symptoms?

Common symptoms are:
- upper abdominal pain (just under the ribs)
- heartburn or indigestion
- 'hunger pain' when the stomach is empty (between meals and at night)
- pain relieved by antacids and milk

Uncommon symptoms are:
- back pain (between the shoulder blades)
- bleeding—vomiting blood and blood in motions

Who is prone to ulcers?

Ulcers are common in:
- men
- young to middle-aged adults
- those who constantly take certain drugs (e.g. aspirin, cortisone, NSAIDS)
- heavy smokers
- heavy alcohol drinkers
- those who suffer constant stress and anxiety

What are the risks?

Most ulcers are relatively easy to cure or control. Bleeding can result in anaemia or can be sudden, and this is an emergency. Perforation or blockage of the duodenum can occur. Cancer rarely occurs with a gastric ulcer.

What is the treatment?

Self-help

- Do not smoke.
- Drink alcohol only in moderation.
- Do not swallow aspirin or antiarthritic drugs unless really necessary.
- Follow a normal healthy diet with 3 balanced meals a day.
- Do not skip meals, eat irregularly or have late-night snacks.
- Avoid any foods that make your symptoms worse.
- Continue your normal activities, but aim for a non-stressful lifestyle.
- Take antacid tablets or medicines to relieve symptoms.

Medical help

Your ulcer problem should be managed with the advice of your doctor. Antacids may not be enough, and special drugs are now available to heal ulcers These modern drugs reduce the output of gastric juice and counteract *Helicobacter pylori* (usually with triple therapy), and need to be taken exactly as instructed. If all these things fail, an operation can be very successful.

Note

- Peptic ulcers are now very treatable with excellent modern drugs, and so any suffering should not be necessary.
- Report any sudden severe stomach pain or vomiting or passing of blood.

Pityriasis rosea

What is pityriasis rosea?

It is a skin rash thought to be caused by a virus. It commonly occurs in young adults (especially aged 15–30) but might occur at any age. It is not considered to be contagious.

What are the symptoms?

The rash

The rash usually starts with a large spot on the trunk called a 'herald' patch because it heralds the onset of a widespread rash several days later. The spots then break out over the body to cover the trunk and upper arms (a 'T-shirt' distribution) and the upper legs. Rarely, the rash can cover the neck and face. The spots become oval patches (about the size of a coin) of salmon-red or copper-coloured skin with scaly margins.

Other symptoms

Patients are not ill, although there may be some minor discomfort from itching. Some patients have no itching at all, while some can have considerable itching.

What are the risks?

There are no risks attached to pityriasis rosea, but you should visit your doctor to make sure that you do not have some other similar skin disorder such as ringworm. No scarring will result from the skin rash unless there is a complicating infection. Second attacks are rarely seen.

How long does the rash last?

Pityriasis rosea usually runs a natural course of 4–10 weeks. There are no medicines or treatments available to shorten this course.

What is the treatment?

There is no special treatment for pityriasis rosea. You should lead your normal active life. If possible, expose the skin to moderate amounts of sunlight, as this tends to lessen the rash, but you must avoid sunburn. Otherwise, ultraviolet light therapy 3 times a week is helpful.

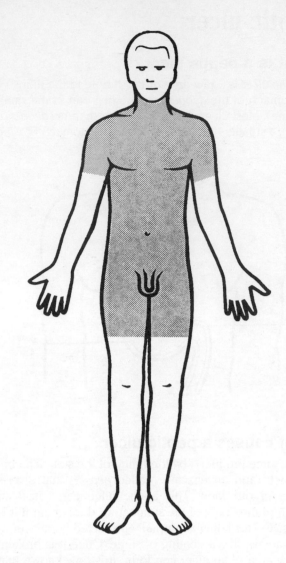

Typical distribution of the rash of pityriasis rosea

Bathe and shower as usual, but use a mild soap such as Dove or Neutrogena. If itching is a bother, use some soothing lotions or creams. These include calamine lotion or calamine lotion with 1% phenol or urea cream. If itching is severe, your doctor will prescribe special medication.

John Murtagh, *Patient Education*, Second edition, McGraw-Hill Book Company

Pruritus ani

What is pruritus ani?

Pruritus ani simply means 'itch of the anus' or 'itchy backside'. It is a very common disorder of the skin surrounding the anus. In children threadworms may be suspected; however, it is usually seen in adult males with considerable inner drive, often at times of stress and in hot weather when sweating is excessive.

What are the causes and aggravating factors?

It can be caused or aggravated by:
- medical problems such as eczema, threadworms, antibiotic treatment, diabetes and fungal infection
- tinea cruris or 'jock itch', which has to be ruled out
- local anal disorders such as piles, fissures and warts
- poor hygiene
- excessive sweating (e.g. due to tight clothing such as panty hose in summer)
- contact dermatitis caused by dyed or perfumed toilet tissue, soap, powders or clothing
- overwork, both physical and mental
- obesity

Rules of treatment

1. Scratching
Stop—it's taboo! If you scratch at night, wear light cotton gloves to bed.

2. Bathing
Avoid hot water. Excessive showering and scrubbing is also bad for this condition. Use a cream such as bland aqueous cream for cleaning rather than soap.

3. Drying
Keep the area as dry and cool as possible. After washing, dry gently and thoroughly with a soft towel or soft tissue: do not rub. Warm air from a hairdryer is very useful.

4. Bowel movements
Keep bowels regular and smooth by eating plenty of high-fibre foods such as bran, fresh carrots and apples. Some doctors claim that your bowel actions should be so smooth and complete that toilet paper should not be necessary.

5. Toilets
Clean gently after bowel movements. Use soft paper tissue (avoid pastel tints), then clean with tufts of cotton-wool with aqueous cream or bland soap and water. The best way is to use cottonwool wetted with warm water only.

6. Soaps and powder
Do not use perfumed soaps and talcum powder, including baby powder. A neutral soap such as Dove or Neutrogena is preferable.

7. Clothing
Wear loose clothing and underwear. In men, boxer shorts should be used in preference to jockey shorts. Cottons should be used. Let the air circulate in the area. At times a skirt but no underpants (in women) is desirable. Avoid panty hose if possible.

8. Topical creams
Do not use ointments or creams unless your doctor has prescribed them. If a cream has to be used, simple creams may be the most soothing (e.g. toilet lanoline).

Seek your doctor's advice before using 'over-the-counter' prescriptions. Your doctor may prescribe a special cream.

> **Remember**
>
> Pruritus ani will certainly settle with this plan of management.

John Murtagh, *Patient Education*, Second edition, McGraw-Hill Book Company

Psoriasis

What is psoriasis?

It is a chronic skin disorder in which red or deep pink raised patches covered by white scales appear on the skin. It usually causes no discomfort but it can get slightly itchy, especially on the scalp or around the anus. The main problem is the unsightly appearance of the rash, but fortunately it is usually covered by clothing. You may have a single patch or several large ones. The cause of psoriasis is unknown and it shows a tendency to run in families.

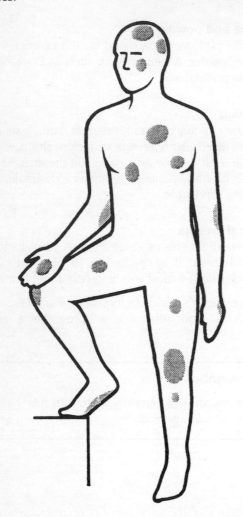

Common sites of psoriasis

What part of the body is usually affected?

Psoriasis commonly affects the elbows, knees and scalp, although patches can surface anywhere on the body, including under the nails of the fingers and toes. It occurs less commonly in the armpits, under the breasts, on the genitals and around the anus.

Is psoriasis common?

Yes; it affects about 1 in 40 people. It appears most often between the ages of 10 and 30, and most cases are mild.

How does it happen?

The skin in the patches of psoriasis is growing much faster than normal skin. As your skin is worn away, it is replaced by cells produced beneath the surface. In psoriasis the normal rate of cell production is speeded up, and this does not allow the cells to manufacture a substance called *keratin* that gives skin its hard surface. The result is unsightly flaking of the skin.

Is it serious?

No; it does not usually affect general health. Some people (about 5% of those with psoriasis) can develop a painful arthritis in the joints.

How is psoriasis diagnosed?

A doctor can make a diagnosis on the appearance of the rash without the need for tests. If there is any doubt, a piece of skin can be removed for examination (a biopsy).

What are other important facts about psoriasis?

- It is worse in winter, due to the relative lack of sunlight.
- An outbreak is often triggered by a period of mental stress.
- Yellow blisters can occur in patches on the soles and palms.
- It is most unlikely to appear on the face.
- It should not prevent you from enjoying a normal life.
- It can temporarily disappear, especially during summer.
- It tends to flare up around puberty and the menopause in women.

What is the treatment?

There are many treatments, depending on the severity of the condition and the nature of your skin. It is best to keep the treatment as simple as possible. It is worth noting that no special diet has proved successful as a treatment for psoriasis.

For many people, careful sunbathing or using an ultraviolet lamp helps clear up psoriasis. However, if you have sensitive skin you must take care not to become sunburnt, because this can make the condition worse. The use of coal tar is a time-honoured treatment for psoriasis. Some patented preparations are messy, but patients should persevere with this effective and safe treatment.

Your doctor will be able to advise you about the best drugs to treat your condition. A cautious approach is advised.

> **Note**
>
> - Psoriasis is not an infection and is not contagious.
> - No one has a cure for psoriasis—beware of quack 'cures'.
> - Avoid sunburn.

John Murtagh, *Patient Education*, Second edition, McGraw-Hill Book Company

Schizophrenia

What is schizophrenia?

It is a disorder of the mind that results in disorganisation or normal thinking and feeling. Schizophrenia, which literally means 'split mind', is often thought of as a split or double personality (the 'Dr Jekyll and Mr Hyde' perception), but this is a false impression.

Schizophrenia can come in various forms with different symptoms and outcomes. The common type is described here.

What is the cause of schizophrenia?

The cause or causes are not yet fully understood, but we know that there is a malfunction or breakdown in some cells in the brain most likely due to a chemical imbalance or deficiency. This problem can be triggered by very stressful circumstances, illness, major surgery and childbirth. It is not caused by family upbringing or other parental influences. However, there is a genetic factor involved.

What are the symptoms?

The 'attacks' may come on suddenly or, as is more usual, gradually with a withdrawal from daily activities and the onset of unusual or strange behaviour. The symptoms include:
- mixed-up thinking (called *thought disorder*)
- mixed-up feelings (feeling 'unreal')
- hallucinations, especially hearing things
- delusions (a fixed wrong belief)
- loss of energy and initiative
- inappropriate emotions
- withdrawal from social activities
- slow or unusual movements
- bizarre behaviour
- deterioration in work and study performance
- tension, anxiety or depression

The hallucinations are typically auditory, such as hearing strange voices in the head or in the air. Visual hallucinations (seeing things) and tactile hallucinations (feeling things) are uncommon.

What does the onlooker notice?

The affected person appears to become withdrawn, vague, 'flat', unable to converse normally and logically, unable to answer questions normally (may be blank) and lacking in feeling.

His or her emotions will appear flat and inappropriate (such as laughing at something sad or serious and crying without cause). The person may start neglecting his or her personal appearance.

If the schizophrenia is severe, the person will seem very disturbed and irrational.

How does the sufferer feel?

The person feels confused, lonely and afraid. He or she may be aware of loss of control of thinking and behaviour. The person may feel that he or she is being controlled from outside and perhaps may feel under threat from people who actually love him or her. The person may feel great tension and anger.

How common is schizophrenia and who gets it?

About 1 person in 100 has it to some degree while about 4 in 1000 will be suffering from it at a given point in time. It is typically seen in young adults—most people develop it between the ages of 15 and 25. Men and women are equally susceptible. Anyone can develop it, but it does tend to run in families.

What are the risks?

The main risks occur during severe attacks, when sufferers can do physical harm to themselves and others. This applies especially to the older paranoid schizophrenic. They also may try to commit suicide.

What should relatives or friends do?

Medical care is vital for these people—if you suspect someone in your family has the problem, persuade him or her to visit the doctor, whom you should contact beforehand to explain your observations. The person can be most unco-operative and upset, but must not be left alone—medical help must be obtained. The person will have little or no insight into the problem and will often claim that there is nothing wrong. A lot of family support is needed.

What is the treatment?

Effective treatment is available in the form of major tranquillising drugs, psychotherapy and rehabilitation. Sometimes electroconvulsive therapy may be required. Once the problem is under control, the patient needs ongoing supervision. Support is available from various organisations. Ask about support groups.

What is the outlook?

Most people recover and lead normal lives but may require regular checks or constant medication. Times of extreme stress create risk of relapse. There are varying degrees of schizophrenia, from mild to severe. The mild cases usually 'bounce back' to normality, while the severe ones can have problems most of their lives, especially if unsupervised.

Skin cancer

Skin cancer is usually found in fair-skinned people who are exposed to too much sun.

What are the main types of skin cancer?

Basal cell carcinoma
- the commonest and least dangerous type
- usually appears on the face and neck
- is easily treated

Squamous cell carcinoma
- is quite dangerous
- appears on hands, forearms, face and neck
- can spread to other parts if left untreated too long

Melanoma
- the rarest and most dangerous type
- usually starts in a mole
- can occur anywhere on the body

What are the signs of skin cancer?
- crusty non-healing sores or 'sunspots'
- a persistent small lump that is red, pale or pearly in colour
- a new spot, freckle or mole that has changed colour, thickness or shape over months

> - Dark spots (dark brown, black or blue-black) need special attention.

What are the causes?

The main cause is exposure to the harmful ultraviolet rays of the sun over a long time. Exposure to some chemicals, such as arsenic and polycyclic hydrocarbons, can cause skin cancer.

What are the areas to watch?

Watch your face, ears, neck, shoulders, arms and the backs of your hands. However, melanoma is an exception and can appear anywhere on the body.

Who is at risk?

Fair-skinned people living in hot, sunny climates are most at risk. People with freckles and fair skin are especially at risk. It is most common in people of Celtic (Scottish, Irish and Welsh) background. It is not as common in people with very dark skin (of African, Indian and Asian origin). It is rare in Australian Aborigines.

The darker the skin, the lower the risk of developing skin cancer. Those with fair, sensitive skin who burn easily and rarely tan are at greatest risk.

Sunspots (*solar keratoses*) are dry, rough, persisting spots on the skin, which can change into skin cancer and need to be watched.

How is it prevented?

Protect yourself from the sun:
- Try to avoid direct sunlight when the sun is strongest (from 10 am to 3 pm standard time, i.e. from 11 am to 4 pm daylight-saving time).
- Always wear a broad-brimmed hat, T-shirt and baggy shorts when in the sun.
- Be wary of reflected sun on cloudy days and wind that dries the skin.
- Use a factor 15+ sunscreen on exposed skin and renew it regularly.
- Make sure you protect yourself at high altitudes.
- Wear a shirt or dress with sleeves.
- Protect children from sunburn. Their skin is more sensitive than adults' skin to sunlight.

Early detection

The earlier you detect skin cancer, the simpler the treatment. The outlook for most skin cancers is excellent.

> **Remember**
>
> You are the best person to check your skin—no one knows it as well as you.

What should be done?

Go to your doctor without delay if you develop a skin lump. The doctor may want to remove part or all of it for examination in the laboratory.

John Murtagh, *Patient Education*, Second edition, McGraw-Hill Book Company

Sleep problems

How much sleep do we need?

Many people are not aware that the amount of sleep we need for normal health varies with our age. Also, adults are different in the amount of sleep they need; for some, 4 hours a night is ample; for others, 10 hours is not enough. The average sleep for a 50-year-old is 7 hours a day.

What is a sleep problem?

There is a problem when lack of sleep or too much sleep interferes with your activities during the day. The commonest cause is *insomnia*, which may be caused by anxiety or depression. There are other problems that can interfere with sleep, including problems of your bed mate. These problems include restless legs, sleep apnoea (brief periods of not breathing) and snoring.

What is insomnia?

Insomnia is a lack of adequate sleep, which may be difficulty getting off to sleep, difficulty staying asleep or waking early. It is a temporary problem in most instances and is usually due to a passing personal problem; however, sometimes it just happens for no reason.

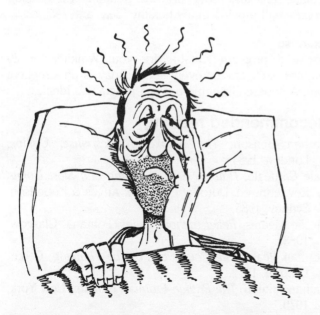

What can I do to settle to sleep?

If you have difficulty going to sleep, the following guidelines might be useful:
- Do not try too hard in attempting to go to sleep.
- Establish a routine to follow before going to bed.

- Go to bed to sleep (not to read, eat or watch television).
- Only lie down to go to sleep when you feel sleepy.
- Try to settle down before going to bed. Do not try to sleep immediately after a heavy meal, after difficult work that required a lot of concentration, after strenuous exercise or after an emotional upset or argument.
- Try to recognise what helps you settle best. The following are useful to some people: glancing through a magazine, listening to the radio, having a warm (not too hot) bath or shower, or some other relaxation technique. You might find something else that works better for you.
- Often, having a warm milk drink as you retire to bed will help.
- Many people find that drinks containing caffeine (such as tea, coffee and cocoa) make it difficult to go to sleep.
- Alcohol can stop many people from settling to sleep and can cause others to have disturbed sleep.
- Decide the hours during which you want to sleep and try to sleep only within that period. Repeated 'naps' during the day will make sleep at night difficult.
- In general, you will come to no harm if you do not sleep at all for one or two nights; you will catch up later.
- Find a settling-down routine that works best for you. Even if it seems only partly effective, the fact that you have a routine will eventually assist your sleep.
- Undertake a relaxation program such as meditation. Don't take your worries to bed.

What about sleeping tablets?

Doctors prefer you to work at getting a natural sleep by the various relaxation techniques. However, sometimes drugs can help you over a difficult period and may help you get into a pattern.

Some hypnotic drugs are suitable, but should be taken for a short time (say 2–3 nights) and taken in the lowest effective dose. Most people seem to make a prescription of 25 tablets last for 3–6 months, and this is sensible.

Rarely, some people with chronic insomnia manage best with regular use of sleeping tablets and cannot manage without them. In such instances, long-term use of sleeping tablets is justified.

A special tip

Special sleep disorder units to help your problem are present in most major cities. Ask your doctor about them.

Stress: coping with stress

What are the effects of stress?

Abnormal stress can have many troublesome physical and emotional effects on us, but they vary from person to person. Common problems are tiredness, fatigue, anxiety, sleep disturbance, poor concentration, restlessness and irritability.

Stress-related illnesses include depression, drug abuse (including problem drinking), irritable digestive system, peptic ulcers, headache, mouth ulcers, impotence, irritable bladder, dermatitis, heart disease, breast pain and cancer.

What are important causes?

We are constantly under some form of stress in our lives and generally cope very well. The most stressful circumstances leading to ill health have been shown to be death of a spouse or close family member, divorce and marital separation, imprisonment, personal injury or illness, marriage, retirement, sex difficulties, pregnancy, guilt over a wrongdoing and similar traumas. However, many of us feel unduly stressed over modern living and we need help.

What can you do to cope?

- Talk it over with someone.
- Look for solutions: stop escaping.
- Practise relaxation.
- Develop healthy hobbies.
- Practise a sensible healthy diet.
- Exercise.
- Avoid smoking and other drugs and limit alcohol.

Talking it over

'Getting it off your chest' is more important than you realise. Talk to someone you admire and trust. Going to a minister of religion or your doctor can be powerful, especially if you can feel forgiven and if any guilt is relieved. The traditional Christian sacrament of confession or reconciliation is noted to be very powerful in helping stressed guilty people.

Relaxation

Practising relaxation is vital for the uptight person. Meditation is excellent and classes are available, but you can practise yourself.

Make a commitment to yourself to spend some time every day practising relaxation. About 20 minutes twice a day is ideal, but you might want to start with only 10 minutes.

- Sit in a quiet place with your eyes closed, but remain alert and awake if you can. Focus your mind on the different muscle groups in your body, starting at the forehead and slowly going down to the toes. Relax the muscles as much as you can.

- Pay attention to your breathing: listen to the sound of your breath for the next few minutes. Breathe in and out slowly and deeply.
- Next, begin to repeat the word 'relax' silently in your mind at your own pace. When other thoughts distract, calmly return to the word 'relax'.
- Just 'let go': this is a quiet time for yourself, in which the stresses in body and mind are balanced or reduced.

Try to practise when your stomach is empty: before breakfast and before the evening meal are ideal times.

During the day, check yourself frequently for tension: take a few long, deep breaths and breathe away the tension.

Practise positive thinking. If you catch yourself thinking negative thoughts about your illness, silently say over and over to yourself: 'Every day, in every way, my health is getting better and better.'

Note: Prayer is an excellent form of meditation and relaxation.

Health through nutrition

A sensible approach to your diet can make you feel marvellous. *Increase* the amount of complex carbohydrates and fibre (vegetables, fruit, whole-wheat products, brown rice, fish, cereals, etc.) in your diet. Drink plenty of water. *Decrease* salt, total fats (butter, cream, meat fats, cheese, peanut butter, etc.), refined carbohydrates (sugars, sweets, cordials, ice-cream, cakes, etc.) and caffeine (coffee, tea and cola drinks). Reading *The Pritikin Promise* will provide many healthy ideas and recipes.

Exercise

Devise a program suitable for you. Walking for 20 minutes each day or every second day is an excellent start. A good callisthenic or yoga program is ideal.

Recommended reading

Herbert Benson, *The Relaxation Response*, Collins, London, 1984.

Dale Carnegie, *How to Stop Worrying and Start Living*, Rev. edn, ed. Dorothy Carnegie, Angus & Robertson, Sydney, 1985.

Ainslie Meares, *Relief without Drugs*, Fontana, Glasgow, 1983.

Norman Peale, *The Power of Positive Thinking*, Cedar, London, 1972.

Nathan Pritikin, *The Pritikin Promise*, Bantam, New York, 1979.

Claire Weekes, *Self-Help for Your Nerves*, Angus & Robertson, London, 1976.

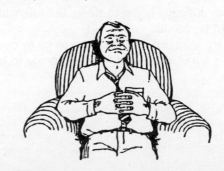

Sunburn

Sunburn is inflammation or redness of the skin caused by overexposure to the ultraviolet rays of the sun or to sun lamps. It is more likely to occur in people with light coloured skin.

What are the symptoms?

The effects of sunburn can vary from mild to severe.

Minor sunburn
- The skin is only mildly red.
- There is only mild discomfort for about 2 days.

Moderate sunburn
- The skin is red, hot and tender.
- Discomfort develops in only a few hours and settles in 3–4 days.
- There is some peeling of the skin.

Severe sunburn
- The skin is red, hot, painful and swollen.
- Blisters develop.
- If the sunburn is very severe, there may be headache, fever, nausea and possibly delirium.

What are the traps?

Sunburn is not caused only by exposure to the direct rays of the sun in the cloudless sky. It can also occur on hazy or overcast days, as thin clouds and light smog do not fully trap the effect of ultraviolet rays. Sunburn can also be caused by rays reflected off water, sand, snow and concrete. Taking various drugs (such as some antibiotics, hormones and tranquillisers) can increase the risk of sunburn.

What are the risks?

Severe sunburn can cause dehydration and skin loss, which may result in poor healing. Repeated sunburn or constant overexposure to the strong sun causes premature ageing of the skin with wrinkling and can lead to skin cancer.

What skin areas are most at risk?

The nose, cheeks, ears, back of neck and backs of the legs are most likely to be sunburnt.

How can you prevent sunburn?
- Avoid the direct sun from 10 am to 3 pm (11 am to 4 pm in daylight-saving time).
- Use a sunscreen with a minimum of SPF 15+.
- Use natural shade. Beware of reflected light from sand or water and light cloud.
- Wear broad-brimmed hats and protective clothing.
- Wear muted colours such as light tan in preference to whites and bright colours.
- Use zinc oxide ointment for maximum protection.

What about sun tanning?

If this is necessary, restrict sun exposure to 5–10 minutes each side on the first day. Increase this by 5 minutes per side each day. Use a sunscreen (*not* suntan) lotion until tanning is underway.

What is the treatment?
- Hydrocortisone 1% cream or ointment is helpful for more moderate to severe sunburn. It should only be used in the first 24 hours and not on broken skin.
- Cold compresses ease heat and pain: dip gauze or towels in cold water and lay these on the burnt areas.
- Soak in a water bath containing oil (baby oil) or baking soda. Pat the skin dry afterwards.
- Oily calamine lotion can soothe after bathing.
- Aspirin or paracetamol relieves pain and any fever.
- Increase your fluid intake, especially for severe burns.
- Do not sunbathe until the redness and tenderness has disappeared.

John Murtagh, *Patient Education*, Second edition, McGraw-Hill Book Company

Tension headache

What is the cause of tension headache?

Overactivity of muscles of the scalp, forehead and neck causes tension headache. A dull ache or tightness in these areas, like a tight band around the head or a heavy weight on top, results from this overactivity.

Trigger factors

- increased tension or stress (both mental and physical), for example:
  - excessive worry
  - all work—no play
  - long periods of study, typing or other concentration
  - perfectionism
- increased tension in the neck muscles, for example:
  - poor posture
  - injuries to the spine
- repressed hostility, anger or frustration
- a poor, scrappy diet, for example eating on the run (combined with stress)

What is the treatment?

Drugs

A mild pain-killer such as aspirin or paracetamol can help stop the pain, but avoid stronger drugs (including tranquillisers) unless directed by your doctor.

Self-help

The best treatment is to modify your lifestyle in order to eliminate or reduce the trigger factors. For example:

- Learn to relax your mind and body.
- During an attack, relax by lying down in a hot bath or spa with a warm dry cloth (or even a cold wet cloth) over the aching area.
- You could attend special relaxation courses such as yoga or meditation classes.
- Be less of a perfectionist; do not be a slave to the clock.
- Do not bottle things up. Stop feeling guilty. Approve of yourself. Express yourself and your anger.
- If your neck is aching, massage or mobilisation followed by special exercises should help.

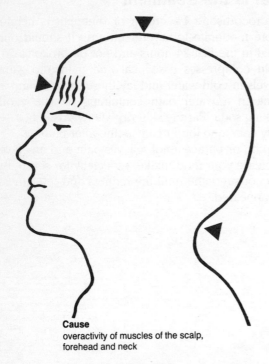

Cause
overactivity of muscles of the scalp, forehead and neck

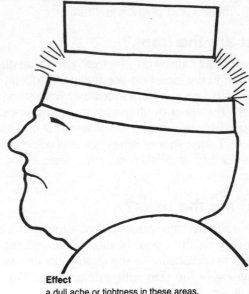

Effect
a dull ache or tightness in these areas, like a tight band around the head or a heavy weight on top

The cause and effect of tension headache

John Murtagh, *Patient Education*, Second edition, McGraw-Hill Book Company

Travel: air travel

Flying has revolutionised travel. Air travel is safe and comfortable; however, 'air sickness' and jet lag are problems that face many travellers.

What is jet lag?

This is the uncomfortable aftermath of a long flight in which the person feels exhausted and disoriented, has poor concentration, insomnia and anxiety. The problem on arrival is poor concentration and judgment during daytime.

Other symptoms that may occur include anorexia, weakness, headache, blurred vision and dizziness.

Jet lag is a feature of flying long distances east–west or west–east through several time zones, causing the person's routine daily rhythm of activity and sleep to get out of phase.

What factors influence jet lag?

General factors
Noise, vibration, air humidity and sitting still for long periods can influence jet lag.

Specific factors
Duration of the flight, time of departure, changes in climate and culture at the destination affect the severity of jet lag. The problem is aggravated by:
- stress of the pretrip planning
- last-minute rushing and anxiety
- lack of sleep during the trip
- overeating and excessive alcohol during the flight
- smoking

How can you minimise the problem?

Careful planning and a few simple hints observed during and after the flight can ease jet lag.

Before the flight
- Allow plenty of time for planning.
- Plan a 'stopover' if possible.
- If possible, arrange the itinerary so that you are flying into the night.
- Ensure a good sleep the night before flying.
- Ensure a relaxed trip to the airport.
- Take along earplugs if noise (75–100 decibels) bothers you.

During the flight
- *Fluids*: Avoid alcohol and coffee. Drink plenty of non-alcoholic drinks such as orange juice and mineral water.
- *Food*: Eat only when hungry and even skip a meal or two. Eat the lighter, more digestible parts of your meal.

- *Dress*: Women should wear loose clothes (e.g. long skirts, comfortable jeans, light jumpers) and avoid girdles or restrictive clothing. Wear comfortable (not tight) shoes and take them off during flight.
- *Smoking*: Reduce smoking to a minimum. Non-smokers should seek a non-smoking zone.
- *Sleep*: Try to sleep on longer sections of the flight (give the movies a miss). Close the blinds, wear special eye 'masks' and ask for a pillow. Consider using sedatives such as temazepam (Euhypnos or Normison).
- *Activity*: Try to take regular walks around the aircraft and exercise at airport stops. Keep your feet up when resting, and exercise by flexing the major muscles of the legs. Avoid resting the calves of your legs against the seat for long periods.

At your destination
Take a nap for 1–2 hours if possible.

Wander around until you are tired and go to bed at the usual time. It is good to have a full day's convalescence and avoid big decision-making soon after arrival. Allow about 3 days for adjustment after the London to Australia flight.

Who is fit to fly?

Patients with these problems should avoid flying:
- upper airways congested by infection, including influenza
- severe respiratory disease (emphysema, chronic bronchitis, pneumothorax)
- unstable heart failure
- severe anaemia (below 70 g/L)
- pregnancy beyond 200 days (28 weeks)
- previous violent or unpredictable behaviour
- within 4 weeks of a myocardial infarction (coronary or heart attack)
- within 14 days of a cerebrovascular accident (stroke)
- within 14 days of major surgery
- brain tumour or recent skull fracture
- recent eye surgery

Special precautions are required by travellers with:
- *Colostomy*: Patients should wear a large colostomy bag and take extra bags.
- *Varicose veins*: Wear supportive stockings and exercise frequently.
- *Plaster casts*: Those with broken limbs in plaster should be careful of swelling.
- *Pacemakers*: Those with pacemakers may have a problem with X-rays at some overseas airports. Mention it to officials before passing through security equipment.
- *Epilepsy*: Medication should be increased on the day of travel.
- *Diabetes*: Diabetics should discuss their therapy and control with their doctor.

Travel: guide for travellers

Travellers to countries that have low standards of health and hygiene risk contracting infectious diseases. Most problems are caused by contaminated food and water and by mosquitoes, which transmit malaria, yellow fever, dengue and Japanese encephalitis.

Prevention is better than cure; the advice that follows is designed to minimise the chance of contracting a serious disease while travelling overseas.

Food and drink

Diseases that can be picked up from eating and drinking contaminated food include travellers' diarrhoea, hepatitis A, cholera and typhoid.

While visiting countries at risk, drink only boiled water and reputable commercially bottled beverages. Avoid ice, dairy products, salads, uncooked foods, ice-cream, raw seafood, shellfish and food from street vendors.

You can purify water by boiling it or adding iodine tablets.

Vaccinations

Important recommended vaccinations are shown in the table. Your doctor will advise you on which vaccinations you will need. Other diseases to consider are rabies and typhus.

Malaria

One sting from an infected mosquito can cause serious illness. Malaria is common in many African, South American and South-East Asian countries. To prevent malaria, protect yourself from mosquitoes and take anti-malarial drugs prescribed by your doctor.

Avoid rural areas after dusk. Use insect repellents that contain diethyltoluamide (such as Rid or Repellem). Wear protective light-coloured clothing with long sleeves and legs, and sleep in screened rooms or use mosquito nets. Avoid using cologne, perfume and aftershave.

Antimalarial drugs should be taken before exposure and up to 4 weeks after exposure to give maximum protection.

Malaria that resists drug treatment with chloroquine occurs in many countries. Your doctor will prescribe another drug as well as or instead of the usual chloroquine if you are at risk of exposure to this type of malaria.

> Drugs cannot guarantee 100% protection. If you develop an unexplained fever, sore throat or severe rash, seek medical advice.

Your destination

Different countries have different vaccination requirements. For advice about the country you intend to visit, contact your own doctor.

Diarrhoea

There are several ways to relieve and treat travellers' diarrhoea:

1. Avoid solid foods and drink small amounts of fluids often. (Remember: use only boiled water or safe commercial beverages.)
2. Rest.
3. Take antidiarrhoeal tablets as directed (for mild cases).
4. When the diarrhoea has settled, eat light foods such as rice, bread or biscuits.

> ### Some golden rules
> - Never carry a parcel or baggage to oblige a stranger.
> - Avoid casual sex. If not, use a condom.
> - 'If you can't peel it, boil it or cook it, *don't eat it*.'
> - Never walk around barefoot at night in snake-infested areas (and use a torch).
> - Prevent mosquito bites.

A guide to vaccination for travellers for important diseases (in rural areas of high risk countries)

Vaccination	Duration	Comments
Tetanus	10 years	}
Diphtheria	10 years	Essential for travelling.
Polio	10 years	
Yellow fever	10 years	Compulsory if visiting certain central African or South American countries.
Cholera	3 months	Not recommended by WHO; still required if epidemic.
Typhoid	2–3 years	Recommended for all developing countries.
Hepatitis A	varies	}
Hepatitis B	5 years	Might be advisable if you are visiting rural developing countries:
Tuberculosis	life	ask your doctor.
Measles	life	
Meningococcus	3–5 years	Consider for visits to endemic areas if in close contact with locals.
Japanese encephalitis	1–4 years	Consider in certain Asian countries for trips longer than 12 months or during an epidemic.
Rabies	1 year	Recommended for long stays in high risk areas.

John Murtagh, *Patient Education*, Second edition, McGraw-Hill Book Company

Travel sickness

Who gets travel sickness?

Almost everyone is sick when sailing on rough seas. However, some people—especially children—suffer sickness from the effect of motion on a boat, in a car or in a plane. The larger the boat, plane or car, the less is the likelihood of sickness; travel by train rarely causes sickness.

Nearly all children grow out of the tendency to have travel sickness, but many adults remain 'bad' sailors.

What are the symptoms?

Nausea, vomiting, dizziness, weakness and lethargy are the main symptoms. Early signs are pallor and drowsiness, and sudden silence from an active, talkative child.

What causes it?

The problem arises in the semicircular canals of the inner ear. They are set deep in the thick skull bone and are the body's balance mechanism.

They are affected by the movement and vibration of travel. Some people have sensitive inner ear canals and are prone to sickness, especially on certain types of journeys (e.g. winding roads through hills) and in certain vehicles.

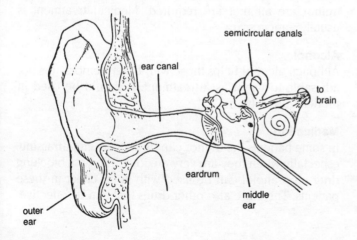

What is the treatment?

1. Keep calm and relaxed before and during travel.

   With children, avoid excitement and apprehension about the travelling. Encourage activities such as looking at distant objects; discourage activities such as reading and games that require close visual concentration.

2. Lie down, if possible, because this rests the inner ear canals and reduces the urge to vomit. If travelling by car, stop regularly for breaks. Passengers should use the front seat if possible.

3. Do not have a large meal a few hours before the journey or during it; avoid milk and fried or greasy foods.

   Do not travel with an empty stomach: have a light, simple meal about an hour before and do not drink too much. Glucose drinks such as lemonade are suitable, as are glucose sweets and biscuits while travelling.

Medication

Many medicines are available for travel sickness either as oral preparations or skin patches.

Tablets

These are good for mild travel sickness. It is desirable to take oral medication for travel sickness 60 minutes before the trip. During a long trip this can be repeated 3–4 times a day to prevent the symptoms.

Some medicines such as antihistamines make you drowsy, so take care: this sedative effect may be good for children or for those travelling long distances by plane.

Skin patches

Scopolamine adhesive patches are the most widely used medication for long-term travel, especially sea travel. One patch should be applied to dry unbroken hairless skin behind the ear 5–6 hours before travel. It should be left on for 3 days but removed immediately the trip is over.

Wash the hands thoroughly after applying and removing the disc—be careful not to touch your eyes with your fingers after doing this.

Tremor: essential tremor

What is essential tremor?

It is a tremor that mainly affects the hands and head and possibly the voice and legs. It can come on at any age.

It is also called *juvenile tremor* (if it comes on in children), *senile tremor* (if it comes on in the elderly), *benign tremor* (because it is not serious) and *familial tremor* (because it tends to run in families).

Is it similar to Parkinson's disease?

Essential tremor often gets confused with Parkinson's, but it is different in that it is most marked when the arms are held out while the tremor of Parkinson's is most marked with the hands resting and tends to disappear when the hands are used to do things. Walking is normal with essential tremor but abnormal with Parkinson's.

What are the symptoms of essential tremor?

- A slight tremor begins in one hand and then spreads to the other.
- The tremor may also affect the head, chin, tongue and only rarely the legs.
- The head tremor has a 'yes–yes' nodding action but can also have a 'no–no' shaking action. It can be stopped by supporting the head.
- It interferes with writing and handling cups of tea, spoons and other objects.
- Anxiety makes the tremor worse.
- Alcohol tends to make it better.
- Some cases are so mild that it is not diagnosed while in others it can be quite severe.

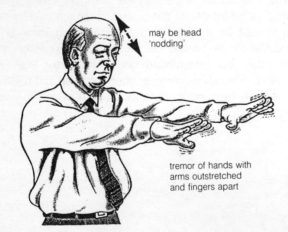

may be head 'nodding'

tremor of hands with arms outstretched and fingers apart

Symptoms of essential tremor

Who gets essential tremor?

It is a relatively common problem (affects about 4 per 1000) and has a tendency to run in families. It can come on at any age, although it usually comes on in early adulthood, even in adolescence.

What is the cause?

The cause is not exactly known, but certain chemicals that transmit nerve impulses are thought to be present in smaller quantities than normal.

Does it need special investigation?

Special expensive investigations are not necessary and are not likely to show up any abnormality. Essential tremor can be usually diagnosed upon observation.

What are the risks?

Essential tremor is not a serious illness and most people cope normally throughout life without any disability, even if it comes on in childhood. Very rarely some patients can become disabled and surgery may be needed to help them.

What is the treatment?

Explanation and reassurance

Because most patients cope with essential tremor throughout life, reassurance and education about the tremor are all that are required. Medical treatment is usually unnecessary.

Alcohol

Although alcohol helps those with faster tremors, it is not advisable to use it as a treatment. It should be used in moderation only.

Medication

In some patients the tremor can be socially embarrassing, especially when they are very anxious. The beta-blocking drug propranolol can be used with good effect in these patients. There are also other drugs that can be effective.

John Murtagh, *Patient Education*, Second edition, McGraw-Hill Book Company

Urticaria

What is urticaria?

Urticaria, also known as *hives*, is a common allergic disorder in which a red, itchy, lumpy skin rash appears 'out of the blue'. These skin lumps, which are known as *weals*, can develop anywhere on the body, including the palms and soles. The weals, which have pale centres and red margins, can spread out and join up to form large irregular patches. They are usually about 1 cm to 5 cm across. These weals can rapidly change shape and come and go over a period of minutes or hours. Urticaria can be *acute* in onset (in which the cause is often known and the disorder settles within 6 weeks) or *chronic* (where it lasts longer).

What causes urticaria?

Urticaria is a type of allergy resulting from a release of a chemical called *histamine*. The cause of this histamine release is often unknown, but common causes are foods, drugs and infestations. Sometimes the cause is very obvious, such as when urticaria appears minutes after eating.

Check list of possible causes

- foods: eggs, nuts, shellfish, other fish, cheese, oranges, chocolate, caffeine, strawberries and others
- food colourings (e.g. tartrazine)
- drugs: penicillin, sulpha antibiotics, aspirin, codeine, vaccines and others
- insect bites: bees, wasps, sandflies, fleas, mosquitoes and others
- azo dyes
- plants: nettles, poison ivy and others
- animals: cats, horses and others
- infection: viral, bacterial or fungal
- infestation: parasites
- exposure to heat and cold
- exposure to sunlight
- underlying chronic disease (e.g. lupus, lymphoma)
- pregnancy ((last trimester)

> **Note**
>
> Tension and stress usually make urticaria worse.

What is angio-oedema?

This is a serious form of urticaria in which the face, especially the lips and skin around the eyes, suddenly swells. It can be serious if the throat swells. You should contact your doctor immediately if this develops.

How is the cause found?

You may be asked to keep a food diary and note any associations. You may also have to undergo patch testing of your skin to find out what you may be allergic to.

What is the treatment?

- Antihistamines, usually taken by mouth, are used to relieve the rash and itching. Avoid taking aspirin or other drugs not prescribed for you.
- Itching can be relieved by daubing with calamine lotion.
- Cold water compresses such as soaking a towel in cold water can also relieve itching. Avoid hot baths or showers during the acute phase—keep it cool!
- Decrease your activity during the acute phase. It is better not to get hot and sweaty.
- Avoid alcohol and caffeine-containing drinks, especially if there is a possibility of these being a trigger factor.

Varicose veins

What are varicose veins?

They are twisted and swollen veins caused by faulty valves in the system of veins in the leg. The failure of the valves to close properly causes blood returning to the heart to pool in the veins.

How do they form?

Blood is collected from the leg in a network of superficial veins (just under the skin, on the surface of muscles). These veins are connected with deep veins in the muscles by perforating veins. When the muscles of the leg contract they pump the blood up these veins, which have one-way valves to prevent blood flowing back into the superficial veins.

When the valves do not close properly the blood tends to flow into the superficial veins, causing them to swell with the 'pooled' blood.

There are two main types of faulty systems:

1. faulty valves in the groin, which cause the typical long knobbly veins along the leg

2. faulty valves in the perforating veins, which cause problems mainly around and above the ankle

The latter problems are the more troublesome.

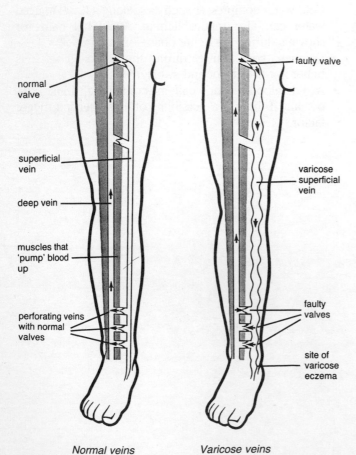

Normal veins   Varicose veins

What are the symptoms?

The usual first sign is the appearance of prominent bluish swollen veins in your leg when you stand up. The usual site is either at the back of the calf or the inside of the leg from the ankle to the groin. At first they are not painful, but as the veins get larger they may become tender to touch and the skin above them or at the ankle may begin to itch.

With severe varicose veins the whole leg may ache and the skin, especially at the ankle, may become brownish. This discoloured skin is called *varicose eczema*.

What are the risks?

Varicose veins are usually annoying and unsightly rather than disabling. Serious complications include the development of an ulcer in the skin (usually after an accident), inflammation of the vein or a clot in the vein.

Sometimes a knock or cut over a vein can cause severe bleeding. If this happens, put your leg up above your body and wrap a firm bandage around the bleeding vein.

What is the treatment?

Self-help

- Keep off your feet as much as possible.
- Whenever possible, sit with your legs up on a footstool.
- Buy or get a prescription for support tights or stockings and put them on before you get out of bed every day.
- Do not scratch itchy skin over your varicose eczema.
- See your doctor if you develop eczema or an ulcer.

Surgery

The most satisfactory answer to the problem of varicose veins is through surgery. The operation generally has good results, as the veins with the faulty valves are tied off or stripped away. It is possible to operate without leaving large scars.

After surgery varicose veins tend to come back, usually in a different place, in about 10% of treated patients.

John Murtagh, *Patient Education*, Second edition, McGraw-Hill Book Company

Vertigo: benign positional vertigo

What is benign positional vertigo (BPV)?

BPV or *positional vertigo* is a spinning sensation of the head (*vertigo*) brought on by a certain position of the head, usually sudden changes of position. The word 'benign' means that it is not a serious condition and is likely to eventually get better.

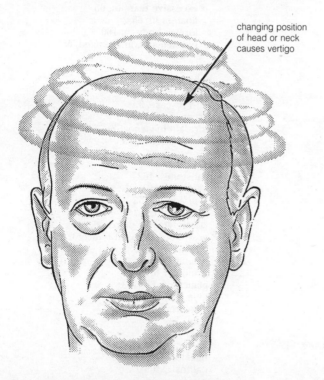

changing position of head or neck causes vertigo

What is the cause of BPV?

In most people the cause is unknown, but it can follow accidents causing neck or head injuries in some people.
There are two theories to explain BPV:

1. A problem exists in the neck, usually a 'kink' in some of the swivel joints of the neck. The neck is connected to the balance centre by special nervous pathways.

2. There are tiny pieces of floating debris in the balance centre of the inner ear (the *labyrinth*). These little bits of sediment somehow upset the balance centre when disturbed.

What are the symptoms?

- a brief attack of severe dizziness (vertigo), usually for about 10–30 seconds, that comes on a few seconds after a certain head movement
- quickly subsiding dizziness

The changing head positions that provoke an attack can be:

- tilting the head backwards
- changing from a lying to a sitting position
- lying on one ear or the other
- turning the head to the side with the neck injury

Who gets BPV?

Although it can occur at all ages, the elderly are affected most. It is the commonest cause of vertigo in the elderly. Women are twice as likely as men to get it. BPV is a surprisingly common problem.

How long do the bouts of BPV last?

Each attack usually lasts less than 30 seconds but can last 60 seconds or so. The attacks tend to come in bursts but usually settle within a few weeks and most people are able to return to work within a week. The bouts tend to come back after months or years, but some people only ever have one attack.

What are the effects of BPV?

There are usually no ill effects in the long run. Unlike some other causes of severe dizziness, there is usually no vomiting, tinnitus (ringing in the ears) or deafness. One has to be careful with driving.

What is the treatment?

There is no special treatment. Drugs are not effective at preventing the attacks. It is basically a matter of allowing the bouts to run their course, but there are some things that may help:

- Avoid head positions that provoke the attack.
- Do special neck exercises.
- Obtain mobilisation treatment to the neck by a qualified therapist.

Sometimes it may be necessary to be referred to a specialist to make sure it is just BPV and not a problem with the circulation to the brain.

Index

for influenza, 92
for measles, 26, 28
for mumps, 26, 29
for polio, 26
for rubella, 26, 33
for tetanus, 26
of travellers, 192
for tuberculosis, 192
for whooping cough, 26
impotence, 58
incontinence of urine, 47
infant colic, 27
infertility
in couples, 172
in men, 85, 95
in women, 50, 85, 95
influenza, 92
ingrowing toenails, 173
insomnia, 187
iron deficiency anaemia, 174
irritable bowel, 175

J
jet lag, 191

K
knee
exercises for, 104
osteoarthritis of, 63

L
leg ulcers, 67
lice
head, 93
pubic, 94
loneliness
in babies, 19, 31
during retirement, 70

M
malaria, 192
marijuana, 138
marital trouble, common causes of, 3
marriage, making it work, 3
mastitis, 7
measles, 28
melanoma, 176
Ménière's syndrome, 177
menopause, 48
menstrual cycle, understanding the, 42
middle ear infection, 20, 25
migraine, 178
miscarriage, 8
mumps, 29
muscles
strained, 118
torn, 118

N
nappy rash, 30
neck
exercises for, 106
pain in, 110
postaccident pain in, 111
nipples
cracked, 9
inverted, 9
sore, 9
non-specific urethritis, 95
nose, stuffy and running, 179
nosebleed, 180
nutrition, 77
in pregnancy, 4

O
obesity, 78
osteoarthritis, 112
in elderly, 63
of hip, 63
of knee, 63

osteoporosis, 48, 68
otitis externa, 156
otitis media, 21

P
pain
in back, 102, 117
in breasts, 7, 49
in neck, 110, 111
Parkinson's disease, 69
pelvic inflammatory disease, 50
pelvic muscle exercises, 47
peptic ulcer, 181
pharyngitis, 96
pill, contraceptive, 51
pityriasis rosea, 182
plantar fasciitis, 113
plantar warts, 101, 136
plaster instructions, 114
polio, immunisation against, 26, 192
postnatal blues, 10
postnatal depression, 10
pregnancy, 4
premenstrual syndrome, 52
presbycusis, 66
presbyopia, 65
prostate
enlargement of, 59
operation for, 60
pruritus ani, 183
psoriasis, 184
pubic lice, 94

R
rash
eczema, 12
nappy rash, 30
pityriasis rosea, 182
psoriasis, 184
seborrhoea, 34
viral, 39
rearing a happy child, 31
reflux
in adults, 169, 170
in infants, 32
relaxation
for anxiety, 127
for stress, 188
retinal disorders of eye, 65
retirement planning, 70
rheumatoid arthritis, 115
rubella, 33

S
scabies, 97
schizophrenia, 185
school exclusion
for chickenpox, 15
for measles, 28
for mumps, 29
for rubella, 33
sciatica, 116
seborrhoea in infants, 34
sex
and AIDS, 80
and gonorrhoea, 85
and herpes, 89
and non-specific urethritis, 95
safe, 80
shingles, 91
shoulder, exercises for, 107
sixth disease, 39
skin cancer, 176, 186
skin tests in atopic eczema, 12
sleep problems, 187
smear test, 54
smoking
and bronchitis, 81
and emphysema, 158
quitting, 79

as a risk factor, 76, 79
snake bites, 134
snuffling infant, 35
specific learning disabilities, 20
spider bites, 134
spondylosis
of cervical spine, 110, 111
lumbar, 117
sports injuries, first aid for, 118
sprained ankle, 119
steam inhalations, 179
sterilisation
female, 55
male, 62
stings, 134
stress
coping with, 188
and heart attacks, 76
stroke, 71
sunburn, 189
with acne, 40
with psoriasis, 184

T
technique
breast examination, 53
testicular examination, 61
teething, 36
temporomandibular joint dysfunction, 120
tennis elbow, 121
tension headache, 190
testicular self-examination, 61
tetanus, immunisation against, 26, 192
thoracic spine, exercises for, 108
thrush, vaginal, 56
thumb sucking, 37
tinea pedis, 98
tinnitus, 72
tonsillectomy, 99
tonsillitis, 99
transient ischaemic attack, 71
travel
by air, 191
guide for travellers, 192
travel sickness, 193
tremor
essential, 194
Parkinson's, 69, 194
triglycerides, 75
tubal ligation, 55

U
ulcer
aphthous, 128
leg, 67
peptic, 181
umbilical hernia, 38
urethritis, 85, 95
urine, incontinence of, 47
urticaria, 195

V
vaccination, *see* immunisation
vaginal thrush, 56
varicose veins, 196
vasectomy, 62
vertigo, benign positional, 197
viral infection, 100
viral skin rashes, 39
vitamin C
for chronic bronchitis, 81
for common cold, 82
for influenza, 92

W
warm-up exercises for legs, 122
warts, 101, 136
weight, losing it wisely, 78
whooping cough, immunisation against, 26

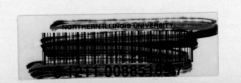